Signal and Acoustic Modeling for Speech and Communication Disorders

Speech Technology and Text Mining in Medicine and Health Care

Edited by
Amy Neustein

Volume 5

Published in the Series

Ganchev, *Computational Bioacoustics*, 2017
ISBN 978-1-61451-729-0, e-ISBN 978-1-61451-631-6,
e-ISBN (EPUB) 978-1-61451-966-9

Beals et al., *Speech and Language Technology for Language Disorders*, 2016
ISBN 978-1-61451-758-0, e-ISBN 978-1-61451-645-3,
e-ISBN (EPUB) 978-1-61451-925-6

Neustein (Ed.), *Speech and Automata in Healthcare*, 2014
ISBN 978-1-61451-709-2, e-ISBN 978-1-61451-515-9,
e-ISBN (EPUB) 978-1-61451-9607, Set-ISBN 978-1-61451-516-6

Neustein (Ed.), *Text Mining of Web-Based Medical Content*, 2014
ISBN 978-1-61451-541-8, e-ISBN 978-1-61451-390-2,
e-ISBN (EPUB) 978-1-61451-976-8, Set-ISBN 978-1-61451-391-9

Signal and Acoustic Modeling for Speech and Communication Disorders

Edited by
Hemant A. Patil, Amy Neustein,
Manisha Kulshreshtha

DE GRUYTER

Editors
Dr. Hemant A. Patil
APSIPA Distinguished Lecturer 2018-2019,
Room No. 4103, Faculty Block-4,
Near Indroda Circle,
DA-IICT Gandhinagar
PIN- 382 007, Gujarat State- INDIA.
hemant_patil@daiict.ac.in

Dr. Amy Neustein
Linguistic Technology Systems, Inc.
800 Palisade Avenue Suite 1809
Fort Lee NJ 07024
USA
amy.neustein@verizon.net

Dr. Manisha Kulshreshtha
33 Linda lane
Niskayuna
NY 12309
USA
manramk@gmail.com

ISBN 978-1-61451-759-7
e-ISBN (PDF) 978-1-5015-0241-5
e-ISBN (EPUB) 978-1-5015-0243-9
ISSN 2329-5198

Library of Congress Control Number: 2018942854

Bibliographic information published by the Deutsche Nationalbibliothek
The Deutsche Nationalbibliothek lists this publication in the Deutsche Nationalbibliografie;
detailed bibliographic data are available on the Internet at http://dnb.dnb.de.

© 2019 Walter de Gruyter GmbH, Berlin/Boston
Typesetting: Integra Software Services Pvt. Ltd
Printing and binding: CPI books GmbH, Leck
Cover image: MEHAU KULYK / SCIENCE // PHOTO LIBRARY / Agentur Focus

www.degruyter.com

Foreword

For Signal and Acoustic Modeling for Speech and Communication Disorders

This fine collection of articles from 10 renowned research groups across the world brings together work related to the analysis and detection of relevant conditions and behavior of humans via use of their speech.

Recent advances in the technology of speech signal processing have the potential to assist in the detection and treatment of a vast range of human disorders, most notably in areas of speech and communication. Until recently, speech analysis has been largely dedicated to coding and recognition applications, for example, the vast network of cellular telephony and the many products and services that allow users to communicate with computers via voice. Such services almost always assume normal speech communications, that is, the user employs a normal voice. However, in the medical field, there is a great need to diagnose various abnormal conditions in humans, and their vocal output has been a largely untapped resource. Surely, various medical tests such as X-rays, temperature, and blood pressure readings, etc., serve as a primary window to human conditions. Nonetheless, one's speech is a very simple indicator of the state of one's health. Till recently, analysts relied only on their intuition as to how to interpret a patient's speech. With recent advances, we can expect to give useful computer analysis tools to such personnel. The set of speech difficulties that one can hope to assist cover the range of congenital defects, developmental disorders, degenerative diseases, and disabling neuromotor conditions.

This anthology brings together researchers from leading universities and laboratories across five continents. The contributors to this volume examine acoustic modeling across a wide range of communication disorders. Causes include Parkinson's, Autism Spectrum Disorder, cleft palate, intellectual disabilities, neuromotor disorders (e.g., dysarthria), stroke, tumors, brain injury, and reactions to medication. The works here use advanced innovations to show how recent speech technology can benefit healthcare.

The methods described are non-invasive and cost-effective, as they can detect, monitor, and gauge speech, language, and communication disorders, without any effect on patients and with minimal equipment (i.e., microphone and computers).

This book has three sections. The first section discusses how specific developments in speech signal processing can be highly instrumental in diagnosing and treating speech and communication disorders, as well as in detecting early signs of medical problems that may impair neuromotor functioning and compromise speech intelligibility.

The first chapter analyzes whispered speech – a common type of vocal output that has been little examined in the past. People with vocal cord problems often

https://doi.org/10.1515/9781501502415-201

resort to whispering, and others employ such when trying to speak very softly. Study of whispering may help detect heart-related problems.

The second chapter examines hypernasality – a speech quality owing to defective velopharyngeal closure; speech analysis can estimate the degree of congenital abnormality of the lip and palate, and assist in assessing neuro-muscular and hearing problems.

The third chapter in the first section of the book examines recent advances in automatic acoustic analysis toward diagnosis of speech disorders. One area of recent work deals with analysis of prosody (intonation, i.e., the durations, pitch and intensity of speech), for which behavior of normal and disordered speech often differs, for example, in speaking rate. The method discussed in this chapter has been successfully tested in several European languages. This chapter also delves into chaos theory, exploiting such aspects of speech to distinguish normal and pathological voices.

The second major section of the book examines how speech relates to cognitive, affective, and developmental disorders. The first chapter in this section compares the speech of children and adults with intellectual disability, to the speech of normal speakers. While language impairments as detected by professionals are a primary way to discover language problems, there is great variability in the acoustic nature of such abnormalities, leading to much difficulty of proper diagnosis, that is, it is easy for even professionals to miss subtle acoustic signs that automatic analysis may find.

Speakers use, in complex ways, both prosody and spectro-temporal features to communicate all sorts of information via speech, most notably, they communicate ideas to humans listening. This occurs via the syntactic, semantic, and pragmatic content of their words. However, the speech signal contains far more information, encoded in highly complex ways, for example, cues to who is speaking, what emotional and medical state they are in, and what language they are speaking.

This section's first chapter shows a speech classification system that differentiates reliably between speakers with an intellectual disability and those with normal cognitive functioning. The next two chapters deal with Autism Spectrum Conditions (ASC). One provides a survey of autism and speech, language, and emotion. People with ASC vary their spoken content in ways often different from normal speech. The second chapter on autism examines clinical applications of speech technology.

The third major section of the book presents studies in the assessment and quantification of speech intelligibility in patients with anatomical defects, disabling conditions, and degenerative diseases. The studies in this section cover both congenital and acquired speech disorders. The first chapter in this section does automatic assessment of consonant omission and speech intelligibility in cleft palate speech, for 530 participants speaking Mandarin.

Next is a study of distinctive auditory-based cues and rhythm metrics to assess the severity of patients with dysarthria, from either acquired or congenital neuromotor communication disorders that affect their speech intelligibility. The diagnosis method in this chapter uses a model simulating the outer, middle, and inner parts of the ear. Relevant auditory-based cues are combined with Mel-Frequency Cepstral Coefficients (MFCCs) and rhythm metrics. MFCC has been used for decades as a standard way to analyze speech in automatic speech recognition (ASR).)

The Nemours and Torgo databases of dysarthric speech are used. Standard methods of ASR, such as Gaussian mixture models (GMMs), support vector machines (SVMs), and multinomial logistic regression (MLR) are tested for this dysarthric speech assessment.

The third section of the book concludes with an analysis of how wireless sensor networks and embedded systems can be used to measure the motor defects of patients suffering from Parkinson's disease. This chapter shows how data fusion between a sensor network and an embedded system can help quantify the disease. This is particularly relevant today, as healthcare systems increasingly use ubiquitous and pervasive computing to monitor patients at a distance.

The editors of this volume have done a fine job in reviewing recent international work in this field. They have presented here the most current and advanced research findings in signal and acoustic modeling of speech pathologies. The target audience for this book is speech scientists, clinicians, and pathologists.

Prof. Douglas O'Shaughnessy
(Ph.D. MIT USA, IEEE Fellow and ASA Fellow),
McGill University,
Canada

Acknowledgments

This coedited book volume is furthered by the stellar contributions of authors across the globe, including three IEEE fellows, Professors John H. L. Hansen and Bjorn Schuller, and Professor Douglas O'Shaughnessy who wrote the foreword. Special thanks are due to Professor Joshua John Diehl for contributing a solo chapter to this volume.

In addition, special thanks go to authorities of DA-IICT Gandhinagar and members of Speech Research Lab at DA-IICT, whose steadfast encouragement has sustained us throughout the lengthy project. Special thanks are due to series editor, Dr. Amy Neustein, whose patience, trust and confidence in the research capabilities of both the authors and the editors helped bring this challenging book project to fruition. We also acknowledge the excellent support from the editorial team and production staff at De Gruyter without which this book project would not have been possible.

Prof. Hemant A. Patil, DA-IICT Gandhinagar, Gujarat
APSIPA Distinguished Lecturer (DL) 2018–2019

https://doi.org/10.1515/9781501502415-202

Contents

Part I: **Applying New Developments in Speech Signal Processing in the Diagnosis and Treatment of Speech and Communication Disorders and in the Detection of Risk to Neuro-Motor Functioning**

Part II: **Using Acoustic Modeling in the Detection and Treatment of Cognitive, Affective, and Developmental Disorders**

List of Contributors

Plínio A. Barbosa
State University of Campinas, Brazil
pabarbosa.unicampbr@gmail.com

Achraf Benba
Electronic Systems Sensors and
Nanobiotechnology (E2SN), ENSET
Mohammed V University, Morocco
achraf.benba@um5s.net.ma

Zuleica A. Camargo
Catholic University of São Paulo, Brazil
zuleica.camargo@gmail.com

Joshua John Diehl
LOGAN Community Resources, Inc.,
and the William J. Shaw Center for Children
and Families
University of Notre Dame, USA
jdiehl@logancenter.org

Florian Eyben
audEERING GmbH, Germany
eyben@tum.de

Jia Fu
School of Electrical Engineering
and Information
Sichuan University, China

Sumanlata Gautam
The NorthCap University, India
sumanlatagautam@ncuindia.edu

Ahmed Hammouch
Electronic Systems Sensors and
Nanobiotechnology (E2SN), ENSET
Mohammed V University, Morocco
hammouch_a@yahoo.com

John H.L. Hansen
Erik Jonsson School of Engineering
and Computer Science
The University of Texas, USA
John.Hansen@utdallas.edu

Ling He
School of Electrical Engineering
and Information
Sichuan University, China
ling.he@scu.edu.cn

Hua Huang
School of Electrical Engineering
and Information
Sichuan University, China

Abdelilah Jilbab
Electronic Systems Sensors and
Nanobiotechnology (E2SN), ENSET
Mohammed V University, Morocco
a_jilbab@yahoo.fr

Kamil L. Kadi
Université de Moncton, Canada
kkadi@usthb.dz

Sandra Madureira
Catholic University of São Paulo, Brazil
sandra.madureira.liaac@gmail.com

Erik Marchi
audEERING GmbH, Germany
Technische Universität München
Germany
erik.marchi@tum.de

T.A. Mariya Celin
SSN College of Engineering, India
mariyacelinta@ssn.edu.in

https://doi.org/10.1515/9781501502415-203

T. Nagarajan
SSN College of Engineering, India
nagarajant@ssn.edu.in

Tanvina B. Patel
Dhirubhai Ambani Institute of Information
and Communication Technology (DA-IICT),
India
tanvina.patel@gmail.com

Hemant A. Patil
Dhirubhai Ambani Institute of Information
and Communication Technology (DA-IICT),
India
hemant_patil@daiict.ac.in

Fabien Ringeval
audEERING GmbH, Germany
Université Grenoble Alpes, France
fabien.ringeval@imag.fr

Björn Schuller
audEERING GmbH, Germany
Imperial College London, UK
University of Augsburg, Germany
schuller@tum.de

Sid Ahmed Selouani
Université de Moncton, Canada
selouani@umcs.ca

Latika Singh
The NorthCap University, India
latikasingh@ncuindia.edu

P. Vijayalakshmi
SSN College of Engineering, India
vijayalakshmip@ssn.edu.in

Xiyue Wang
School of Electrical Engineering
and Information
Sichuan University, China

Huijun Yan
School of Electrical Engineering
and Information
Sichuan University, China

Heng Yin
Hospital of Stomatology
Sichuan University, China
phoebeyin@126.com

Chi Zhang
Erik Jonsson School of Engineering
and Computer Science
The University of Texas at Dallas, USA
chi.zhang@utdallas.edu

Yue Zhang
Technische Universität München, Germany
Imperial College London, UK

Introduction

Signal and Acoustic Modeling for Speech and Communication Disorders is a compilation of studies and literature reviews demonstrating how some of today's most advanced technology in speech signal processing can be instrumental in early detection and successful intervention when treating speech and communication disorders. We are using "disorders" in its broadest sense to include a panoply of speech difficulties stemming from congenital defects, developmental disorders, degenerative diseases, and disabling neuromotor conditions found in older adult populations or among those who have been seriously injured.

This anthology brings together researchers and academicians from a number of leading universities and speech labs in the USA, Canada, the UK, Germany, Morocco, India, China, and Brazil. The contributors to this volume, through a variety of research studies and literature reviews, have closely examined signal and acoustic modeling across a broad spectrum of speech and communication disorders. The causes of such disorders include Parkinson's disease, Autism Spectrum Disorder, cleft palate, intellectual disabilities, neuro-motor communication disorders (manifested as dysarthria) – resulting from stroke, brain tumor, traumatic brain injury, or severe reaction(s) to medication. Utilizing some of the most advanced, innovative, and experimentally sound methods in signal and acoustic modeling, the contributors show how such advances in speech technology can greatly inure to the benefit of healthcare and to society writ large – availing patients of noninvasive, cost-effective methods to successfully detect, monitor, and gauge their speech, language, and communication disorders. Given that early intervention is crucial for managing and controlling speech and communication disorders, a better understanding of the speech signal and, more generally, the wide range of acoustic properties of such disorders potentiates intervention and perhaps, someday, a cure for congenital and/or acquired maladies of speech. Paradoxically, what most of us take for granted remains a Sisyphean battle for those with speech and language disorders, who struggle every day to make themselves heard and understood. It is our hope that the illuminating chapters in this collection will encourage further empirical studies and stimulate discussion among speech scientists, system designers, and practitioners on how to marshal the latest advances in signal and acoustic modeling to address some of the most challenging speech and communication disorders.

This book is divided into three sections.

The first section of the anthology discusses in close detail how specific developments in speech signal processing can be highly instrumental in diagnosing and treating speech and communication disorders, as well as in detecting early signs of

https://doi.org/10.1515/9781501502415-001

medical problems that may impair neuromotor functioning and compromise speech intelligibility. The section opens with a comprehensive analysis of whispered speech, which is important because as a diagnostic tool, alone, advances made in the study of "whispered" speech can help clinicians detect early signs of cardiac insufficiency and other heart-related problems, which often show high rates of co-morbidity with *stroke*. The authors show how using metrics that point to the percentage of whispered speech within patients' total daily speech can serve as a very important alternative diagnostic method. No doubt, using whispered speech as a diagnostic indicator is less costly and certainly less invasive to the patient than traditional diagnostic methods.

The whispered speech chapter is followed by an intriguing look at how advances made in the study of "hypernasality" – a speech resonance disorder that occurs due to improper velopharyngeal closure, which causes too much air leakage from the nose thereby introducing an improper nasal balance – can serve as a valuable (and cost-effective) diagnostic tool for speech disorders. The authors show how this is particularly useful for measuring the degree of congenital abnormality of the lip and palate, as well as in the assessment of neuro-muscular problems and hearing impairments. As with whispered speech, hypernasality metrics provide a sensible alternative to invasive methods that cause pain and discomfort to patients while placing an economic burden on an overextended healthcare system.

The next chapter in this section looks at how some of the most important advances in acoustic-based tools and scripts for the automatic analysis of speech have proven essential for diagnosing speech disorders. By examining Praat-scripts developed for analyzing prosodic acoustic parameters as an aid for acoustic science on prosody modeling, speech scientists are able to determine the correlation in prosody and perception in normal and pathological speech. This occurs because the SG detector script assist in language-mediated, semi-automatic identification of syllable-sized normalized duration peaks to investigate prominence and boundary marking. By making such scripts freely available, this novel method has been successfully tested in French, German, Swedish, English, and in (Brazilian and European) Portuguese.

Oftentimes, the differences between the normal and pathological voices can be so subtle that it requires methods that are painstakingly precise. As such, the section is rounded out by an eye-opening view into chaos theory and its application to speech and communication disorders. The authors examine in close detail how one can apply a novel chaotic titration-based approach to detect and quantify the amount of chaos that exists in the speech signal. They show how by titrating the speech signal with noise, which is similar to titrating acid with a base in the chemical titration process, the amount of chaos measured is related to the noise added to titrate the speech signal. This innovative approach yields a significant amount of relevant information in terms of the chaotic behavior of the speech sample, helping to classify normal and pathological voices.

The second section of the book takes a close look at cognitive, affective, and developmental disorders and their manifestations in speech and communication abnormalities. The section opens with a fascinating study of 30 children and adults with mild-to-moderate Intellectual Disability, with 52 age-matched controls. The authors rightly point out that though health professionals use language impairments as one of the main diagnostic criteria to diagnose Intellectual Disability, the acoustic nature of such abnormalities and their diagnostic power is currently underestimated, particularly in early detection of such disorders. The authors meet this challenge by showing how one may quantify speech abnormalities using acoustic parameters including fundamental frequency (Fo), intensity, and spectro-temporal features encoded at different time scales in speech samples. Here, the spectro-temporal features are extracted, as these features provide the phonological basis of speech comprehension and production. Using these research parameters, the authors found significant differences in these measures between the experimental and control groups. Building upon these differences, the authors designed a classification system that can differentiate between the speech of those with an Intellectual Disability and those with normal cognitive functioning in the control group, yielding a 97.5 percent accuracy. The authors show how their study is a step toward developing speech-based markers for contributing to the early diagnosis of mild-to-moderate Intellectual Disability.

The second section follows with two chapters on Autism Spectrum Disorders.

The first chapter on autism provides an excellent survey of autism and speech, language, and emotion. The authors discuss how individuals with Autism Spectrum Conditions (ASC) show difficulties in social interaction, communication, and restricted interests and repetitive behavior. They show how those suffering from ASC also experience difficulties in modulating and enhancing spoken content through expressiveness at different communication levels – in particular, speech, language, and emotion. The chapter provides a comprehensive look at the peculiarities of ASC manifestations in both speech and language and as related to emotion as well. The authors explore the interests and challenges of using speech technology for individuals with ASC by examining these different aspects of communication.

The second chapter on autism explores clinical applications of speech technology for Autism Spectrum Disorder (ASD). The author demonstrates how individuals with ASD show considerable variability in their speech deficits, ranging from functional linguistic/affective uses of prosody to more subtle differences in the manner in which prosody is used in communicating with others.

The chapter elucidates how technological developments show promise for early identification of vocal deficits in ASD and the potential for speech technology to improve treatment of this disorder. In doing so, the author explores a number of uses of speech technology in clinical therapeutic settings, and, in particular, how theoretical applications, such as voice modeling, hold a lot of promise. With an emphasis on the importance of a healthy interdisciplinary collaboration between speech scientists and clinicians, the chapter illuminates the most pressing areas that are in need of rigorous research.

The third section of the collection presents rigorous studies in the assessment and quantification of speech intelligibility in patients with anatomical defects, disabling conditions, and degenerative diseases that produce speech impediments and pathological speech. The studies in this section cover both congenital and acquired speech disorders.

We open the section with an informative study of automatic assessment of consonant omission and speech intelligibility in cleft palate speech. The authors show how crucial it is to use the most effective methods for assessing cleft palate speech in clinical practice. They propose two algorithms to automatically detect the consonant omission and assess the speech intelligibility in cleft palate speech. Using robust methods, the cleft palate speech database contains 530 participants, with a large vocabulary size that encompasses all initial consonants and the most widely used vowels in Mandarin. Based on the differences between vowels and initial consonants in Mandarin, their work combined the short-time autocorrelation function and the hierarchical clustering model to realize the automatic detection of consonant omission. The authors found that the recognition accuracy of automatic speech recognition system is proportional to speech intelligibility.

This chapter on cleft palate speech is followed by a study of distinctive auditory-based cues and rhythm metrics to assess the severity level of dysarthria. The authors point to the large population of children and adults that suffer from acquired or congenital neuromotor communication disorders that affect their speech intelligibility. They propound the importance of automatic characterization of the speech impairment to improve the patient's quality of life and assist experts in the assessment and treatment of the speech impairment. In their chapter, the authors present different techniques for improving the analysis and classification of disordered speech to automatically assess the severity of dysarthria. A model simulating the external, middle, and inner parts of the ear is presented. The model provides relevant auditory-based cues that are combined with conventional Mel Frequency Cepstral Coefficients (MFCCs) and rhythm metrics to represent atypical speech utterances. The experiments are carried out using data from the Nemours and Torgo databases of dysarthric speech.

Gaussian mixture models (GMMs), support vector machines (SVMs), and multinomial logistic regression (MLR) are tested and compared with the context of dysarthric speech assessment. The experimental results showed that the MLR-based approach using multiple and diverse input features offers a powerful alternative to the conventional assessment methods.

The third section is concluded by a forward-looking analysis of the use of wireless sensor networks and embedded systems to measure the motor defects of patients suffering from Parkinson's disease. In the quantification of Parkinson's disease, the authors explore how a medical cyber-physical system can gauge in addition to motor defects, using EMG and blood pressure sensors, the degradation of the patient's condition by analyzing the patient's voice signal to extract descriptors that characterize Parkinson's disease. They show how data fusion between the sensor network and the embedded system can quantify the disease process and evolution to better assist the patient in a treatment plan suited for the patient's condition. Given the emerging science of ubiquitous/pervasive computing in healthcare, the authors truly show prescience in their use of wireless sensor networks and embedded systems for tracking, among other physiological functions, the subtle changes in voice production as indications of disease progression in the patient suffering from Parkinson's disease.

As editors of this volume, we have endeavored to make this book, appearing in the Series in *Speech Technology and Text Mining in Medicine and Health Care*, a comprehensive collection of studies, expositions, and literature reviews that present the most current and advanced research findings in signal and acoustic modeling of speech pathologies across as broad a spectrum as possible. This anthology is aimed at speech scientists, system designers, and clinicians and speech pathologists whose *weltanschauung* is to bring to the patient the most advanced and effective methods for early intervention and optimal care, especially in a world where healthcare access is often inadequately available to those who need it most. Perhaps, this work will illuminate, inspire, and galvanize healthcare institutions to avail themselves of more advanced methods in detecting, monitoring, and treating speech and communication disorders. We are deeply humbled by the contributions of this book and are grateful to have the opportunity to work so assiduously with the authors, as well as with each of our co-editors, to bring this tome to fruition.

Part I: **Applying New Developments in Speech Signal Processing in the Diagnosis and Treatment of Speech and Communication Disorders and in the Detection of Risk to Neuro-Motor Functioning**

Chi Zhang and John H.L. Hansen

1 Advancements in whispered speech detection for interactive/speech systems

Abstract: While the challenge of non-neutral speech is attracting more research attention in recent years, the specific speaking style of "whisper" is of particular interest in both speech technology and human-to-human communication, especially for hearing-impaired individuals. Whisper is a common mode of natural speech communication, which is an *alternative* speech production mode, used in public circumstances to protect content privacy or identity, or potentially a common speaking style for individuals with speech production limitations. The *spectral* structure of whispered speech is dramatically different from that of neutral speech. This profound difference between whisper and neutral speech is caused by the fundamental differences in production mechanisms of these two speech modes. Given these differences, the performance of current speech-processing systems, which are designed to process neutral speech, degrades significantly. In this chapter, challenges of speech processing for whispered speech will be reviewed. Next, the requirement of front-end whispered speech detection for speech-processing applications will be introduced. An overview of current advancements for both unsupervised/model-free whispered speech detection and model-based distant-whispered speech detection will be presented. Finally, a brief summary and conclusion is followed by a discussion on directions for future work.

Keywords: Whispered speech, neutral speech, whispered speech detection, whispered speech processing, speech recognition

1.1 Introduction

Speech production based on vocal effort can generally be categorized into five modes: (i) whispered, (ii) soft, (iii) neutral, (iv) loud, and (v) shouted, based on how much effort is put on vocal folds when speech is produced. Neutral speech is a modal speech produced at rest. In neutral speech, voiced phonemes are produced by a periodic vibration of the vocal folds, which regulates airflow into the pharynx and oral cavities. However, for whispered speech, the shape of the pharynx is adjusted such that the vocal folds do not vibrate, resulting in a continuous air stream or turbulence without periodicity [1–4]. Whispered speech is the speech mode with results in reduced

https://doi.org/10.1515/9781501502415-002

perceptibility and a significant reduction in intelligibility. In general, whispered speech can occur in a variety of settings with the physiological speech production change from neutral of a complete absence of vocal fold vibration. As a natural mode of speech for communication, whispered speech can be employed by people in public situations to protect the content of the speech information, or in some settings to reduce the probability of being able to identify the speaker. For example, when an automated phone answering system is requesting people to provide their credit number, bank account details, or other personal information, speakers using a cell phone in public situations may prefer to speak in a whisper mode. Alternatively, as a para-linguistic phenomenon, some circumstances would prohibit neutral speech, such as in a library or a formal setting like a conference or performance in a theatre. In these situations, whisper will be employed to convey information between the speaker and the listener to avoid being overheard by other people nearby. Furthermore in some voice pathology cases, changes in the vocal fold structure or physiology or muscle control due to disease of the vocal system, such as functional aphonia, laryngeal cancer, functional voice disorder or alteration of the vocal folds due to medical operations or reduced forced vital air capacity of the lungs, may result in the speaker employing whisper as their communication style [5–7]. In one of the recent studies conducted in health-related acoustic domain [8], vocal perturbation and speech-breathing characteristics were computed from patient speech as an early indicator of heart failure. Therefore, the existence and percentage of whispered speech within the patients' daily speech may also help to serve as an alternative diagnosis methods.

Current speech-processing algorithms are primarily developed based on an assumption that the speech signal to be processed is in neutral mode rather than any of the other four vocal effort modes. Previous work [9, 10] has shown that speech produced across different vocal effort levels has a profound impact on speech technology, and in particular, speaker recognition systems. Vocal effort here refers to whisper, soft, loud, and shouted speaking conditions based on speaker-identification systems trained using speech produced under neutral conditions. While the NATO RSG-10 study [11] was the first to show that closed set speaker identification performance under stress, including soft and loud spoken speech, was impacted, the study by Zhang and Hansen [10] represents one of the first, which performed analysis on the production differences and quantified the loss in performance using a well-organized speech corpus. While soft, loud, and shouted speech all result in significant mismatch between neutral speech conditions, whisper is more pronounced due to the fundamental differences in physical speech production.

To maintain performance of current speech-processing systems for whispered speech, feature and algorithmic advancements are necessary to ensure consistent performance to that experienced for neutral speech. This chapter aims to explore this space and provide both a summary of recent advancements as well as insight into directions for future research in the field.

1.2 Background and analysis

Due to the fundamental differences between the production mechanisms of neutral versus whispered speech, these altered characteristics of whispered speech result in degraded performance of speech-processing systems, including speech recognition, speaker identification, language ID, speech coding, and other speech/language technologies. Therefore, in recent years, several research studies have focused on whispered speech processing. The investigation foci of whispered speech include a theoretical point of view in speech production and perception [12–18], and for practical reasons in whispered speech recognition [19–23]. While these studies have considered an analysis of speech production under whisper and assessing the impact of whisper speech on speech technology, little, if any, systematic effort has been reported on how to effectively detect and locate whispered speech within input audio streams. These studies have focused on pure homogenous whispered speech data, or they are assuming prior knowledge of the location of whispered speech within the audio stream. However, whispered speech detection is crucial, since for subjects with healthy vocal systems, it is expected that whisper mode will occur in mixed neutral/whisper combinations depending on the information content within the audio stream (e.g., it is generally the case that normal speakers cannot sustain whisper mode for extensively long periods of time, within the range of 10 mins-to-hours) [24]. To utilize speech-processing techniques that address whispered speech, the locations of whispered speech must first be identified within the audio stream.

To fulfill this crucial task of detecting whispered speech within a neutral phonated audio stream, a brief review of whispered speech production is first considered. Figure 1.1 [19] shows the dramatic differences between neutral and whispered speech waveforms for the sentence "She is thinner than I am" from the same speaker. It can be seen that the whispered speech waveform is much lower in the overall amplitude contour, lacks any periodic segments, and is generally more aperiodic in nature.

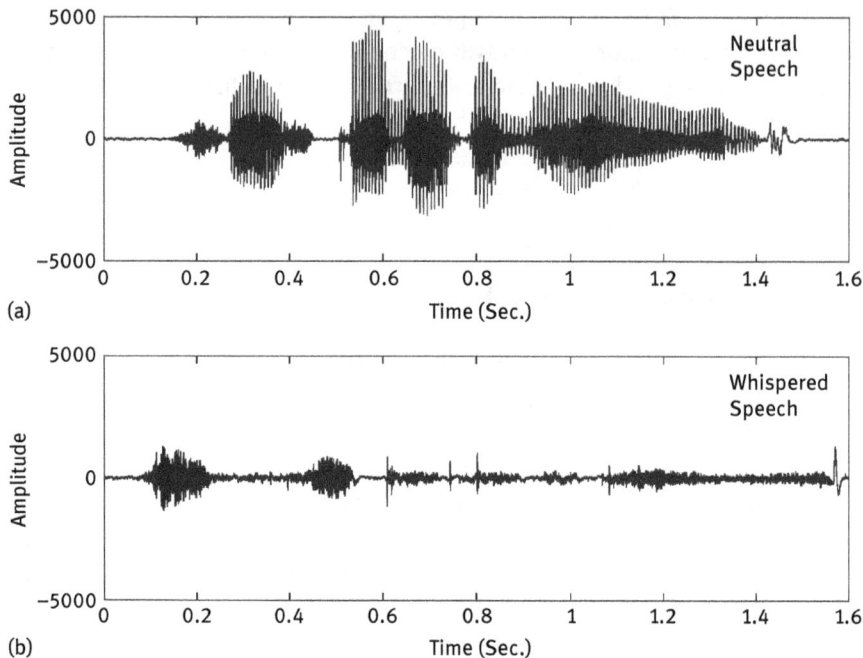

Figure 1.1: Waveforms of (a) neutral, and (b) whispered speech [24].

The whispered speech is different from neutral speech in both time and frequency domains. Due to the alternative speech-production mechanism, the
resulting speech spectra between whisper and neutral speech are significantly
different. The differences between whispered and neutral speech include the
following [20, 21, 25–27]:
- A complete absence of periodic excitation or harmonic structure in whispered speech;
- A shift for the lower formant locations;
- A change in the overall spectral slope (becomes flatter, with a reduction from
  the low frequency region);
- A shifting of the boundaries of vowel regions in the F1–F2 frequency
  space; and
- A change in both energy and duration characteristics.

Given these temporal and spectral differences between whispered speech and
neutral speech, developing algorithms, which are sensitive to these differences, may provide a solution to detect whispered speech within an input

audio stream. Effective whispered speech detection should provide knowledge of both the existence and accurate starting and ending points of whispered segments. This information would also play a significant role for concatenated speech applications. As a front-end step, whisper detection may help indicate when a whisper-dedicated algorithm or whisper adaptation of a neutral trained system should be employed. With knowledge of locations of whispered speech, the cell phone system may apply an enhancement or even a transformation to the whisper audio segment, to improve intelligibility to listeners. When whispered segment locations are obtained from a preceding whisper detection algorithm, an automatic speech recognition (ASR) system, for example, the one used by any automated phone answering service, can either choose the whisper-adapted acoustic models or apply an alternative feature extraction method for whispered segments to achieve more robust recognition results. For healthcare-related speech-processing applications, when the speech is from individuals with vocal fold pathologies, those with lung problems with insufficient lung capacity for vocalization of speech, or individuals with full laryngectomies, whispered speech detection will be necessary to alert these applications to engage processing algorithms designed for whispered speech. Even the percentage of whispered speech detected from speech can be a potential indicator of the recovering progress for those subjects who are participating in medical treatment for their larynx diseases. Furthermore, since whisper has a high probability of conveying sensitive information, with the help of a whisper detection algorithm, a speech document retrieval system or call center monitor system can identify, where potential confidential or sensitive information occurs within a neutral speech audio stream.

1.3 Advancements in unsupervised whispered speech detection

In this section, an unsupervised model-free framework for effective whispered speech detection is introduced to identify, where whisper is located within a given neutral speech audio stream. The algorithm is developed using an entropy-based feature set: Whisper Island Detection (WhID), which is an improvement of the 4-D WhID feature set [24]. The WhID feature set is integrated within T^2-Bayesian Information Criterion (BIC) segmentation algorithm [28] for vocal effort change point (VECP) detection and utilized for whispered speech detection. Figure 1.2 shows the high-level flow diagram of the whispered speech detection algorithm.

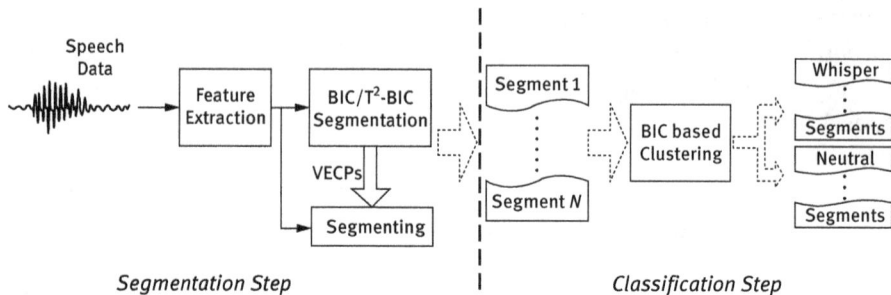

Figure 1.2: Flow diagram of whispered speech detection [30, 36].

1.3.1 Algorithm development for whispered speech detection

The potential VECPs of the input speech data embedded with whispered speech are first detected in the segmentation step (left part of Figure 1.2). Based on the sequence of potential-detected VECPs, the speech stream is divided into segments. An improved T^2-BIC algorithm [24] previously described is incorporated to detect the potential VECPs between whisper and neutral speech. The T^2-BIC algorithm, developed by Zhou and Hansen [28] and also described in previous works [10, 20, 29], is an unsupervised model-free scheme that detects acoustic change points based on the input feature data. A range of potential input features for the T^2-BIC algorithm can be used to detect input acoustic changes within the audio stream. Here, the T^2-BIC algorithm is considered as a potential method to detect the VECPs between whisper and neutral speech if an effective feature for vocal effort change is employed.

In the classification step (right portion of Figure 1.2), unlike using a previously proposed gaussian mixture model (GMM) classifier [24], a BIC-based clustering phase is deployed to group the segments. Based on the fact that the averaged spectral information entropy (SIE) of whisper is larger than that of neutral speech, after the segments are grouped into two clusters, the segments can be identified based on vocal effort by comparing the averaged SIE between the two clusters.

1.3.2 WhID feature set

Unlike the previous study [24], the formulation of the WhID feature set for each 20 ms speech frame is modified as follows:
1) Based on the comparison of the averaged power spectrum density between whisper and neutral speech, the frequency bands with the largest and smallest

differences are selected to calculate the one-dimensional SIE ratio. Based on the manually labeled vocal effort information of the speech data used in previous study [24], the utterances from 59 speakers are segmented into blocks having consistent vocal effort. The difference between the averaged power spectral density (PSD) of whisper segments to that of neutral speech segments is depicted in Figure 1.3, with the maximum and minimum differences marked with circles.

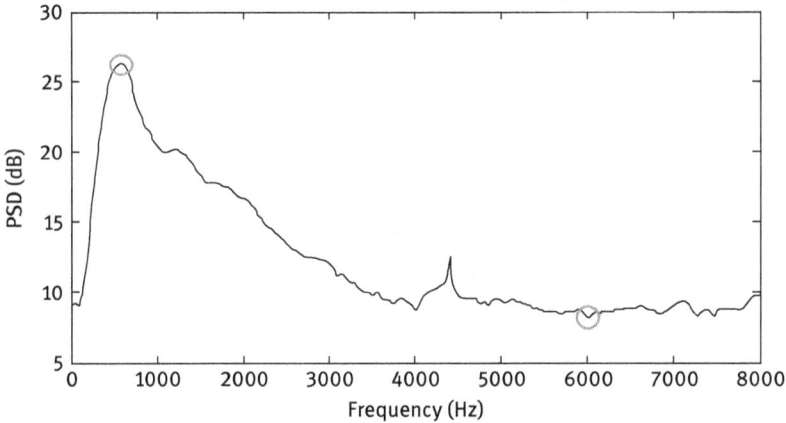

Figure 1.3: Difference between averaged PSD of whispered and neutral speech [30].

2) The SIE is calculated within the frequency range of 300–3,500 Hz, which is the normal telephone speech range, while not using the frequency range above 3,500 Hz, since the SIE in that region is similar for whisper versus neutral speech. The selection of the frequency range of 300–3,500 Hz is further supported by the maximum KL distance between the estimated distributions of SIE of whisper and neutral speech. Therefore, the SIE is calculated within the range of 300–3,500 Hz.
3) The spectral tilt is calculated for each speech frame and used to form the three-dimension of the WhID feature set.

Histograms of each of the dimensions of the 3-D WhID feature are compared between whispered and neutral speech in Figure 1.4. In mathematical statistics, the Kullback–Leibler divergence, also called relative entropy, is a measure of how one probability distribution diverges from the second expected probability distribution [31]. In this work, we use the Kullback–Leibler divergence to measure the discriminant property of each feature

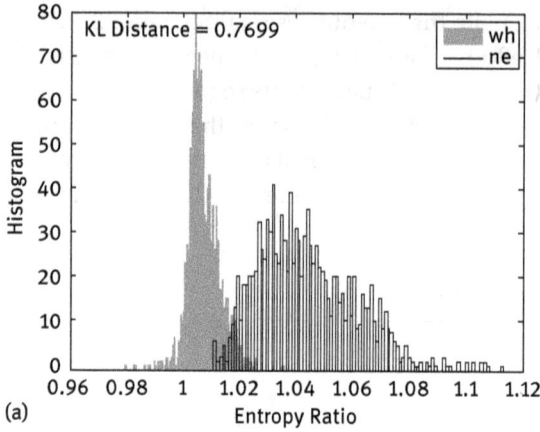

(a)

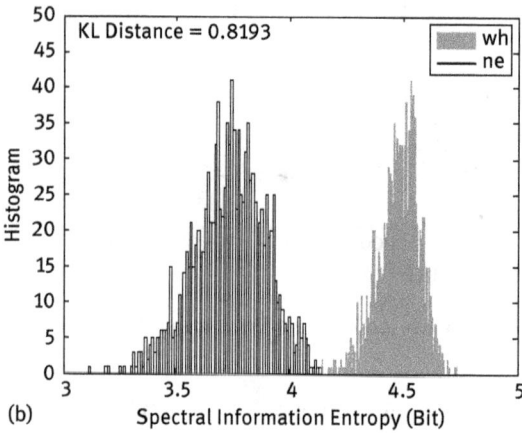

(b)

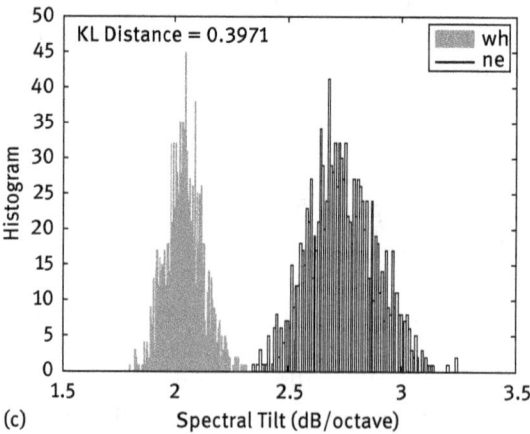

(c)

Figure 1.4: (a) Histogram of 1st dimension of improved 3-D WhID feature set: Whisper vs. neutral speech: entropy ratio (5,900–6,100 Hz vs. 478–678 Hz); (b) histogram of 2nd dimension of improved 3-D WhID feature set: Whisper vs. neutral speech: spectral information entropy (300–3,500 Hz); and (c) histogram of 3rd dimension of improved 3-D WhID feature set: Whisper vs. neutral speech: spectral tilt.

dimension between whisper and neutral speech. The Kullback–Leibler divergence between the estimated distributions of whispered and neutral speech for each dimension of the features is listed in the corresponding figure to further support the modification of the WhID feature set. The details of SIE are explained in our previous work [30].

1.3.3 T^2-BIC segmentation and BIC clustering algorithms

The segmentation task can be reformulated as a model selection task between two nested competing models. The BIC, a penalized maximum likelihood model selection criterion, is employed for model selection [32]. The segmentation decision is derived by comparing BIC values. As a statistical data processing method, BIC requires no prior knowledge concerning the acoustic conditions, and no prior model training is needed. Instead of choosing a hard threshold for the segmentation decision, BIC statistically finds the difference in the acoustic features of the input frames to determine a point, which can separate the data within the processing window into two models. Due to the quadratic complexity of the BIC-based segmentation algorithm [28], the T^2 value (Hotelling's T^2-statistic is a multivariate analog of the well-known t-distribution [33]) was calculated to find candidate boundary frames. Next, BIC value calculations are performed only around the frames in the neighborhood of candidate boundary frame to find the best frame breakpoint and verify the decision of the boundary as is typical in the original BIC algorithm [24]. Here, the T^2-statistic was integrated within the BIC algorithm in this manner for processing shorter audio streams, while the traditional BIC algorithm was used to process longer duration blocks. The BIC algorithm was used for a process window larger than 5 s, and T^2-BIC was used when a process window is less than 5 s By utilizing the 3-D WhID feature set, which was shown to be discriminative between whisper and neutral speech, the T^2-BIC algorithm can detect possible VECPs between whisper and neutral speech.

After obtaining the possible VECPs from the T^2-BIC algorithm with the WhID feature set incorporated into the segmentation step, the classification of vocal efforts can be performed by deploying the BIC clustering algorithm [30, 36]. The BIC-based clustering algorithm was proposed and utilized as a clustering technique in applications for speaker segmentation and clustering [32, 34, 35]. With VECP detection results, the speech audio was over-segmented into several vocal effort consistent segments. If we suggest that each acoustically homogeneous segment can be modeled as one multivariate Gaussian process, for each pair of segments, there are two hypotheses:

H_0: both segments are under same vocal effort and

H_1: the two segments are under different vocal efforts.

Here, hypothesis H0 assumes that all samples from these two segments are distributed as a single Gaussian, which means these two segments should be clustered together. Hypothesis H1 assumes that the frame samples of one segment are drawn from one Gaussian, while those frame samples of the second segment are drawn from a separate Gaussian. With these assumptions, if BIC favors H0 then the data are assumed to be homogeneous in terms of vocal effort, otherwise these two segments should be separated.

The BIC value of the two hypotheses are calculated and compared to form a metric to decide whether the two segments should be clustered. Using the BIC scores based on the above assumption, a hierarchal routine is utilized to cluster the segments based on their vocal efforts. After VECP detection, assuming there are M segments, each segment is treated as a node. Based on the assumption in above paragraph, the BIC scores for each possible pair of segments are calculated. The pair of nodes with the highest positive BIC score are clustered together to form a new node, resulting in M-1 remaining nodes. The same procedure is performed on the rest M-1 nodes till there are only two nodes (whisper and neutral speech) left or the BIC score is less than 0.

After obtaining the two final clusters, the averaged 3-D WhID feature for each cluster can be calculated. With the knowledge that the averaged SIE of whisper is larger than that of neutral speech as was shown in Figure 1.4(b), and/or the fact that the averaged spectral tilt of whisper is flatter than that of neutral speech [9], the two clusters are easily labeled in terms of vocal effort by comparing the averaged WhID features. In addition, the false alarm error from VECP detection is compensated by clustering successive segments, which have the same vocal effort together.

1.3.4 Whispered speech detection performance

In our previous study [10], the multi-error score (MES) was developed and introduced to evaluate the performance of acoustic features for detection of VECPs. The MES consists of three error types for segmentation mismatch: miss detection rate (MDR), false alarm rate (FAR), and average mismatch in milliseconds normalized by adjacent segment duration. To ensure that the metric unit of these three error types are consistent, the error type mismatch in milliseconds are measured as a percentage of the mismatch over the total duration of the two consecutive segments, such that the metric unit of all the three error types are, therefore, in percentage. Figure 1.5 illustrates these three types of error.

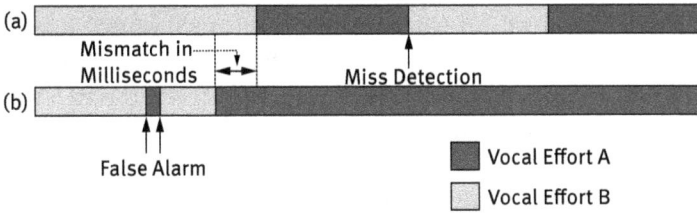

Figure 1.5: Three types of segmentation error [36].

The calculation of MES can be illustrated by the following equation, with FAR, mismatch rate (MMR), and MDR weighted by 1, 2, and 3, respectively:

$$MES = 1 \times \text{False Alarm Rate} + 2 \times \text{Mismatch Rate} + 3 \times \text{Miss Detection Rate}. \quad (1.1)$$

The weight of three chosen here is to emphasize the increased cost for miss detection of a whisper island (largest cost). The weight of two for false alarms was chosen since false alarm errors are not as troubling, and there are potential post-processing steps, which could reduce these false positive segments. The MMR is obtained by calculating the percentage of the mismatch in milliseconds versus the total duration of the two segments corresponding to the actual breakpoints. More details concerning the MES can be found in our previous study [20].

For the case of vocal effort segmentation, the false alarm error rate can be compensated by merging two very close segments of common vocal effort, or by merging two adjacent segments classified as the same vocal effort in a later vocal effort classification step. Hence, false alarm errors have less impact than the miss detection errors in the overall evaluation of segmentation (i.e., this is the reason for a weight of "1" in equation (1.1)). Furthermore, the average mismatch between experimental and actual break points is an important norm, which reflects break point accuracy for the features and data. The MMR is obtained by calculating the percentage of mismatch in milliseconds versus the total duration of the combined two adjacent segments corresponding to the actual breakpoint. The MDR and MMR are more costly errors for whispered speech detection, so these errors are scaled by 3 and 2, respectively, in equation (1.1).

Next, we consider the meaning of the resulting MES scores, including an upper and lower bounds on performance. The ideal whisper/neutral segmentation has a zero FAR, zero MDR, and 0 mismatch in milliseconds (or 0%, which occurs when: $(0 \text{ ms})/(T_{total}) \times 100\%$ is calculated), and thus the MES will be zero in the ideal/lower-bound case. For the case where the MMR, FAR, and MDR are all no greater than 10%, the resulting MES will be no greater than 60, which denotes "fair" performance for whisper segmentation. If the FAR is at 10%, however the MDR and MMR are at 15%, the MES increases to 85, which suggest that segmentation is collectively considered to be performing "poorly". In the worse case scenario, with a 100% FAR, 100% MDR, and 100% MMR, the MES will have an upper bound of 600. Therefore, the goal of the segmentation phase is to achieve an MES as low as possible.

To illustrate the advantage of modifying WhID formulation as well as assess performance of the model-free whispered speech detection algorithm, an assessment was performed with experimental results tabulated using the MES. Speech audio consisting of 41 TIMIT sentences were alternatively read in whisper and neutral mode by 59 subjects from the UT-VE II corpus (i.e., UTDallas vocal effort II corpus [24]) and transcript files containing manually labeled vocal effort information for these audio files were used in the experiments. Each TIMIT sentence is 2 to 3 s long in duration. Within the speech audio from each subject, the 10th and 11th sentences are read in whisper mode to form a 4–6 s of long whispered speech segment. Audio files from 59 subjects were used to extract the modified 3-D WhID feature sequence and evaluated with the proposed model-free algorithm for whispered speech detection. The experimental results in terms of MES and detection accuracy are compared with the results obtained using the previously formulated four-dimensional (4-D) WhID feature and classification algorithm [24]. The MES score and detailed error scores using the current proposed feature set and classification algorithm are compared with the results from [24] in Table 1.1.

Table 1.1: Evaluation for vocal effort change points detection

Feature type	MDR (%)	FAR (%)	MMR (%)	MES
4-D WhID [24]	0.00	8.13	1.69	11.51
3-D WhID	0.00	4.95	1.45	7.86

By using the BIC/T^2-BIC algorithm [24] for VECP detection, due to the reduced dimension, the proposed modified WhID feature has less computational complexity than the previous 4-D WhID feature set. Furthermore, improved VECP detection is achieved with a 0% MDR as well as lower false alarm and MMRs than that is seen using the 4-D WhID feature solution, which points to the success of the modified WhID as having better performance in differentiating vocal effort between whisper and neutral speech.

With the results of VECP detection using the modified 3-D WhID feature set, the mode-free vocal effort clustering algorithm is evaluated for whispered speech detection accuracy, which is the percentage of correctly detected whispered speech

Table 1.2: Evaluation for overall whispered speech detection.

Feature	Detected number	Detection rate (%)
3-D WhID	1,182	100

segments versus the total number of whispered speech segments. The detection accuracy of the proposed algorithm is summarized in Table 1.2.

Unlike that algorithm requiring prior knowledge of vocal effort for the training data [24], the proposed model-free vocal effort solution deploys an effective discriminative property of the 3-D WhID feature and BIC-based model selection theory, which is also used in VECP detection, to differentiate, cluster, and label the segments with different vocal effort and achieves the same 100% whispered speech segment detection rate as the previous 4-D feature algorithm.

1.3.5 Robustness evaluation

Although good VECP detection and whispered speech detection were achieved, which are indicated by the low MES and 100% detection rate, a further assessment of the robustness of proposed algorithm is warranted, given that it must be effective in actual whisper speech audio streams. These results were obtained by the model-free algorithm using the modified WhID feature, due to the existence of in-stream audio interference, such as background noise, channel distortion, and environmental distortions in the real word, the robustness of the proposed feature and algorithm need to be explored. Several experiments were carried out to assess the performance of the proposed algorithm under different levels of background white noise.

Additive white noise was generated and added to the test utterance used in Section 3.4 under scenarios with Signal-to-Noise Ratio (SNR) values of −5, 0, and 5 dB. The SNR value is calculated as the overall energy ratio between whisper-embedded neutral speech and the additive white noise. Therefore, for the whisper segments within the audio stream, the SNR value would be even worse. The VECP detection performances for each of the SNR scenarios are shown in Table 1.3.

It can be observed that, although the VECP detection performance improves as SNR increases, indicated by the lower MES scores, as long as the SNR increases, the existence of miss detection and high FAR and even the high MMR will degrade the detection rate of whispered speech in the subsequent classification step.

Table 1.3: Evaluation for vocal effort change points detection under noise existence (3-D WhID).

SNR (dB)	MDR (%)	FAR (%)	MMR (%)	MES
−5	1.39	16.89	3.50	28.06
0	0.65	12.69	2.43	19.50
5	0.34	9.53	2.07	14.72

The interference in the real world may be more complicated than that is seen for this white noise scenario, thus features or algorithm advancements, which are more robust to environmental factors, are needed. This fact serves as the basic motivation to develop a model-based whispered speech detection algorithm described in the following section.

1.4 Advancement in distant whispered speech detection

While detecting whisper speech in a traditional audio stream is difficult, a more challenging task is to detect whispered speech from a distance-based speech capture platform, where the whispered speech is recorded via a far-field microphone in a controlled environment. In real-world conditions, although practical whisper speech typically takes place in quiet environments, for example in a library, there exists environment distortion, such as background/room noise or reverberation that can impact performance. Furthermore, when whispered speech is produced at a distance, the radiation channel characterized by the room acoustical property may influence the acoustical property of both whisper and neutral speech in the frequency domain. In addition, it becomes more difficult to determine whether the distant speech is just normally phonated speech with a lower volume stemming from a distant microphone capture or whether the distant talker is actually whispering. In our previous study [37], a preliminary study was conducted to detect distant-based whispered speech using a microphone array-based speech enhancement technique. Although the microphone array-based enhancement improved VECP detection and whispered speech detection rate, there were still relevant whispered speech segments not detected due to the environmental noise or capture channel influence for the acoustical features. In this phase of the study, a vocal effort likelihood (VEL) feature set, which is discriminative between vocal efforts considering both environmental and capture channel effects, is proposed to detect the distant whispered speech within neutral speech audio.

In the previously developed framework [10, 20, 24], the acoustic feature set was extracted directly from each speech frame and submitted to the T^2-BIC segmentation algorithm to detect VECPs between whisper and neutral speech as shown in Figure 1.6(a). Next, the speech feature sequence was segmented according to the detected VECPs and compared with the GMMs of whisper and neutral speech to classify the vocal effort of each segment. As illustrated in Figure 1.6(b), instead of directly using the acoustic feature for VECP detection as in the frameworks presented in our previous works [10, 20, 24] and Section 3, the proposed algorithm uses the frame-based VEL scores as the discriminative feature set to detect the VECP between whisper and neutral speech.

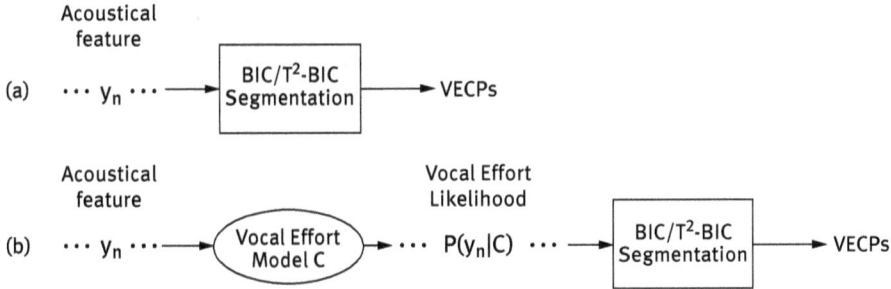

Figure 1.6: (a) Acoustical feature-based VECP detection and (b) Vocal effort likelihood-based VECP detection.

Although a proper acoustic feature may be sensitive to the vocal effort change between whisper and neutral speech, the changes in content of the speech may introduce variations, which are not dependent on the vocal effort change within the feature. By comparing the speech feature of the current frame with the mono-vocal-effort GMM, which is modeling the vocal effort, the output score can be viewed as the likelihood of the current speech frame being the specific vocal effort modeled by the GMM. In this case, the fluctuation of the feature, which consists of the likelihood scores of speech frames from the whisper and neutral GMMs, is highly dependent on the vocal effort of the speech frames. Therefore, the feature set VEL may be viewed as a discriminative feature space across vocal effort. In this study, to detect whispered speech, the VEL is calculated for both whisper and neutral speech to form a two-dimensional (2-D) VEL feature set.

Furthermore, the feature set VEL, compared with the acoustic feature set used to train the GMMs, has a reduced feature dimension. Although the traditional BIC algorithm has been improved, resulting in BIC/T^2-BIC to reduce the computational costs, the covariance matrix calculation and update for the BIC/T^2-BIC algorithm can still be costly if we use a high-dimensional feature. By deploying the VEL 2-D feature set compared with the 4-D feature WhID, 13-D feature Mel-Frequency Cepstral Coefficients (MFCC) [24] and even the 3-D modified WhID feature in Section 3, the computational costs will be reduced using the BIC/T^2-BIC segmentation scheme.

1.4.1 Feature set: Vocal effort likelihood

In this phase of the study, the speech data employ a 20 ms frame length with 50% overlap between the consecutive frames. For each frame, a 13-D MFCC feature is extracted. For the jth frame, the feature $\mathbf{y}_j$ is compared with the GMMs of both whisper and neutral speech, respectively, to estimate the VEL of each vocal effort given the feature vector, $\mathbf{y}_j$:

$$\begin{aligned} \text{VEL}_{\text{whisper}} &= p\left(C_{\text{whisper}}|\mathbf{y}_j\right) \\ \text{VEL}_{\text{neutral}} &= p\left(C_{\text{neutral}}|\mathbf{y}_j\right), \end{aligned} \tag{1.2}$$

where $\mathbf{C}_{\text{whisper}}$ and $\mathbf{C}_{\text{neutral}}$ represent the GMMs trained with the corresponding acoustical feature for either whisper or neutral speech, respectively; $p(\mathbf{C}_{\text{whisper}}|\mathbf{y}_j)$ and $p(\mathbf{C}_{\text{neutral}}|\mathbf{y}_j)$ represent the output scores obtained from the comparison between the current frame and GMMs of both whisper and neutral speech, respectively. Next, the VEL feature vector can be formed as,

$$VEL = \begin{bmatrix} \text{VEL}_{\text{whisper}} \\ \text{VEL}_{\text{neutral}} \end{bmatrix}. \tag{1.3}$$

Since GMMs trained with an appropriate acoustical feature can be viewed as a viable representation of the acoustic space of either whisper or neutral vocal effort [24], $p(\mathbf{C}_{\text{whisper}}|\mathbf{y}_j)$ and $p(\mathbf{C}_{\text{neutral}}|\mathbf{y}_j)$ will, therefore, represent the probability of the current frame being either whisper or neutral speech. For example, for a given frame which is known to be whisper, the probability score $p(\mathbf{C}_{\text{whisper}}|\mathbf{y}_j)$ should be much larger than the $p(\mathbf{C}_{\text{neutral}}|\mathbf{y}_j)$. Furthermore, the variations between phonemes, which may influence the acoustical feature, are normalized in the VEL set by comparing the feature of each frame with the GMMs.

1.4.2 System description

The framework for the proposed algorithm is illustrated in Figure 1.7.

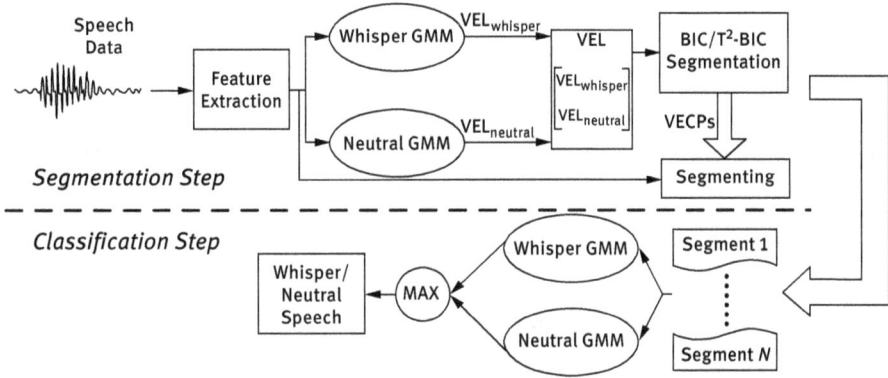

Figure 1.7: Flow diagram of the framework for model-based distant whispered speech detection. [30, 36]

In the segmentation step, the acoustic features are compared with the GMMs of both whisper and neutral speech to obtain the 2-D VEL feature set. The VEL feature set is smoothed using a sliding average window and then submitted to the BIC/T^2-BIC algorithm for detection of VECPs within the audio stream. Unlike the previous algorithm [24], model information of vocal effort is employed in both segmentation and classification steps (i.e., this approach is, therefore, supervised). Given that the training data of each GMM for vocal effort are acquired in the environment in which the distant whisper-embedded neutral speech was collected, the environmental and distance characteristics are included in the GMMs.

1.4.3 UTDallas distant whisper speech corpus: UT-VE-III

To verify the environmental robustness of the proposed distant whispered speech detection algorithm, in addition to the vocal effort/whisper corpora of UT-VE-I and UT-VE-II collected under controlled environmental conditions [24], the corpus named UT-VE-III, consisting of neutral and whispered speech produced at different distances in a real-world environment, was developed [30, 36].

The corpus was collected in a rectangular conference room using an 8-channel TASCAM US-1641 USB audio interface with two SHURE PG185 condenser wireless Lavalier microphones and a 6-channel microphone array.

The corpus consists of both conversational speech and read speech, which contain both contain whisper embedded within neutral speech audio streams. The Lavalier microphones are worn by both subjects and clipped in front of their chests. Since the Lavalier microphones are worn by both subjects at all capture distances, the distance between Lavalier microphone and subject was kept relatively unchanged. Therefore, the speech data collected through the Lavalier microphone reflect the change of capture channel, while the speech data collected through the distant microphone array contain both environmental effects and change of capture channel. The table setting of data collection is depicted in Figure 1.8. All conversations and readings in the collection were recorded by a 6-channel microphone array located at the center of the short side edge of the table and the two wireless Lavalier microphones worn by data collector and subject (all synchronously recorded). The ultimate aim of this corpus is to enroll 30 subjects (15 males and 15 females) in data collection. It should be noted here

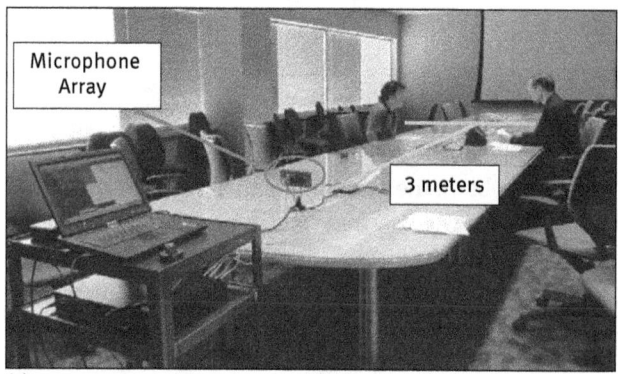

(a)

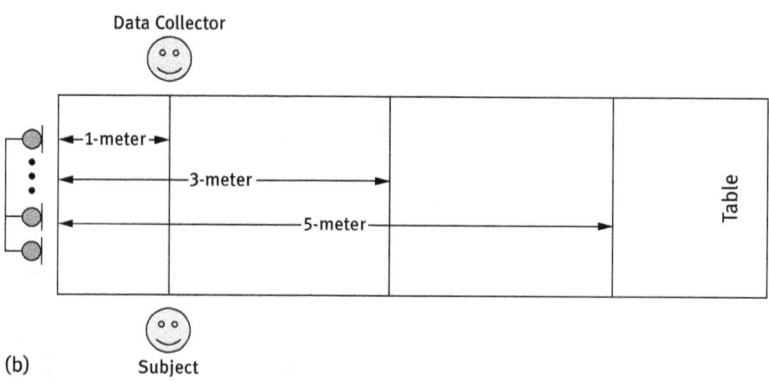

(b)

Figure 1.8: Meeting table setting of data collection for UT-VE-III, (a) data collection scene and microphone array position, (b) table setting in data collection [30].

that the distance from the subject (i.e., person who is the speaker) and subject (i.e., data collector) is maintained across the three distance positions. Therefore, the same level of vocal communications between the two subjects would be maintained as the perpendicular distance to the microphone array is increased. Further details concerning the data collection settings and content of corpus are included in our previous works [30, 36]. In this section, the read speech consists of subjects who read 40 TIMIT sentences alternatively between whisper and neutral mode for experiments. The reading speech was repeated by each subject at 1, 3, and 5 m, from the microphone array position, however still facing the same listener/data collector.

1.4.4 Distant whispered speech detection performance

Several experiments were carried out to assess the performance of the proposed model-based whispered speech detection algorithm for distant whispered speech–embedded neutral speech. The audio streams consists of 41 TIMIT sentences alternatively read in whisper and neutral mode by 10 females subjects at three distances (1, 3, and 5 m) in these experiments. Each audio stream was manually labeled for VECPs and vocal effort in the transcript files. The transcript files of these audio streams were used to compare with VECP detection results obtained from the different experimental scenarios, so that the MES could be calculated. The speech audios recorded from the Lavalier microphone, (Lavalier channel) worn by the subject, from one of the microphone arrays (distant channel) were used for whispered speech detection. In total, six experimental scenarios were performed in this study. For each scenario, two GMMs for whisper and neutral speech were trained using a round-robin scheme to obtain open test speaker and open set test speech. The experimental results in MES for each scenario are shown in Table 1.4 for each scenario.

Table 1.4: Evaluation for vocal effort change points detection for distant whispered speech (VEL).

Distance (m)	Channel	MDR (%)	FAR (%)	MMR (%)	MES
1	Distant	0.00	9.85	3.36	16.56
	Lavalier	0.00	8.85	3.38	15.61
3	Distant	0.00	8.24	4.37	16.98
	Lavalier	0.00	8.02	3.09	14.20
5	Distant	0.00	17.37	4.27	25.92
	Lavalier	0.00	8.88	3.23	15.34

The MDR, FAR, MMR, and MES results shown in Table 1.4 are much better than the previously discussed results [37]. In our previous study [37], as microphone to subject-pair distance increases, although enhanced by the microphone array-processing technique, the performance of VECP detection for speech data collected through distant microphone decreased as long as the distance increased. However, as shown in Table 1.4, for the distant channel without any array-processing enhancement, as long as the distance increases, the performance of VECP detection remains consistently good with 0.00% MDR and lower FAR and MMR than those obtained in our previous work [37]. It can be seen that up to 3 m, the difference in VECP detection from distant microphone to close-talk (Lavalier) microphone is small. At 5 m, VECP detection breaks down, especially for the FAR measure. Finally, given improved/consistent VECP detection performance, detection rate results for each scenario are listed in Table 1.5. Again, whisper detection performance is outstanding with this algorithm configuration.

Table 1.5: Evaluation for distant whispered speech detection.

Distance (m)	Channel	Detection Rate (%)
1	Distant	100
	Lavalier	100
3	Distant	100
	Lavalier	100
5	Distant	100
	Lavalier	100

1.5 Conclusions and directions for future research

Whispered speech detection, especially within a distant whispered speech detection scenario, is a challenging research problem, which has received little attention in the speech research community. There are profound differences in speech production under whisper (e.g., no voicing) for all speech, which renders speech system technology virtually ineffective (e.g., ASR, speaker ID, voice coding, etc.). Effective whispered speech detection is the first step needed to ensure that subsequent engagement of effective speech-processing steps could be employed to address whisper. In this study, we have proposed a 3-D discriminative WhID feature set combined with a previously formulated BIC/T^2-BIC algorithm [24], which was shown to have a smaller MES with 0% MDR, meaning that all VECPs between whisper and neutral speech within the audio streams were correctly detected. Next, the segments partitioned according to the detected VECPs were correctly labeled based on vocal effort using a model-free BIC-based clustering approach. The experimental results indicated that degraded performance of the proposed model-free framework with 3-D WhID in the case where there are noise-corrupted audio streams. This result indicated that further research into robust acoustical features for whispered speech detection was necessary.

To cope with the distortion of the discriminative property of WhID caused by environmental factors as well as any changes in channel effects due to voice capture, a VEL feature set with a model-based whispered speech detection algorithm was also developed (Section 4). With environmental and channel characteristics enrolled into the GMMs of vocal effort, the VEL depicted the probability of the current speech frame being from the specific vocal effort represented by the GMMs. Therefore, this solution can effectively discriminate the vocal effort of whisper *versus* neutral speech, when employed with the BIC/T^2-BIC algorithm in VECP detection. The model information of vocal effort was deployed also in classifying vocal efforts. Given the availability of training data for a vocal effort model with environmental effects, the proposed model-based algorithm has been applied successively for detection of distant-based whispered speech within continuous audio streams.

The resulting effective whispered speech detection frameworks in this study, therefore, offer potential benefits for many speech applications, which can improve the given reliably whispered speech detection results. Due to the profound differences in speech production under whisper, the existence of whispered speech within the training data for the model for a speaker, a language, or dialect, will blur that accurate modeling. Therefore to improve system performance for whisper-embedded data, it should be possible to not only detect and exclude the whispered speech segments from the input data but also utilize the whispered speech detection to purify the training data or development data for more accurate acoustic modeling.

One nature of naturally occurring whispered speech is to convey sensitive information. The content of sensitive information can usually be identified by some keywords. A keyword-spotting system could, therefore, also be used to detect whether the input speech audio contains the interested keywords. A modified keyword-spotting system [30], which is equipped with whispered speech detection as a front-end along with whisper-specified acoustical models, could then be deployed to retrieve the desired speech audio content containing interested sensitive information.

In the health domain, the relation among speech mode and lung, larynx, and throat diseases have been found and studied for years [5–7]. Whispered speech and speech under other vocal efforts would exist before/after the treatment of such diseases. The detection and analysis of whispered speech or speech under other vocal efforts may therefore be used as a diagnosis tool for those diseases. Recently, even the relation between speech mode and heart failure has been studied [8]; collectively, the proposed feature sets and algorithms can be modified to work as a front-end processing step for those studies to obtain the speech under the desired mode in daily speech analysis.

References

[1]   Gavidia-Ceballos L. Analysis and modeling of speech for laryngeal pathology assessments, RSPL: robust speech processing laboratory, Ph.D. Thesis, Duke University, Durham, North Carolina, 1995.

[2]   Gavidia-Ceballos L, Hansen JHL Direct speech feature estimation using an iterative EM algorithm for vocal fold pathology detection. IEEE Trans Biomed Eng 1996; 43(4):373–383.

[3]   Meyer-Eppler W. Realization of prosodic features in whispered speech. J Acoust Soc Am 1957;29(1):104–106.

[4]   Thomas I. Perceived pitch of whispered vowels. J Acoust Soc Am 1969;46(2B):468–470.

[5]   Stetson ARH. Esophageal speech for any laryngectomized patient. Arch Otolaryngol 1937;26(2):132–142.

[6]   Jürgens U, von Cramon D. On the role of the anterior cingulate cortex in phonation: a case report. Brain Lang 1982;15(2):234–248.

[7]   Hess DR. Facilitating speech in the patient with a tracheostomy. Respir Care 2005;50 (4):519–525.

[8]   Murton OM, Hillman RE, Mehta DD. Acoustic speech analysis of patients with decompensated heart failure: a pilot study. J Acoust Soc Am 2017;142(4):EL401.

[9]   Zhang C, Hansen JHL. Analysis and classification of speech mode: whispered through shouted. INTERSPEECH-07, Antwerp, Belgium, Aug. 2007:2289–2292.

[10]   Zhang C, Hansen JHL. Effective segmentation based on vocal effort change point detection. IEEE/ISCA ITRW Speech Analysis and Processing for Knowledge Discovery, Aalborg, Denmark, June 4–6, 2008.

[11]   Hansen JHL, Swail C, South AJ, Moore RK, Steeneken H, Cupples EJ et al. The impact of speech under 'stress' on military speech technology. Published by NATO Research & Technology Organization RTO-TR-10, AC/323(IST)TP/5 IST/TG-01, March 2000 (ISBN: 92-837-1027-4).

[12]   Jovicic S, Saric Z. Acoustic analysis of consonants in whispered speech. J Voice 1997; 22(3):263–274.

[13]   Ito T, Takeda K, Itakura F. Analysis and recognition of whispered speech. Speech Commun 2005;45:139–152.

[14] Kallail K. An acoustic comparison of isolated whispered and phonated vowel samples produced by adult male subjects. J Phonetics 1984;12:175–186.

[15] Eklund I, Traumuller H. Comparative study of male and female whispered and phonated versions of the long vowels of Swedish. Phonetica 1996;54:1–21.

[16] Gao M. Ones in whispered chinese: articulatory features and perceptual cues. MA thesis, Dept. of Linguistics, University of Victoria, British Columbia, Canada, 2002.

[17] Schwartz M, Rine H. Identification of speaker sex from isolated whispered vowels. J Acoust Soc Am 1968;44(6):1736–1737.

[18] Lass K, Hughes K, Bowyer M, Waters L, Bourne V. Speaker sex identification from voiced, whispered and filtered isolated vowels. J Acoust Soc Am 1976;59:675–678.

[19] Fan X, Hansen JHL. Speaker identification within whispered speech audio streams. IEEE Trans Audio Speech Lang Process 2011;19(5):1408, 1421.

[20] Zhang C, Hansen JHL, An entropy based feature for whisper-island detection within audio streams. INTERSPEECH-08, Brisbane, Australia, 2008:2510–2513.

[21] Ito T, Takeda K, Itakura F. Analysis and recognition of whispered speech. Speech Commun 2005;45(2):139–152.

[22] Fan X, Hansen JHL. Speaker identification for whispered speech based on frequency warping and score competition. INTERSPEECH-08, Brisbane, Australia, 2008:1313–1316.

[23] Fan X, Hansen JHL. Speaker identification for whispered speech using modified temporal patterns and MFCCs. INTERSPEECH-09, Brighton, UK, 2009:896–899.

[24] Zhang C, Hansen JHL. Whisper-island detection based on unsupervised segmentation with entropy-based speech feature processing. IEEE Trans Audio Speech Lang Process 2011;19 (4):883–894.

[25] Morris RW, Clements MA. Reconstruction of speech from whispers. Med Eng Phys 2002;24 (7–8):515–520.

[26] Jovicic ST. Formant features differences between whispered and voiced sustained vowels. Acustica-acta 1998;84(4):739–743.

[27] Matsuda M, Kasuya H. Acoustic nature of the Whisper. EUROSPEECH-99, Budapest, Hungary, 1999:133–136.

[28] Zhou B, Hansen JHL. Efficient audio stream segmentation via the combined T^2 statistic and Bayesian information criterion. IEEE Trans Speech Audio Process 2005;13(4):467–474.

[29] Huang R, Hansen JHL. Advances in unsupervised audio classification and segmentation for the broadcast news and NGSW corpora. IEEE Trans Audio Speech Lang Process 2006;14 (3):907–919.

[30] Zhang C. Whisper speech processing: analysis, modeling, and detection with applications to keyword spotting, Ph.D. thesis, University of Texas at Dallas, Richardson, TX, 2012.

[31] Kullback S, Leibler RA. On information and sufficiency. Ann Math Stat 1951;22(1):79–86.

[32] Chen SS, Gopalakrishnan PS. Speaker, environment and channel change detection and clustering via the Bayesian information criterion. in Proc. DARPA Broadcast News Transcription and Understanding Workshop, 1998:127–132.

[33] Anderson TW. An introduction to multivariate statistical analysis. New York: Wiley, 1958.

[34] Ajmera J, Wooters C. A robust speaker clustering algorithm. IEEE Workshop on Automatic Speech Recognition and Understanding, ASRU '03, Nov. 2003:411–416.

[35] Cettolo M, Vescovi M. Efficient audio segmentation algorithms based on the bic. 2003 Proceedings of IEEE International Conference on Acoustics, Speech, and Signal Processing (ICASSP '03), 2003;6:537–540.

[36]   Zhang C, Hansen JHL. An advanced entropy-based feature with a frame-level vocal effort likelihood space modeling for distant whisper-island detections. Speech Commun 2015;66:107–117.

[37]   Zhang C, Yu T, Hansen JHL. Microphone array processing for distance speech capture: A probe study on whisper speech detection. 2010 Conference Record of the Forty Fourth Asilomar Conference on Signals, Systems and Computers (ASILOMAR), Nov. 2010:1707–1710.

P. Vijayalakshmi, TA Mariya Celin and T. Nagarajan

2 Selective pole defocussing for detection of hypernasality

Abstract: Speech communication involves coordinated movement of several nerve impulses from the brain to the muscles and articulators that are involved in speech to produce intelligible speech. If the coordination of any of these systems is affected, it results in a disordered speech. Hypernasality is a speech resonance disorder that occurs due to improper velopharyngeal closure. This inadequate closure causes too much of air leakage from the nose thereby introducing an improper nasal balance resulting in an audible air escape through the nose during speech. The causes of velopharyngeal dysfunction (VPD) are many ranging from anatomical causes (e.g., Cleft-lip and palate) to neuromuscular problems and hearing impairment. Clinically, there are wide varieties of invasive instruments available for the assessment of hypernasal speech. These invasive intrusions cause much pain and discomfort. On the other hand, the non-invasive methods are highly expensive and subjective. The focus of this chapter is to discuss a non-invasive, reliable method for detecting hypernasality using signal-processing techniques. The presence of oral-nasal coupling in hypernasal speech enables a periodic glottal flow through the nasal cavity for the voiced sounds, especially vowels. On that note, to begin with, we distinguish the oral vowels, uttered by hypernasal and normal speakers, based on the presence of additional formants, introduced due to oral-nasal coupling, using linear prediction (LP)-based formant extraction technique. For the hypernasal speech, the LP analysis frequently fails to resolve two closely spaced formants. On the contrary, increasing the LP-order may show a spurious peak in the low frequency region of the normal speech as well due to pitch harmonics. To disambiguate this, in the present study, using a higher order LP spectrum, the pole corresponding to the formant peak in the low frequency region around 250 Hz for hypernasal speech and pitch harmonics in the same region for normal speech is defocussed (i.e., pushed towards the origin) and a new signal is re-synthesized. In a spectrum, if a peak is corresponding to a true-formant and not due to pitch harmonics, suppressing it would have a significant difference in the time-domain when re-synthesized. This aspect is used for the detection of hypernasality. The normalized cross-correlation at zero-lag is used to check the similarity between the input and the re-synthesized signal for hypernasal/normal decision. This technique for the hypernasal/normal decision task is performed for the vowels /a/, /i/ and /u/. Further, a Gaussian mixture model (GMM)-based classifier is trained to classify the hypernasal speech from the

https://doi.org/10.1515/9781501502415-003

normal using first formant frequency and the corresponding −3 dB bandwidth as a two-dimensional feature vector, for comparison.

Keywords: Hypernasality, speech resonance disorder, formant extraction, linear predictive, nasalized vowels, Pole Modification, cleft-lip

2.1 Introduction

Speech is an acoustic realization of phonemes produced by time-varying vocal tract system excited by time-varying excitation source. Speech production requires coordinated contraction of several muscles, involving highly complex neuromuscular processes and coordinated movements of several articulators. If the coordination of any of these structures and/or neuromuscular movements is affected, it results in disordered speech, making oral communication ineffective. The effect of these disorders ranges from simple sound substitution to the inability to use the oral-motor mechanism for functional speech.

Speech production system can be sub-divided into three major sub-systems [1], namely, (i) laryngeal, (ii) velopharyngeal and (iii) articulatory sub-systems. Speech disorders may affect a few or all of the sub-systems of speech production mechanism. Some of the representative speech disorders [2] affecting these sub-systems are as follows:
- Laryngeal dysfunction due to polyps, nodules, paralysis of vocal folds, etc.
- VPD caused due to structural problems, peripheral nervous system damage, hearing impairment, etc.
- Articulatory problems due to brain damage or neurological dysfunction, physical handicaps, such as cerebral palsy or hearing loss.
- Dysarthria, a family of neurological problems that affect one or all the three sub-systems of speech depending on the location and severity of the damage in the nervous system.

The sounds that make up for speech communication require a certain vocal tract configuration and excitation. For a person with an anatomic and/or neurological impairment, the required vocal tract configuration and excitation may be compromised. The resulting speech is, therefore, of a reduced quality and may even be unintelligible. Speech sounds can be categorized into nasal and oral sounds. The air passes through the nasal and oral cavities during the nasal sounds and through the oral cavity for the oral sounds. Words involving nasal sounds, such as "mam," "mom," and "man" experiences an air-flow along the nose and mouth during its production, whereas for words such as "pat," "cat" and "bat," air flows along the oral tract alone. It is the closure at the velopharyngeal space that builds the air pressure in the oral or nasal cavity to make the sounds sound either oral or nasalized.

During the velum at rest, as shown in Figure 2.1(a) [3], the velum rests against the back of the tongue for nasal breathing. This allows the air that is inhaled through the nose to go through the throat (pharynx) to the lungs and to exhale. During speech, these structures close off the oral cavity (mouth) from the nasal cavity (nose) as shown in Figure 2.1(b). This allows the speaker to build up air pressure in the mouth to produce various oral sounds with normal pressure and normal oral resonance. When this closure is improper due to structural or neurological difficulties, there are chances for certain oral sounds to sound-like nasal as shown in Figure. 2.1(c) and (d). Figure 2.1(c) shows the abnormality of soft palate that include a short velum (of length 28.1 ± 4.9 mm, whereas the normal velum length is 32.53 ± 3.38 mm [4]), cranial base anomalies, a history of adenoidectomy, surgery for mid-face advancement, enlarged tonsils and

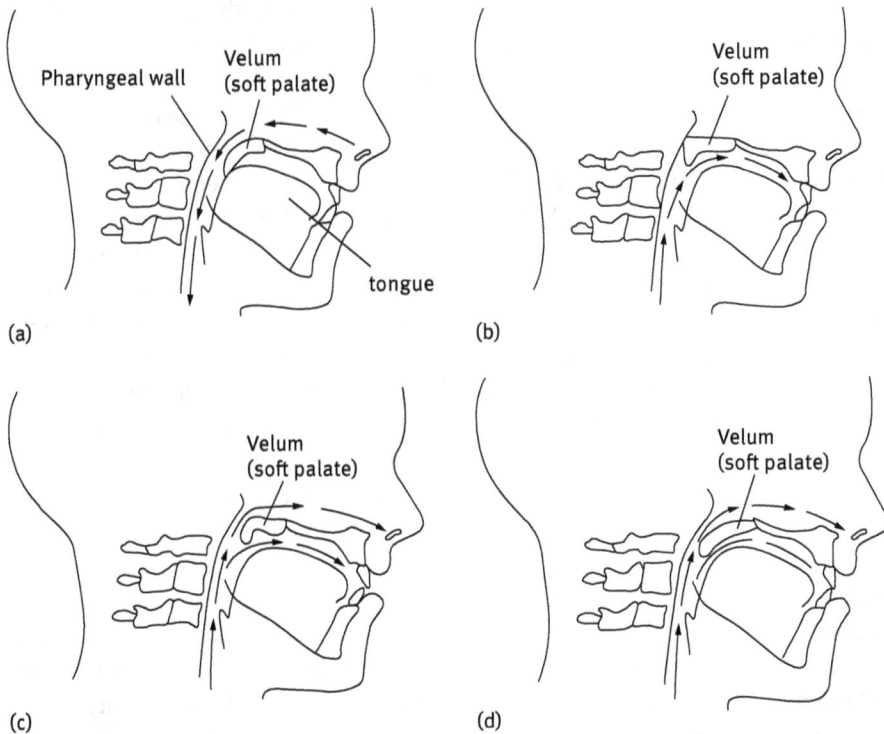

Figure 2.1: Normal velopharyngeal function (a) velum at rest, (b) velum during speech velopharyngeal dysfunction, (c) velum is too short and (d) velum has poor movement (Adapted from [3]).

irregular adenoids. Neuromotor disorders and neuromuscular disorders can cause poor velopharyngeal movement as shown in Figure 2.1(d).

Velopharyngeal is a compound word that comes from the words "velo" and pharyngeal, meaning the connecting tract between the velum or the soft palate and the pharynx or the throat. Any dysfunction along the velopharyngeal port or at its closure leads to VPD [5]. The VPD can be of three types, namely, velopharyngeal insufficiency, velopharyngeal incompetency and velopharyngeal inadequacy. Insufficiency results due to the lack/reduced tissue in the palate or throat, which causes a poor intact or imperfect closure across the velopharyngeal port as shown in Figure 2.1(c). If the velopharyngeal structure cannot produce a full closure, due to neuromuscular malfunction rather than the anatomical deficit, then it is referred to velopharyngeal incompetency as in Figure 2.1(d). Inadequacy is a combination of both insufficiency and incompetency.

The nasal phonemes in the English language (e.g., /m/, /n/, /ng/) are produced with nasal resonance, meaning that the velopharynx must open during their production. The improper closure discussed above either due to anatomical (insufficiency) or neurological problems (incompetency) leads to nasal resonance during speech production of oral consonants or vowels. The consequence of this inappropriate closure, guide to an inadequate escape of the air through the nose during the production of non-nasal or oral sounds leading to a hypernasal speech. Hypernasality is a specific example of a vocal tract dysfunction that causes reduced speech quality, due to a defective velopharyngeal mechanism. Cleft-Lip and Palate (CLP) also lead to hypernasal speech. Children with unrepaired CLP have no separation between the nasal cavity and the mouth, thus the child may not be able to build an air pressure in the mouth as the air escapes through the nasal cavity. Thus, hypernasality can be defined as an abnormal coupling of oral and nasal cavity [6] during speech due to imperfect velopharyngeal closure.

As these speech disorders may result in poor speech quality with a consequent reduction of clarity of speech making it unintelligible, this chapter takes a tour to the methods to assess the VPD through clinical approaches as discussed in the following section and signal-processing approaches discussed in Section 2.3. In Section 2.3, a detailed acoustic analysis on nasal resonances is studied to identify the acoustic cues that primarily contribute to nasalization. The LP-based formant extraction technique is used for this work and its basic principles are discussed in Section 2.4. An acoustic analysis is initially carried out to study on the significant acoustic cue for hypernasal and normal speech in Section 2.5. Further, selective pole defocussing technique proposed for the detection of hypernasality tested using speakers with CLP for vowels /a/, /i/ and /u/ and a GMM-based hypernasal/normal speech classifier is discussed in Section 2.6. This chapter concludes in Section 2.7 with the summary and future scope on the work.

2.2 Clinical methods for the assessment of speech disorders

By treating the hypernasal condition in speech, we try to eliminate or decrease the escape of excessive nasal air during oral sound production. To improve the clarity of speech or to make it intelligible, surgery or speech therapy can be performed. Surgical treatment help in changing the size and shape of the velo-pharyngeal space so that during oral sound production the air and sound will be directed out of the mouth rather than through the nose. A small amount of nasality may still prevail even after surgical treatment, however, perhaps not enough for most people to notice. Before proceeding whether to take a surgical intervention or speech therapy, an assessment and detection of hypernasality is important to help diagnose the seriousness of the problem.

Assessment of speech disorders requires investigation of functioning of the organs involved in the production of speech signal. The clinical methods for the assessment of speech disorders can be classified into two categories, namely, (i) instrumental techniques and (ii) subjective methods. Clinically, a variety of approaches including invasive and non-invasive techniques have been carried out to detect the presence of hypernasality in speech. Invasive approaches, which include static lateral radiographs, multi-view video-fluoroscopy and flexible fiber-optic nasendoscopy, give a direct observation of the velopharyngeal structure. However, to understand hypernasality that arises from oral-nasal coupling, an oral-nasal ratio is measured from devices, such as Nasometer, nasal-oral ratio meter, or accelerometer attached to the nose, along with a microphone positioned in front of the mouth. Though all of these techniques are capable of detecting hypernasality, an extent of physical intrusion is required. In addition, it is extremely difficult to incite a young child with cleft palate to place an accelerometer or a catheter in his/her nose and mouth. It may even be difficult to convince the child to submit to less invasive tools such as Nasometer.

The investigation of functioning of the organs obtained from both invasive and non-invasive instrumental assessment methods is interpreted by the perceptual judgment of experienced listeners. This has been a preferred method by which clinicians judge the speech intelligibility, quality of speech, etc., and define treatments to the speakers affected with speech disorders. Detailed perceptual judgments may not be able to identify accurately the underlying pathophysiological basis responsible for their occurrence [7], due to the following reasons.

- Accurate and reliable judgments are often difficult to achieve as they can be influenced by the skill and experience of the clinician and the sensitivity of the assessment.

- A rater (a judge to make judgments on the perceptual analysis) must have extensive and structured experience in listening prior to performing the perceptual ratings.
- These judgments require significant time and personnel resources, and hence, making it difficult to evaluate the range of potential speech distortion. Especially, when the test database is large, the rater's judgment may not be accurate, due to fatigue.
- These evaluations are frequently hampered by lack of consensus among the listeners [8].
- Perceptual assessments are difficult to standardize in relation to both the patient being rated and the environment in which the speech data are recorded.
- It is possible that a number of different physiological deficits can result in a similar perceptual deviation (e.g., distorted consonants can result from inadequate velopharyngeal functioning or from weak tongue musculature).

Therefore, when crucial decisions are required in relation to optimum therapeutic planning, an over-reliance on perceptual assessment only may lead to a number of questionable therapy directions [7]. Hence, a technique that requires no special measurement apparatus other than a microphone would be preferable to maximize patient comfort without compromising the hypernasality detection accuracy.

2.3 Signal processing and acoustic modeling-based methods for the assessment of hypernasal speech

To overcome the problems due to invasive techniques and to avoid problems in perceptual judgments (which is subjective and depends upon cognitive factors), a reliable, cost-effective, non-invasive and objective measure is required for the assessment of speech disorders. The objective measures produce more consistent results than the subjective judgments and are not affected by the human errors.

One category of objective approaches for the assessment of speech disorders uses signal-processing techniques. This helps to find the deviation of the time or spectral-domain features of disordered speech from the corresponding features of normal speech. These techniques require a good-quality microphone and a computer with A/D converter. Signal-processing techniques are non-invasive, fast, objective, thus making the detection process comfortable, simpler, cheaper and unbiased.

There is a well-developed literature for the signal-processing methods to derive acoustic characteristics of normal speech [9–12]. These acoustic characteristics of speech reflect the physical aspects of speech production, functioning of various sub-systems of speech, etc., which in turn reflect the coordination among various articulators and neuromuscular processes, etc. Some of the acoustic features, signal-processing techniques and their significance in the analysis of speech are described as follows.

Acoustic measures, such as maximum duration of sustained vowels, maximum fundamental frequency (F_0) range and variability of F_0, help in the analysis of loudness, monotony and intelligibility of speech. Acoustic perturbation features, such as jitter, shimmer and the variability in prosody, help to analyze the function of the laryngeal sub-system [2, 13, 14]. Apart from the above measures, F_0 statistics, such as mean, mode, range and standard deviation, F_0 contour for individual utterances, harmonic-to-noise ratio and spectral energy ratio, are some of the measures used to analyze the functioning of laryngeal sub-system [15, 16]. Spectrograms clearly denote the changes that occur in the frequency contours, relative intensity of the segments, prosody, etc., [17]. The information available in the acoustic signal, such as speaking rate, articulatory configuration for vowels and consonants, rates of change in the overall configuration of the vocal tract system help to infer about the articulatory and phonatory behavior of a particular speaker [18], which in turn helps in analyzing intelligibility.

In many cases, the analysis of time-varying resonances of vocal tract system and the analysis of formant transitions are the critical features of interest. The spectral analyses of speech signal for the extraction of formants are based on Fourier transform, LP, cepstrum analysis, etc., [9]. These techniques help in the analysis of inclusion of additional resonances or deletion of actual resonance due to structural or functional variation of the vocal tract system.

These signal-processing methods and the acoustic features help to understand the nature of the normal speech. Disordered speech, as described earlier, is due to in-coordination of articulators, neuromuscular movements, etc. These incoordinations are reflected in the form of deviations from acoustic characteristics of normal speech signal. This provides information about inactive/less-active sub-systems of speech and helps the speech pathologist to interpret the problems non-invasively and to decide the treatment required for the speaker having speech disorder. Though the signal-processing techniques for the analysis and derivation of the acoustic characteristics are extensively utilized for the normal speech, these techniques are not well addressed for the assessment of speech disorders as speech signal processing and biological perspectives of speech disorders are inter-disciplinary.

Researchers have attempted to detect VPD by analyzing the speech of hearing impaired, synthesized hypernasal speech and nasalized vowels of normal speech. The acoustic analysis by Glass and Zue [19, 20] shows that the short-time spectra of nasalized vowels often exhibit extra nasal formants or a broadening of the vowel formants typically in the first formant region. Frequency analysis of Hawkins and Stevens [21] strengthens the above findings. It shows that the main features of nasalization are changes in the low-frequency regions of the speech spectrum, where there is a very low-frequency peak with wide bandwidth along with the presence of a pole-zero pair due to the oral-nasal coupling. Chen [22] has proposed one more parameter, (A1-P0), the difference between the amplitude of the first formant (A1) and the extra peak below first formant (P0), to study the vowel nasalization. Cairns et al. [23] have utilized the sensitivity of a Teager energy operator to multicomponent signal for the detection of hypernasality. Here, the normal vowel is considered as a single component signal and nasalized vowel as a multicomponent signal and they found a measurable difference between low-pass and band-pass profiles of the Teager energy operator for the detection of hypernasality. Niu et al. [24] have proposed an estimation of spectral properties of nasal tract, based on transfer ratio function, computed by the ratio of the transfer admittance functions from the air pressure at the velopharyngeal port to the volume velocity at the lips and at the nostrils. The pole pattern of the transfer ratio function shows the spectral properties of the nasal tract. Vijayalakshmi et al. in [25] described a band-limited group delay spectrum-based technique to resolve the closely spaced nasal and oral formants in the low-frequency region and proposed a group delay-based acoustic measure for the detection of hypernasality. Zero time windowing (ZTW) discussed in [26] distinguishes the nasal formant from the first formant through high temporal resolution, that multiplies the speech signal by a highly decaying impulse-like window of size approximately a pitch period. A two-stage CLP speech enhancement is discussed in [27] where the first stage involves removal of nasal formant followed by a formant enhance-ment technique. Perceptual evaluation shows that the enhanced speech signal has better quality in terms of reduced nasality.

The CLP speech therapists are more interested in automatically finding out different levels of hypernasality that indicates the velopharyngeal gap size. Early work on analyzing the hypernasal speech using acoustic modeling involved a GMM to classify hypernasality based on the severity levels, namely, mild, moderate and severe. Tobias et al. [28] proposed an automatic phoneme analysis in CLP speech using GMM with two systems: one based on the

Maximum *Aposteriori* (MAP) adaptation and the other on feature space-maximum likelihood linear regression (fMLLR) and it is inferred that fMLLR-based system is able to achieve automatic phoneme evaluation for various severity levels and observed to agree with the perceptual ratings. Hypernasality detection using energy distribution ratio and hypernasality level classification using GMM classifier are described in [29] and the classification accuracy using GMM classifier is around 80.74%.

From the above literature survey, it is noticed that the acoustic cues of hypernasal speech are (i) nasalization of oral vowels giving rise to an additional pole-zero pair (formants & anti formants) in the vicinity of first formant region, (ii) widening of formant bandwidth leading to reduction in amplitude of the formant especially in the first formant region and (iii) amplitude variation between the additional formant and actual oral formant. Apart from the intro-duction of new pole-zero pair in the first formant region, nasalization gives rise to changes in the spectrum in the high-frequency region as well.

However, none of these acoustic cues listed above are argued as consistent acoustic cue for the detection of hypernasality. As mentioned earlier, during the production of vowel sounds, due to oral-nasal coupling, in addition to the oral-formants, few nasal formants are also introduced. However, the influ-ence of each of these newly introduced resonances in nasalization may not be uniform. For the detection of hypernasality, instead of considering all the possible nasal resonances, if the focus is given only to the consistent and the highly influencing formant, the detection process can be made more accurate. Considering this, the further discussion will concentrate only on the first acoustic cue alone for the analysis and detection of hypernasality. Especially, the focus is given to analyze the effect of each of the additional nasal resonances introduced into the vowel sounds and to derive a consistent acoustic measure for the detection of hypernasality. Towards this end, spectral analysis of speech signal for the extraction of resonances (formants) is carried out using LP-based formant extraction technique. A brief note on basic principles of LP is discussed in the following section. A detailed description can be found in [9], [30].

2.4 Basic principles of linear predictive analysis

The idea behind LP is that a sample of a signal, $x(n)$, can be predicted based on the preceding samples. More specifically, a linear predictor approximates the current sample of a signal as a linear combination of the past samples [9], as shown below:

$$\tilde{x}(n) = \sum_{k=1}^{p} \alpha_k x(n-k), \tag{2.1}$$

where p is the number of past samples that are considered, which is the order of the linear predictor, and α_k is the prediction coefficients.

A speech signal, $s(n)$, can be modeled as the output of a linear, time-varying system/digital filter, excited by $u(n)$, which could either be a sequence of quasi-periodic pulses or random noise. The system/filter could be represented as

$$H(z) = \frac{S(z)}{U(z)} = \frac{G}{1 - \sum_{k=1}^{p} a_k z^{-k}} \tag{2.2}$$

where G is the gain parameter and a_k is the filter coefficients, and these are the parameters that characterize the system.

From Equation (2.2), the speech signal, $s(n)$, can be expressed as

$$s(n) = \sum_{k=1}^{p} a_k s(n-k) + Gu(n). \tag{2.3}$$

The LP can be used to estimate parameters that characterize linear, time-varying systems. In this regard, the speech signal can be estimated as follows:

$$\tilde{s}(n) = \sum_{k=1}^{p} \alpha_k s(n-k). \tag{2.4}$$

The predictor coefficients, α_k, must be estimated such that the prediction error, $e(n)$, which is given by

$$e(n) = s(n) - \tilde{s}(n), \tag{2.5}$$

is minimum. Owing to the time-varying nature of speech signals, the predictor coefficients must be estimated by minimizing the mean-squared prediction error computed over short frames of the signal. If $e_n(m)$ is the prediction error computed over the nth frame, then the short-time average prediction error can be given by

$$E_n = \sum_{m} e_n^2(m) \tag{2.6}$$

For estimating the model parameters, α_k, minimizing the mean-squared error criterion-based autocorrelation and autocovariance methods leads to a set of linear equations that can be efficiently solved using Levinson Durbin's recursion and Cholesky decomposition method, respectively. If α_k is estimated accurately, then $\alpha_k = a_k$, and therefore, the prediction error will be $Gu(n)$, the excitation.

Once the linear prediction coefficients (LPCs) are estimated, formants from the predictor parameters for the voiced section of speech can be estimated by obtaining the spectrum and choosing the formants by a peak picking method. Based on the order of the linear predictor, the number of peaks in the spectrum would vary. As the order is increased, the linear predictor will bear a closer resemblance to the Fourier Transform spectrum of the signal. Therefore, to estimate the formant frequencies, the order of the predictor must be chosen appropriately such that the spectrum contains peaks only at the formant frequencies. Subsequently, the formant frequencies can be estimated from the LP spectrum using a peak-picking algorithm.

The bandwidth of the formants can also be derived from the LP spectrum. The formant bandwidth B_k is related to the radius of the formant r_k and sampling rate f_s as follows:

$$r_k = e^{-\pi B_k/f_s}. \tag{2.7}$$

From the LP spectrum, the formant bandwidths can be derived as the difference between the frequencies at which the magnitude is 3 dB less than that at the formant frequencies.

2.5 Acoustic analysis for the detection of hypernasality

As discussed earlier though there are many acoustic cues for the detection of hypernasality none of them are argued as consistent. The focus of the current section is to analyze the effect of each of nasal resonances introduced onto the oral vowels and to derive a consistent acoustic cue for the detection of hypernasality. Towards this end, acoustic analyses are carried out on nasalized vowels, modified speech and hypernasal speech and are discussed in detail as follows.

2.5.1 Acoustic analysis on nasalized vowels

The current section focuses on acoustic analyses carried out on nasalized vowels, and the perceptual analysis conducted on vowel sounds modified by introducing different nasal resonances and an acoustic analysis on hypernasal speech. Initially, acoustic analysis is carried out on nasalized vowels uttered by the normal speakers. The transition from an oral vowel to nasal consonant or vice versa may involve an intermediate nasalized vowel sound, as the velum lowers before or raises after oral closure [10]. As the velopharyngeal port is open during the production of nasalized vowels, the nasalized vowels can be considered as simulated hypernasal speech. The data analyzed in this study is composed of consonant-vowel-consonant (CVC) units (C-consonant, V-vowel) (/mam/, /min/ and /mun/) with /m/ and /n/ as initial and final consonants, with an intermediate vowel (/a/, /i/ and /u/). For this study, the formant frequencies of pure vowels as shown in Table 2.1 are considered as reference.

Table 2.1: Formant frequencies and −3 dB bandwidth (in Hz) of vowels.

Phonemes	F1	B1	F2	B2	F3	B3	F4	B4
/a/	632	78	1,122	118	2,388	172	3,169	261
/i/	265	74	2,156	164	2,729	184	3,437	190
/u/	359	145	921	282	2,148	320	2,766	461

The spectra of nasalized vowels are analyzed using LP [31]-based formant analysis. Since speech signal is quasi-periodic over a period of 10 to 30 ms [9], the spectral analysis is carried out at 20 ms intervals, with an overlap of

Table 2.2: Formant frequencies (F1–F5) (mean, min. and max. in Hz) of nasalized vowels.

Consonant Vowel Consonant units	Statistics	F1	F2	F3	F4	F5
/man/	Mean	236	746	1,119	1,950	2,577
Nasalized /a/	Min	180	711	1.055	1,732	2,328
	Max	266	766	1,180	1,984	2,741
/min/	Mean	239	524	1,044	2,236	2,728
Nasalized /i/	Min	172	436	945	1,992	2,538
	Max	297	555	1,165	2,454	2,894
/mun/	Mean	241	563	1,042	1,885	2,496
Nasalized /u/	Min	164	461	914	1,847	2,386
	Max	305	711	1,195	2,007	2,592

10 ms, to extract the formants and is shown in Table 2.2. From Table 2.2, it is observed that,

- An additional formant around 250 Hz (refer to F1 in Table 2.2) is introduced into the spectrum of all the three vowels (/a/, /i/ and /u/).
- Due to the introduction of additional nasal formant, first oral formant of the vowels /i/ and /u/, which are already located around 300 Hz gets shifted to a frequency around 500 Hz (refer to F2 of the nasalized vowels /i/ and /u/ in Table 2.2).
- Apart from the above, a formant around 1,000 Hz is observed for the vowels /i/ and /u/ (refer to F3 of /i/ and /u/ in Table 2.2).

The additional formants found in the nasalized vowels may be because of the adjacent nasal consonants. To verify this, acoustic analysis on nasal consonants is performed.

2.5.2 Acoustic analysis on nasal consonants

The speech data analyzed in this study are composed of the words /summer/, /sunny/ and /singing/ collected from 10 healthy speakers. The LP-based formant analysis is performed on the nasal segments of the data (/su**mm**er/, /su**nn**y/ and /si**ng**ing/) to extract formant frequencies and is shown in Table 2.3. It is noticed that the additional formants introduced in the nasalized vowels, as shown in Table 2.2, are almost same as the formants of the nasal consonants given in Table 2.3. Figure 2.2 shows the short-time Fourier spectrum of normal and hypernasal speech. It is observed that the Fourier transform analysis also shows the introduction of additional formant in the low-frequency region of hypernasal speech around 250 Hz. To further cross-verify this, the speech signals of the vowel sounds (/a/, /i/ and /u/) of normal speakers are modified by introducing nasal resonances into the oral resonances as described below.

Table 2.3: Formant frequencies (in Hz) of nasal consonants.

Formants	Mean	Min	Max
F1	219	200	244
F2	947	777	1,111
F3	2,421	2,355	2,533

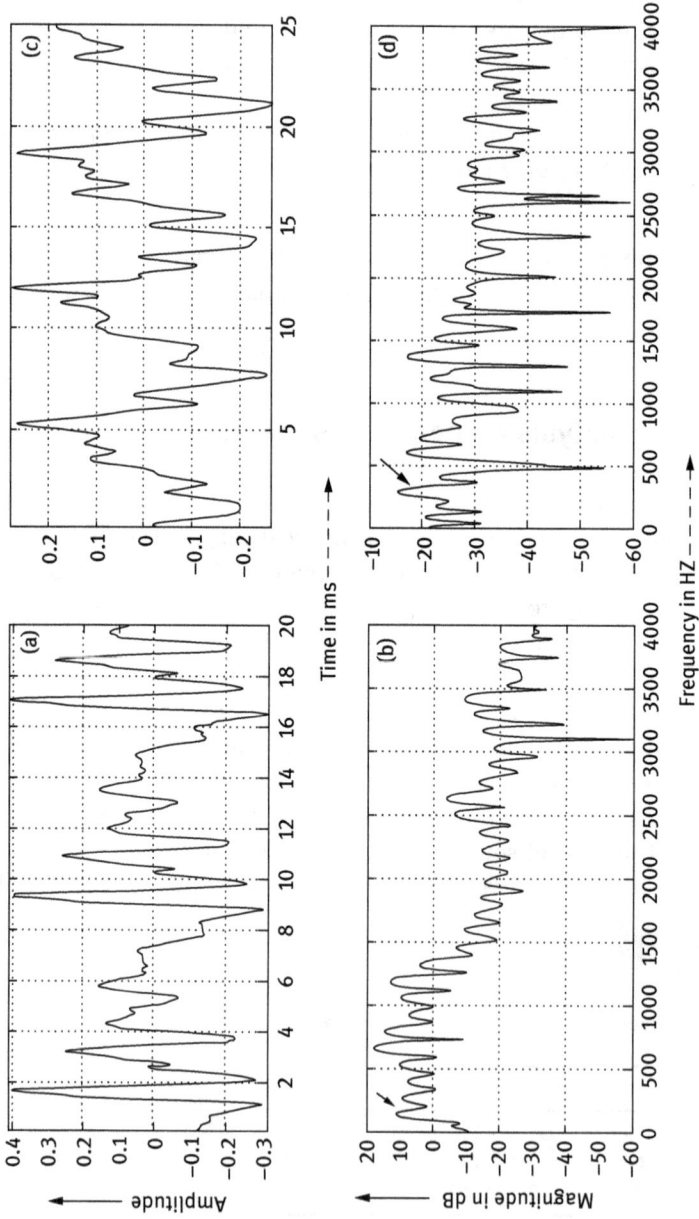

Figure 2.2: A segment of (a) normal speech (c) hypernasal speech, (b) & (d) the corresponding FT- derived magnitude spectra for the sustained vowel /a/.

2.5.3 Generation of modified speech

The modified speech is generated by introducing nasal resonances in addition to the resonances of vowels. From the phonemes /a/, /i/ and /u/ uttered by the normal speakers, LP coefficients, LP residual and gain are extracted. Then, the speech signal of the phonemes /a/, /i/ and /u/ are modified by introducing,

- each of the nasal resonances (250 Hz, 1,000 Hz and 2,500 Hz) separately,
- each pair of nasal resonances (250 Hz and 1,000 Hz, 250 Hz and 2,500 Hz and 1,000 Hz and 2,500 Hz),
- all the nasal resonances and
- all the three nasal resonances with widened formant bandwidths of nasal as well as oral formants.

For each case, separate speech signals are generated after modification. In total, there are eight speech signals for each phoneme after modification and used for perceptual analysis.

2.5.3.1 Perceptual analysis on modified speech signal

For the perceptual experiment, five female and three male listeners, with an average age of 25 years, have participated. The speech and hearing capability of these listeners are certified by a speech pathologist as normal. All are naive listeners, without any past training in perception of nasality. The listeners are asked to rate the modified speech signals for the degree of nasalization and the results are shown in Table 2.4. The test is conducted independent of the

Table 2.4: Scores of perceptual analysis conducted on modified speech signal.

Formants Introduced (in Hz)	Degree of Nasalization			
	No	Mild	Moderate	High
250	–	4	20	–
1,000	–	15	9	–
2,500	22	2	–	–
250 and 1,000	–	–	16	8
250 and 2,500	–	4	20	–
1,000 and 2,500	–	15	9	–
All	–	–	16	8
All (wider BW)	–	–	3	21

phonemes (/a/, /i/, /u/), leading to 24 tests (eight listeners, three phonemes) for each case of the modified speech signal. Each entry in the Table 2.4 indicates the number of tests in favor of a particular rating.

From Table 2.4, it is observed that the introduction of a nasal formant [31],

- at 250 Hz or 1,000 Hz, has moderate influence on nasalization. In particular, introduction of the nasal formant at 250 Hz either alone or combined with other nasal frequencies has more influence on nasalization.
- at 2,500 Hz, does not have any influence on nasality. This is observed when this formant is either introduced separately or as a combination with other two formants.
- at 250 Hz and 1,000 Hz or at all nasal resonant frequencies, have moderate-to-high influence than the other combinations of formant frequencies.
- at all nasal frequencies with increased bandwidth, shows a high degree of nasalization.

Our focus in the current study is to find out the nasal resonances introduced due to oral-nasal coupling rather than the anti-resonances. From this perceptual study, we conclude that out of the three nasal formants, the formants at 250 Hz and 1,000 Hz of nasal consonants have influence on nasalization of vowels and one can expect the same set of formant frequencies in the hypernasal speech as well.

2.5.4 Acoustic analysis on hypernasal speech

The acoustic parameters (formant frequencies and formant bandwidths) that serve as an estimate of nasalization are analyzed in the speech data of 25 speakers with unrepaired cleft palate. The LP spectra of these speakers are examined closely for nasal formants or a widening of formant bandwidth. The LP spectra of phonemes (/a/, /i/ and /u/) of these speakers are analyzed at 20 ms intervals, with an overlap of 10 ms, throughout the vowel to extract the formants, and the average formants over the entire interval for each vowel are found (refer to Table 2.5). From Table 2.5, we observe that

- invariably for all the speakers, there exists a formant frequency around 250 Hz for all the three phonemes /a/, /i/ and /u/. Figure 2.3 shows LP spectra (order 14) for the phoneme /a/ for six hypernasal speakers. From Figure 2.3, it is observed that the first oral formant (around 700 Hz) is not consistently resolved for all the speakers.
- there exists an additional formant frequency around 1,000 Hz for the phonemes /i/ and /u/, as realized in the perceptual analysis described in Section 2.5.3.1 and acoustic analysis on nasalized vowels described in Section 2.5.1.

Table 2.5: Mean formants and −3 dB bandwidths (in Hz) of hypernasal speech.

Phoneme	F1	B1	F2	B2	F3	B3	F4	B4	F5	B5
/a/	253	62	633	78	1,168	130	2,078	172	2,690	250
/i/	244	47	528	55	894	196	1,820	109	2,562	180
/u/	253	46	544	91	1,066	141	1,875	151	2,333	191

Apart from the above observations, it is noticed that in many cases, for the phonemes /i/ and /u/, there is a broadening of the F1 bandwidth. This widening of formant bandwidth may be because of the inclusion of nasal

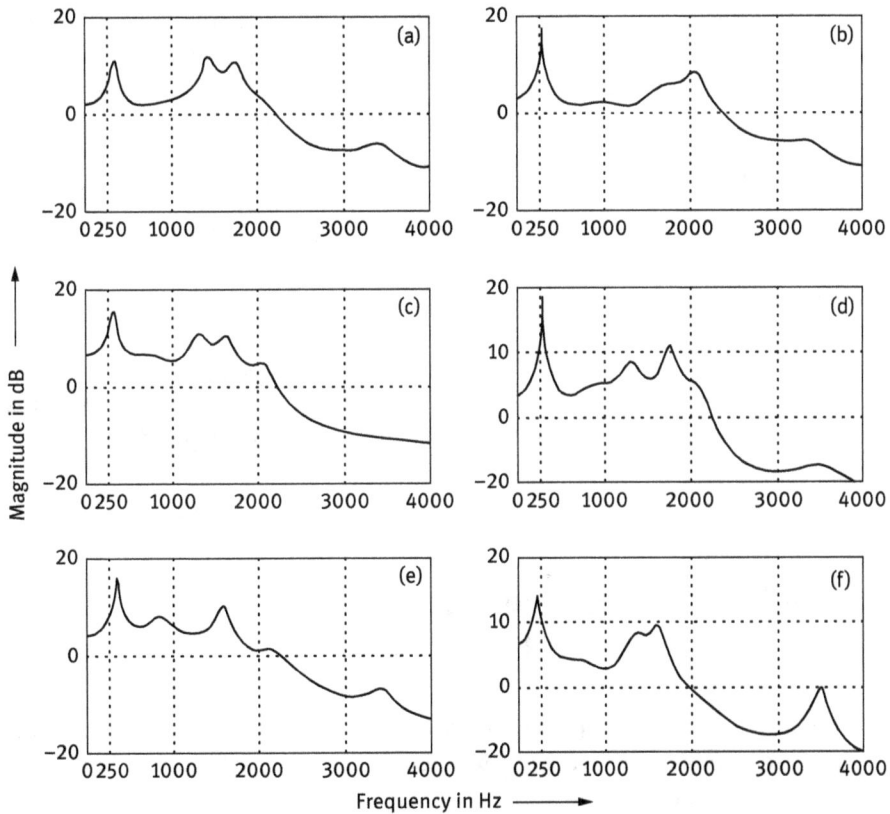

Figure 2.3: LP spectra (order 14) for the phoneme /a/ uttered by six speakers ((a), (b), (c), (d), (e) and, (f)) with hypernasality (refer to formant around 250 Hz in each LP spectrum).

formant frequency, which is very close to F1and resolved only for the higher LP order.

From this, we can conclude that the presence of two or more formants of nasal consonants may be a cue for detection of hypernasality. The perceptual study and acoustic analysis of hypernasal speech and nasalized vowels reveal that nasal formants around 250 Hz and 1,000 Hz play a major role in the nasalization of vowels. Especially, the nasal resonance around 250 Hz that lies below the first formant frequency of all the three phonemes (/a/, /i/ and /u/) is an important and consistent cue for the detection of hypernasality.

To perform the above instinct, a LP-based formant extraction technique can be used for detecting hypernasality. The nasal resonance introduced in the low-frequency region due to oral-nasal coupling for hypernasal speech can be extracted using LP-based technique. However, the major disadvantage of this technique is the vulnerability to the prediction order. Lower-order LP spectrum frequently fails to resolve two closely spaced formants. On the other hand, higher-order LP analysis introduces many spurious peaks in the resultant spectrum. Even for a normal speaker, there are additional peaks below the first oral formant that are due to pitch source harmonics. This leads to an ambiguity if a peak-picking algorithm is used for the detection of hypernasality. To disambiguate this, using a higher order LP spectrum, the pole corresponding to the strongest peak in the low-frequency region below the first oral formant of the vowel is defocussed and a new signal is re-synthesized. In a spectrum, if a peak is corresponding to a true-formant and not due to pitch harmonics, suppressing it would have a significant difference in the time-domain when re-synthesized. This aspect of detecting hypernasality will be used as a focal point for further discussion.

2.6 Selective pole modification technique for detection of hypernasality

Let us consider $q(n)$, the impulse response of the nasal formant alone, and $v(n)$, the impulse response due to the oral formants. Let $h(n)$ be the convolution of $q(n)$ and $v(n)$ as given below:

$$h(n) = q(n)*v(n) \qquad (2.8)$$

$$h(n) = \sum_{k=-\infty}^{k=\infty} q(k)v(n-k) \tag{2.9}$$

The z-transform of $h(n)$, $H(z)$, the system function of the hypernasal speech is given by,

$$H(z) = Q(z)V(z) \tag{2.10}$$

where,

$$Q(z) = \frac{1}{(1-az^{-1})(1-a^*z^{-1})} \tag{2.11}$$

$$V(z) = \frac{A}{\prod_{k=1}^{M}(1-2e^{-B_kT}\cos(\omega_k T)z^{-1}+e^{-2B_kT}z^{-2})} \tag{2.12}$$

In Equation (2.11), a and a^* are the complex pole-pair and B_k in Equation (2.12) is the 3 dB bandwidth of the kth pole, A is the gain of the system, T is the sampling interval and M denotes the total number of poles. Here, impulse and its z-transform are not used for simplicity. To de-emphasize the influence of the nasal formant alone, the poles corresponding to it should be removed. That is,

$$H(z) = V(z) \tag{2.13}$$

Only if,

$$Q(z) = 1 \tag{2.14}$$

This can be ensured in either of the following two ways:
1. Introduce zeros at the same locations of nasal poles (i.e., a and a^*) as given below:

$$Q(z) = \frac{(1-az^{-1})(1-a^*z^{-1})}{(1-az^{-1})(1-a^*z^{-1})} \tag{2.15}$$

2. Reduce the radius of the complex pole 'a' to zero.

For further study, we concentrate on reducing the radius (defocus) of the complex pole in the low-frequency region, below the first oral formant (selective defocussing) and utilize the effect of pole defocussing in the time-domain for the detection of hypernasality.

2.6.1 Selective pole defocussing

Consider a signal, $s(n)$, with sampling period T. Let us presently assume that an all-pole transfer function of $s(n)$ be $S(z)$. Consider a complex pole a_k. Let the radius and angle of a_k in z-domain be r_k and θ_k. Furthermore, the relation between r_k and 3-dB bandwidth B_k, of the corresponding frequency component in the spectrum can be written as $r_k = e^{-\pi B_k T}$. That is, smaller the radius of a pole, broader the bandwidth (lower the gain) of the corresponding resonant frequency in the spectrum. If r_k is reduced without changing θ_k, in the other words, pushing the pole towards the origin (pole-defocussing), causes reduction in the gain (magnitude) of the corresponding frequency component in the spectrum.

To illustrate the effect of pole-defocussing in a system of three poles with different radius and angular frequency [32], the following system is chosen. The system has three complex conjugate pole-pairs with radius r_1, r_2 and r_3 with angular frequencies ω_1, ω_2 and ω_3, respectively (refer to Figure 2.4(a)). The corresponding LP spectrum is shown in Figure 2.4(c). The time-domain behavior of the system is analyzed for the following two cases:

$$\textbf{Case (i): } r_1 > r_2, r_3 \text{ and } \omega_1 < \omega_2, \omega_3 \tag{2.16}$$

In this case, it is observed that the high-frequency components with relatively smaller radius reach steady state earlier than the low-frequency component with higher radius. From Figure 2.4(e), it is observed that the low-frequency component with relatively higher radius suppresses the effect of high-frequency component in the time-domain.

$$\textbf{Case (ii): } r_1 < r_2, r_3 \text{ and } \omega_1 < \omega_2, \omega_3 \tag{2.17}$$

When the pole corresponding to the low-frequency component is pushed towards the origin so that $r_1 < r_2$ and r_3, keep r_2 and r_3 unaltered, as shown in Figure 2.4(b), the high-frequency components, which are concealed earlier due to stronger low-frequency components, are now revealed in the time-domain (refer to Figure 2.4(f)).

In the LP analysis, any sample at time n, $s(n)$, can be expressed as a linear combination of past p samples, such that

$$s(n) = \sum_{k=1}^{p} a_k s(n-k) + Gu(n) \tag{2.18}$$

where $u(n)$ is the normalized excitation source and G is the gain of the excitation. The corresponding all-pole vocal tract transfer function $S(z)$ can be written

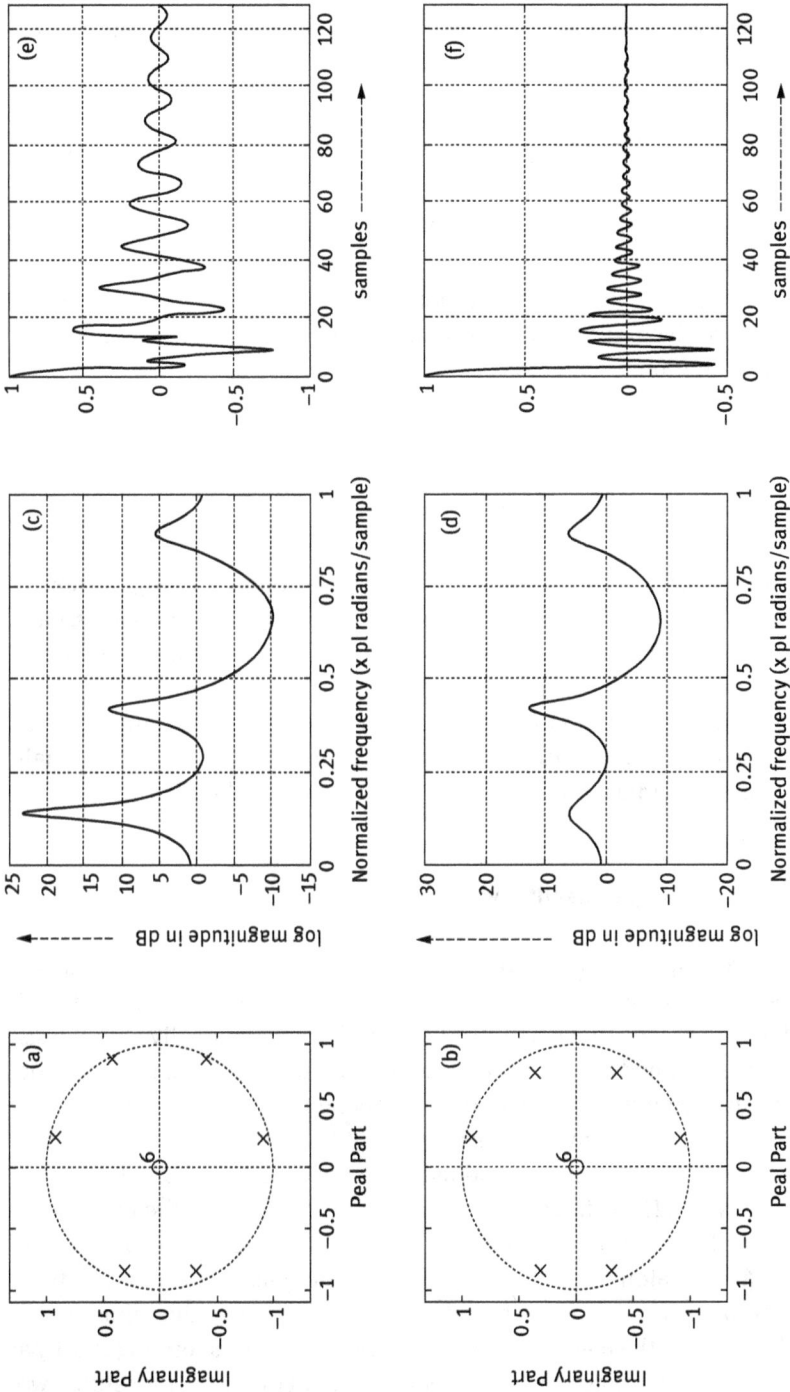

Figure 2.4: Effect of selective pole-defocussing in the frequency- and time-domain of synthetic speech: (a) z-plane with poles at (0.98, 25°), (0.95, 75°), (0.9, 160°), (b) Z-plane with poles at (0.85, 25°), (0.95, 75°), (0.9, 160°), (c) and (d) LP spectra of (a) & (b), respectively and (e) and (f) impulse responses of (a) & (b), respectively.

as $S(z) = 1/A(z)$, where $A(z)$ is the inverse filter transfer function. This can be expressed in terms of roots of a polynomial (y_k) as

$$A(z) = 1 - \sum_{k=1}^{p} a_k z^{-k} = \prod_{k=1}^{p}(1 - y_k z^{-1}) \tag{2.19}$$

Using Equation (2.19), the radius and angle of each of the available resonances (roots) can be computed. This gives us the facility to defocus either the already existing resonances or to introduce additional resonances based on the requirement. Thus, in a given speech signal, defocussing an existing pole helps in analyzing the condition for hypernasal or normal speech.

2.6.2 Analysis on the detection of hypernasality through cleft lip and palate (CLP) speech

To detect the presence of hypernasality using selective pole defocussing, sustained vowels from 25 speakers with unrepaired CLP and 25 normal speakers' speech data are considered for the analysis. As discussed earlier, the consistent cue for the detection of hypernasality is the inclusion of additional formant around 250 Hz. It is to be noted that for the vowel /a/, the first oral formant (F1) is around 750 Hz. However for the vowels /i/ and /u/, the additional formant introduced due to oral-nasal coupling in hypernasal speech, is closer to F1 of the oral vowels /i/ and /u/.

2.6.2.1 Detection of hypernasality (vowel /a/)

For the hypernasal speech (corresponding to vowel /a/), spectrum derived using higher order LP analysis is found to resolve closely spaced nasal and oral formants. For the present study, an LP order 28 is chosen empirically for analysis of all the three sustained vowels. The LP-residual, $e(n)$, and the gain, G, of the speech signal are computed. The frequency components corresponding to all the poles are computed for the given speech signal.

For the hypernasal speech, the radius of the pole corresponding to a nasal resonance below 300 Hz is, in general, greater than the radius of the root due to the pitch source harmonics in the same region. To defocus the pole due to nasal resonant frequency alone, the radius of the low-frequency component with maximum radius below 300 Hz is found automatically. The radius thus found is reduced by dividing the real and imaginary parts of the corresponding root by a factor greater than 1 as shown in Figure 2.5(b) and (c). For the current study, we

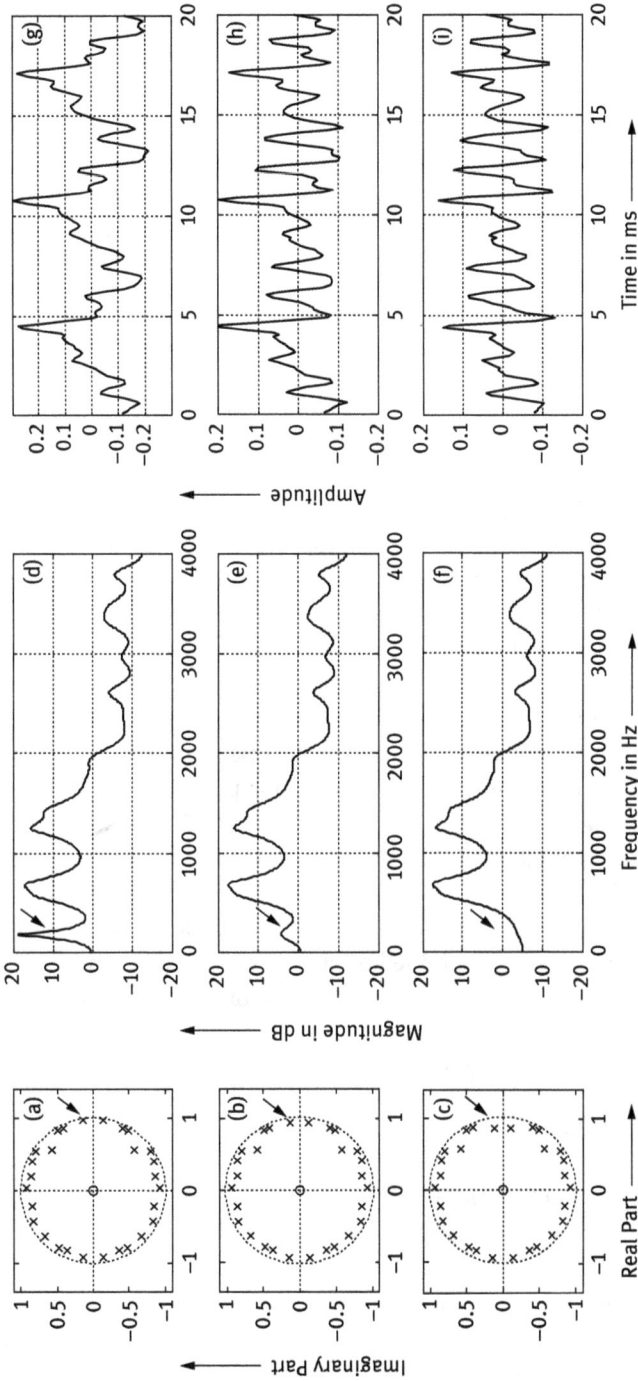

Figure 2.5: Effect of selective pole-defocussing in the frequency- and time-domain for vowel /a/ uttered by hypernasal speaker: (a) Z-plane with poles extracted using LP analysis with order 28 for the speech signal given in (g) and LP spectrum given in (d), (b) and (c) Z-plane after defocussing the pole by factor 1.05 and 1.15, respectively. (e) and (f) LP spectra of (b) and (c), respectively. (h) and (i) speech signal corresponding to (b) and (c), respectively.

empirically observed that dividing the radius by a defocussing factor of 1.15 suppresses the pole considerably without a significant effect on the other portion of the spectrum.

After modifying the available set of roots, a new set of LP coefficients (polynomial), a'_k, are computed. Speech signal is re-synthesized with the new set of LP coefficients, a'_k, keeping $e(n)$ and G, of the input speech signal unaltered. Let the re-synthesized signal, $s'(n)$, be

$$s'(n) = \sum_{k=1}^{p} a'_k s'(n-k) + Ge(n) \tag{2.20}$$

It is observed that, for a hypernasal speech, when the pole due to the additional nasal formant introduced (below 300 Hz) is defocussed, the signal components, which are suppressed due to the strength of the signal component correspond to nasal formant, are disclosed very clearly. Specifically, the signal components between two consecutive excitations that are masked by the signal component due to the nasal resonance are revealed in the speech signal after selective pole-defocussing as illustrated in Figure 2.5(h) and (i). Apart from this, a considerable reduction in the strength of the signal ((0.4 to 0.15) refer to Figure 2.5(g), (h), and (i)) is also observed due to the suppression of the strong nasal formant.

The selective pole-defocussing procedure is performed for the normal speakers as well. For a normal speaker, since the highest peak in the low-frequency region of interest (for the phoneme /a/) is a spurious peak due to pitch source harmonics, defocussing the corresponding pole (refer to Figure 2.6(b) and (c)) does not have a significant effect in the time-domain signal when re-synthesized (refer to Figure 2.6(h) and (i)).

Normalized cross-correlation is used to check the similarity between resultant re-synthesized signal, $s'(n)$, obtained after pole-defocussing and the input signal $s(n)$. The correlation between $s(n)$ and $s'(n)$ is computed as given below:

$$r = \frac{n \sum^{s}(n)s'(n) - \sum^{s}(n)s'(n)}{\sqrt{[n \sum^{s}(n)^2 - (\sum^{s}(n))^2][n \sum^{s'}(n)^2 - (\sum^{s'}(n))^2]}} \tag{2.21}$$

$$r = \frac{Cov(s(n), s'(n))}{Stdevs(n).Stdevs'(n)} \quad \text{for } n = 0....N - 1. \tag{2.22}$$

The maximum of cross-correlation values (normalized) between the input speech signal, $s(n)$, and the re-synthesized speech signal, $s'(n)$, are computed for all the hypernasal and normal speakers. Figure 2.7 shows the distribution of correlation

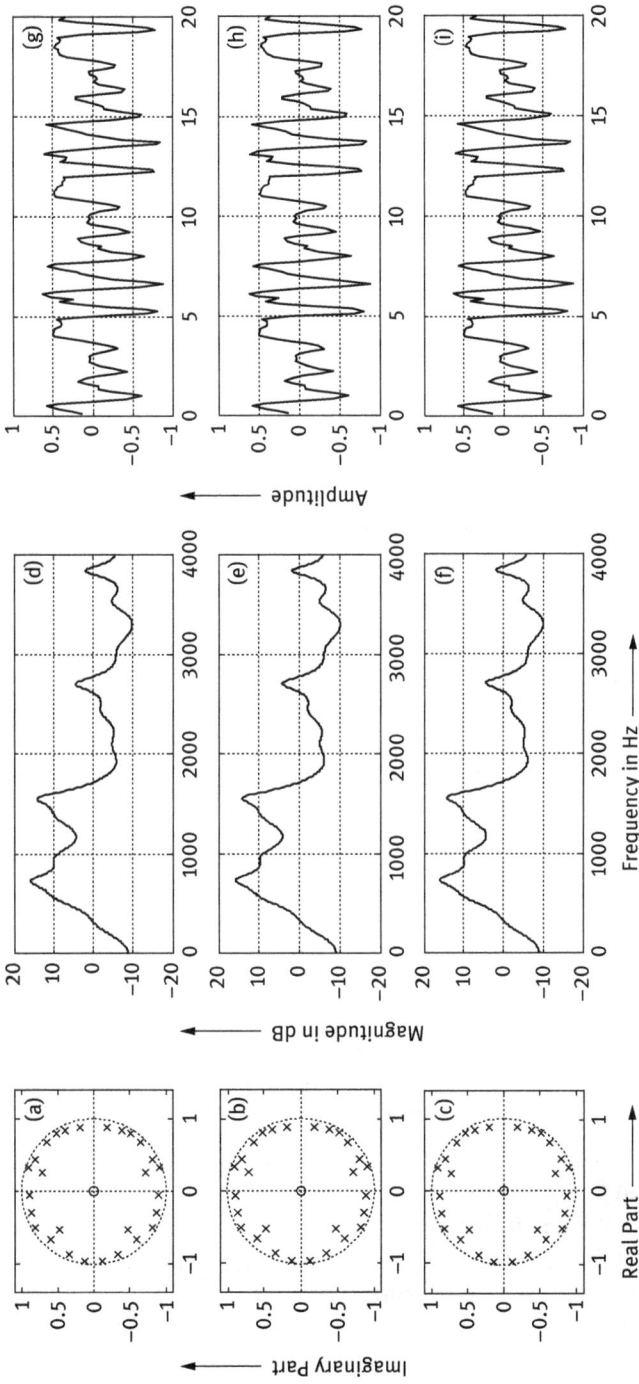

Figure 2.6: Effect of selective pole-defocussing in the frequency- and time-domain for vowel /a/ uttered by normal speaker: (a) Z-plane with poles extracted using LP analysis with order 28 for the speech signal given in (g) and LP spectrum given in (d), (b) and (c) Z-plane after defocussing the pole by factor 1.05 and 1.15, respectively. (e) and (f) LP spectra of (b) and (c), respectively, (h) and (i) speech signal corresponding to (b) and (c), respectively.

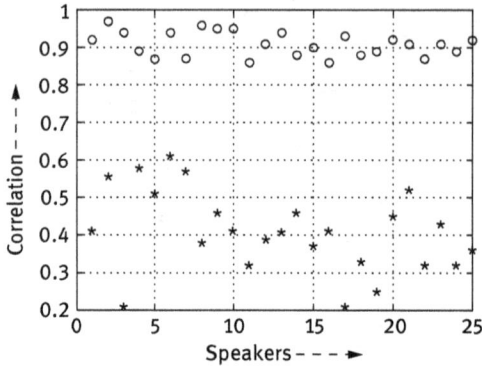

Figure 2.7: Correlation between the input and the re-synthesized speech signals for hypernasal ('*' markers) and normal speakers ('o' markers).

for all the normal and hypernasal speakers. For hypernasal speakers, since the effect of defocussing the strongest pole (nasal formant) in the low-frequency region (below 300 Hz) is significant in the time-domain, the correlation between the input and the modified signal is found to vary from 0.2 to 0.6.

However, for the normal speakers, since only a spurious peak is found in the intended region, suppressing the corresponding pole has relatively less effect on the time domain signal and the correlation is found to be above 0.85 for all the normal speech data. From this analysis, a threshold on correlation is set as 0.65. Using this threshold on correlation, the performance on hypernasal/normal decision task is 100%.

2.6.2.2 Detection of hypernasality (vowel /i/)

For the sustained vowel /i/, the nasal formant around 200–250 Hz is defocussed using the same procedure as discussed in the previous section for hypernasal vowel /a/. The pole (LP order 28) corresponding to the nasal formant is defocussed by a defocussing factor of 1.15. Defocussing the nasal formant in the hypernasal speech selectively shows a significant difference in the time-domain hypernasal speech signal as shown in Figure 2.8(h) and (i). This experiment is repeated for normal speakers with the same LP order and same defocussing factor, however, as expected no prominent effect is observed in the time-domain speech signal when re-synthesized after defocussing as shown in Figure 2.9(g) and (i). The experiment is performed for 25 normal and hypernasal speakers each, and the distribution of correlation between the actual and the re-synthesized speech after defocussing for all the normal and hypernasal speakers is shown in Figure 2.10.

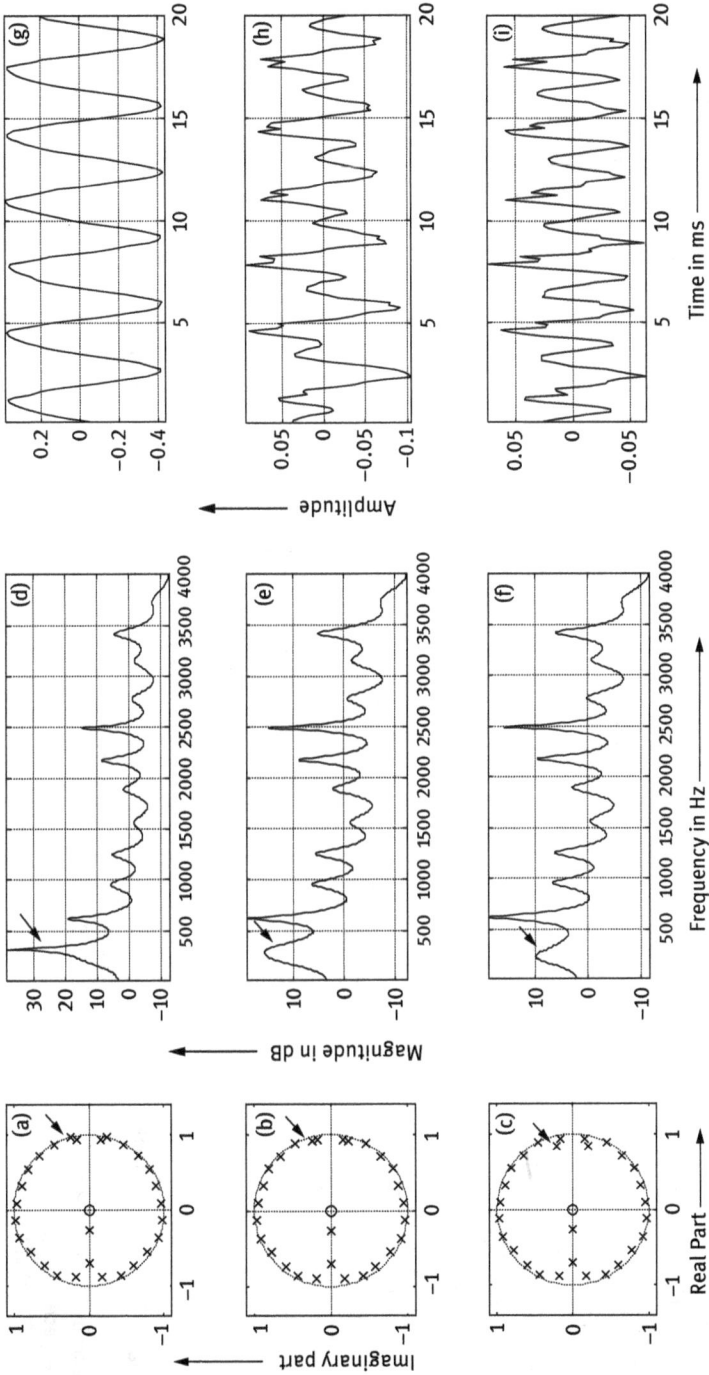

Figure 2.8: Effect of selective pole-defocussing in the frequency- and time-domain for vowel /i/ uttered by hypernasal speaker: (a) Z-plane with poles extracted using LP analysis with order 28 for the speech signal given in (g) and LP spectrum given in (d), (b) and (c) Z-plane after defocussing the pole by factor 1.05 and 1.15 respectively. (e) and (f) LP spectra of (b) and (c), respectively. (h) and (i) speech signal corresponding to (b) and (c), respectively.

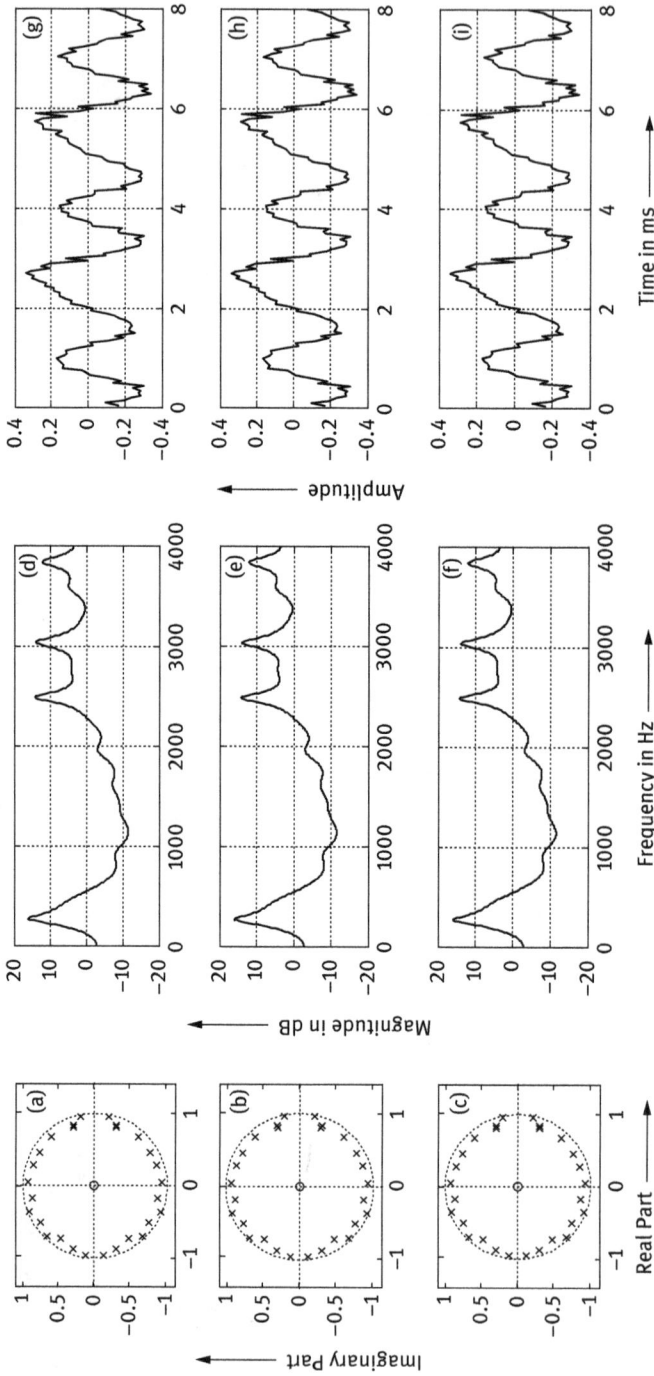

Figure 2.9: Effect of selective pole-defocussing in the frequency- and time-domain for vowel /i/ uttered by normal speaker: (a) Z-plane with poles extracted using LP analysis with order 28 for the speech signal given in (g) and LP spectrum given in (d), (b) and (c) Z-plane after defocussing the pole by factor 1.05 and 1.15, respectively. (e) and (f) LP spectra of (b) and (c), respectively, (h) and (i) speech signal corresponding to (b) and (c), respectively.

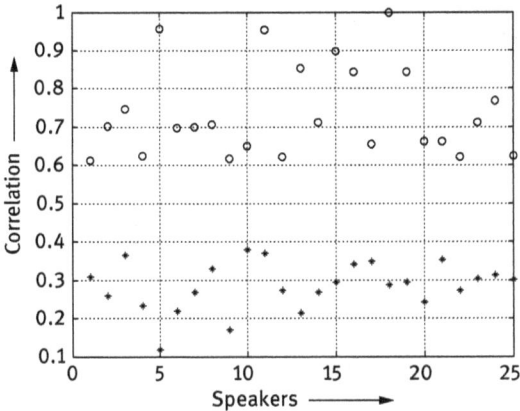

Figure 2.10: Correlation between the input and the re-synthesized speech signals for hypernasal ('*' markers) and normal speakers ('o' markers).

2.6.2.3 Detection of hypernasality (vowel /u/)

For the hypernasal speech corresponding to sustained vowel /u/, the actual formant around 300 Hz is shifted to 500 to 600 Hz as discussed in Section 2.5.1 and the peak around 200–250 Hz corresponds to nasal resonance. Thus, the highest peak around the low-frequency region of interest that corresponds to nasal resonance is defocussed with an LP order of 28 and defocussing factor of 1.15 as discussed for vowels /a/ and /i/ in previous sections. When the pole due to the additional formant is defocussed, the strength due to the nasal formant is suppressed in the time-domain speech signal and clear distinctions are observed before and after defocussing as given in Figure 2.11(h) and 11(i).

The same experiment is repeated for normal speakers with the same LP order and same defocussing factor as shown in Figure 2.12. The experiment is performed for 25 normal and 25 hypernasal speakers and the distribution of correlation between the actual and the re-synthesized speech for all the speakers in both the category is shown in Figure 2.13.

From the above three analyses using sustained vowels (/a/, /i/ and /u/) in hypernasal speech, an additional formant due to nasalization is observed below 300 Hz that is used as an acoustic cue for detecting hypernasality. The radius of the pole corresponding to nasalization is defocussed in all the three sustained vowels with an LP order of 28 and a defocussing factor of 1.15. The hypernasal speech signal after defocussing is re-synthesized, and prominent difference is observed in the hypernasal speech signal before and after

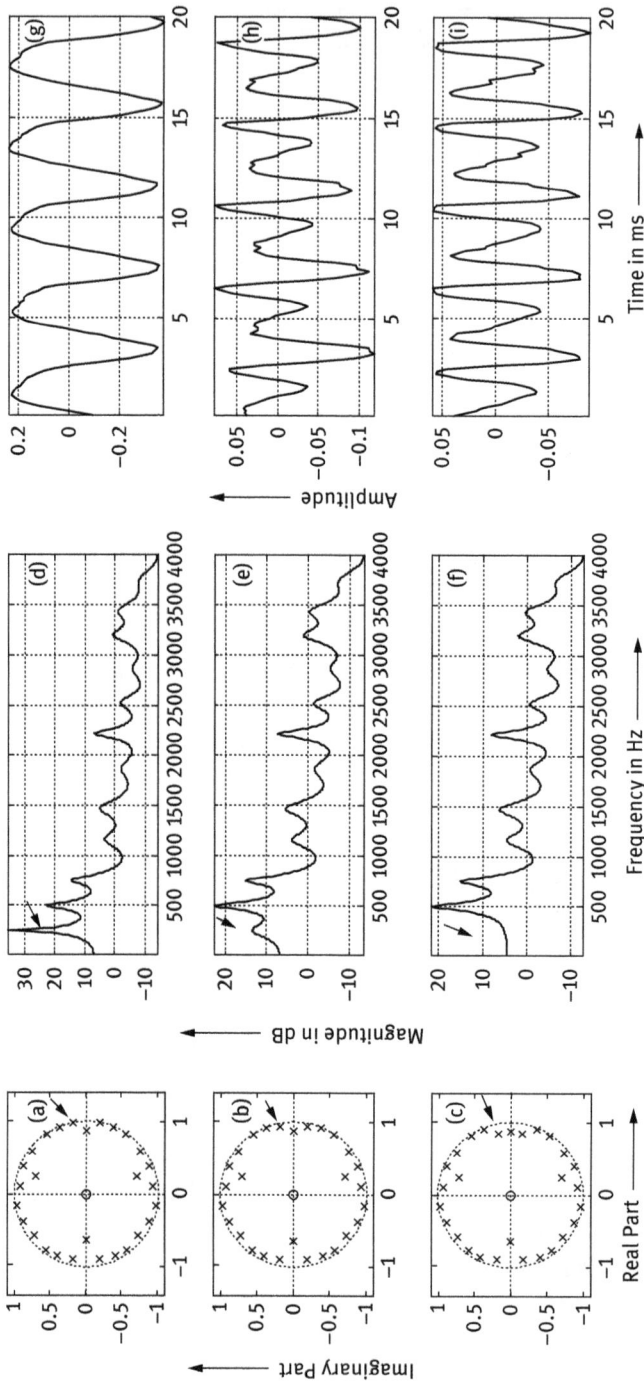

Figure 2.11: Effect of selective pole-defocussing in the frequency- and time-domain for vowel /u/ uttered by hypernasal speaker: (a) Z-plane with poles extracted using LP analysis with order 28 for the speech signal given in (g) and LP spectrum given in (d), (b) and (c) Z-plane after defocussing the pole by factor 1.05 and 1.15, respectively. (e) and (f) LP spectra of (b) and (c), respectively. (h) and (i) speech signal corresponding to (b) and (c), respectively.

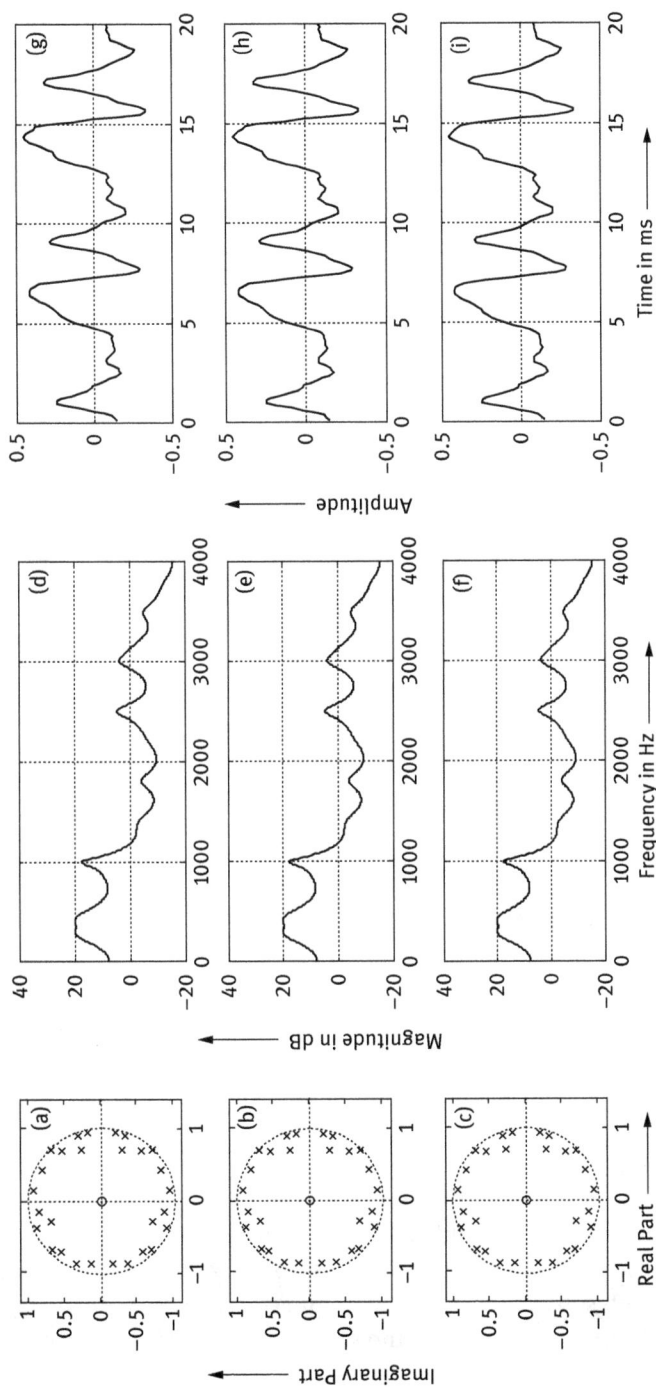

Figure 2.12: Effect of selective pole-defocussing in the frequency- and time-domain for vowel /u/ uttered by normal speaker: (a) Z-plane with poles extracted using LP analysis with order 28 for the speech signal given in (g) and LP spectrum given in (d), (b) and (c) Z-plane after defocussing the pole by factor 1.05 and 1.15, respectively. (e) and (f) LP spectra of (b) and (c) respectively, (h) and (i), speech signal corresponding to (b) and (c), respectively.

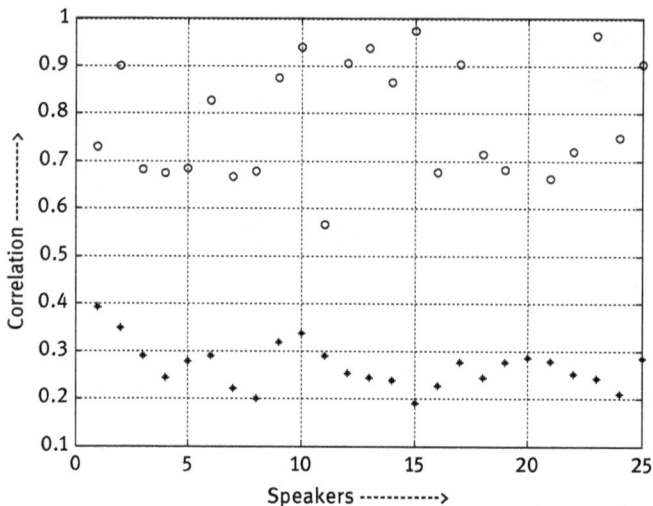

Figure 2.13: Correlation between the input and the re-synthesized speech signals for hypernasal ('*' markers) and normal speakers ('o' markers).

defocussing. This experiment helps in detecting the presence of hypernasality and may help in finding out the degree of hypernasality. Understanding the degree of hypernasality may help in providing proper speech therapy to hypernasal speakers.

2.6.3 GMM-based hypernasal/normal classification

A GMM-based classifier [33] is trained to classify the hypernasal/normal speech using first formant frequency and the corresponding −3 dB bandwidth as a two-dimensional feature vector. The LP-based formant extraction technique is used to extract the first formant frequency and −3 dB bandwidth for the sustained vowels /a/, /i/ and /u/ of hypernasal and normal speech. For the GMM training, 75% of the speech data is used and the remaining 25% of the data are used for testing. During training, using first formant frequency and the corresponding −3 dB bandwidth as a two-dimensional feature vector, GMMs are trained with two mixture components, for each vowel, for hypernasal and normal speech separately. The performance of the GMM-based classifier for hypernasal/normal decision, for the vowels /a/, /i/ and /u/, is found to be 100%.

2.7 Summary and conclusions

This chapter highlighted on speech disorders especially on VPDs due to CLP. The focus primarily was on non-invasive assessment methods for detection of hypernasality through signal processing approach. For the detection of hypernasality, speech data from the speakers with CLP are considered. Since introduction of additional nasal formants and anti-formants is an important cue for the detection of hypernasality, concentration was given to the formant extraction-based acoustic analysis. From the formant frequency-based acoustic analysis on nasalized vowels and hypernasal speech, it is observed that two or more additional formant frequencies, due to nasality, are introduced in addition to actual formants. Among these additional formants, a nasal formant in the low-frequency region around 250 Hz is found to be consistent cue for the detection of hypernasality. To cross-verify the above observation, for the vowels /a/, /i/ and /u/, in addition to their actual formants, nasal formant frequencies are artificially introduced at various frequency locations with different bandwidths and new signals are generated and a perceptual analysis is carried out. All the listeners participated in this perceptual test unanimously agreed that the signal, generated with a nasal formant introduced at the low-frequency range around 250 Hz, is clearly nasalized. Based on these observations, a LP-based selective pole defocussing-based hypernasality detection technique is proposed. For this purpose, a LP-based formant extraction technique is used. Lower order LP analysis frequently fails to resolve two closely spaced formants. On the contrary, increasing the LP order may show a spurious peak in the low-frequency region for the normal speech also that is due to pitch harmonics. To disambiguate this, in this work, the pole corresponding to the peak in the low-frequency region is defocussed and a new signal is re-synthesized. The correlation between the original and the re-synthesized signal is found to be a promising measure for the detection of hypernasality. Further a GMM-based hypernasal/normal classifier is trained and tested using first formant frequency and the corresponding −3 dB bandwidth as a two-dimensional feature vector for the sustained vowels /a/, /i/ and /u/ and is found to classify with a classification accuracy of 100%.

This chapter has focused on additional nasal formant frequency introduced in the vicinity of the first formant due to oral-nasal coupling as a cue for the analysis and detection of hypernasality. Further, the technique can be extended to post-operative CLP speakers to analyze the degree of the nasality after clinical surgery and also for spastic dysarthric speakers who are expected to have hypernasality due to neurological problems. There are diversities among different languages. As the current work is based on vowel nasalization due to oral-nasal coupling, the technique is language-independent.

References

[1] Vijayalakshmi P. Detection of hypernasality and assessment of dysarthria using signal processing techniques, Ph.D. Thesis, Department of applied mechanics, Indian institute of technology, Madras, May 2007.

[2] Hansen JH. Cebellos LG, Kaiser JF. A nonlinear operator-based speech feature analysis method with application to vocal fold pathology assessment. IEEE Trans Biomed Eng 1998;45(3):300–313.

[3] Normal velopharyngeal function and velopharyngeal dysfunction & its types. Available at: https://www.cincinnatichildrens.org/health/v/velopharyngeal. Accessed: 04 May 2017.

[4] Gohilot A, Pradhan T, Keluskar KM. Cephalometric evaluation of adenoids, upper airway, maxilla, velum length, need ratio for determining velopharyngeal incompetency in subjects with unilateral cleft lip and palate. J Indian Soc Pedodontics Preventive Dent 2014;32(4):297.

[5] Kummer AW. Types and causes of velopharyngeal dysfunction. Semin Speech Lang. Thieme Medical Publishers, 2011;32(2):150–158.

[6] Woo AS. Velopharyngeal dysfunction. Semin Plast Surg Thieme Medical Publishers, 2012;26(4):170–177.

[7] Murdoch BE, editor. Dysarthria – a physiological approach to assessment and treatment. Nelson Thornes, Stanley Thornes (Publishers) Ltd., United Kingdom, 1998.

[8] Carmichael J, Green P. Revisiting dysarthria assessment intelligibility metrics. Proceedings of International Conference on Spoken Language Processing (ICSLP), Jeju Island, Korea, Oct. 2004:485–488.

[9] Rabiner LR, Schafer RW. Digital Processing of Speech Signals, 1st ed. Prentice Hall, Englewood Cliffs, New Jersey, USA, 1978.

[10] O'Shaughnessy D. Speech communications: human and machine, 2nd ed. Wiley-IEEE Press, USA, 2000.

[11] Deng L, O'Shaughnessy D. Speech processing – a dynamic and optimization-oriented approach, signal processing and communications series. CRC Press, New York, 2003.

[12] Parsons TW. Voice and speech processing, 1st ed. McGraw-Hill College, New York, 1987.

[13] Wallen EJ, Hansen JH. A screening test for speech pathology assessment using objective quality measures. Proceedings of International Conference on Spoken Language Processing (ICSLP), Philadelphia, USA, Oct. 1996:776–779,

[14] Kasuya H, Ogawa S, Mashima K, Ebihara S. Normalized noise energy as an acoustic measure to evaluate pathologic voice. J Acoust Soc Am 1986;80(5):1329–1334.

[15] Kent RD, Kent JF, Weismer G, Duffy JR. What dysarthrias can tell us about the neural control of speech. J Phonetics 2000;28(3):273–302.

[16] Fry DB. The physics of speech, 1st ed. Cambridge University Press, 1979.

[17] Riley MD. Speech time-frequency representations. Kluwer Academic Publishers, 1989.

[18] Kent RD. Research on speech motor control and its disorders: a review and prospective. J Commun Disord 2000;33(5):391–428.

[19] Glass JR, Zue VW. Detection of nasalized vowels in American English. Proceedings of IEEE International Conference on Acoustics, Speech, and Signal Processing (ICASSP), Tampa, 1985:1569–1572.

[20] Glass JR, Zue VW. Detection and recognition of nasal consonants in American English. Proceedings of IEEE International Conference on Acoustics, Speech, and Signal Processing (ICASSP), Tokyo, 1986:2767–2770.
[21] Hawkins S, Stevens KN. Acoustic and perceptual correlates of the non-nasal-nasal distinction for vowels. J Acoust Soc Am 1985;77(4):1560–1574.
[22] Chen MY, Stevens KN, Kuo HJ, Chen H. Contributions of the study of disordered speech-to-speech production models. J Phonetics 2000;28(3):303–312.
[23] Cairns DA, Hansen JH, Riski JE. A noninvasive technique for detecting hypernasal speech using a nonlinear operator. IEEE Trans Biomed Eng 1996;43:35–45.
[24] Niu X, Kain A, Santen JP. Estimation of the acoustic properties of the nasal tract during the production of nasalized vowels. INTERSPEECH, Lisbon Portugal, Sept. 2005:1045–1048.
[25] Vijayalakshmi P, Ramasubba Reddy M, O'Shaughnessy D. Acoustic analysis and detection of hypernasality using a group delay function. IEEE Trans Biomed Eng 2007;54(4):621–629.
[26] Dubey AK, Mahadeva Prasanna SR, Dandapat S. Zero time windowing analysis of hypernasality in speech of cleft lip and palate children. National Conference on Communication (NCC), IIT Guwahati, India, 2016:1–6.
[27] Vikram CM, Adiga N, Mahadeva Prasanna SR. Spectral enhancement of cleft lip and palate speech. INTERSPEECH, San Francisco, CA, pp. 117–121, 2016.
[28] Bocklet T, Riedhammer K, Eysholdt U, Nöth E. Automatic phoneme analysis in children with cleft lip and palate. IEEE International Conference on Acoustics, Speech and Signal Processing (ICASSP), Canada, 2013:7572–7576.
[29] Ling He, Jing Zhang, Qi Liu, Heng Yin, Margaret Lech. Automatic evaluation of hypernasality and consonant misarticulation in cleft palate speech. IEEE Signal Process Lett 2014;21(10):1298–1301.
[30] Makhoul J. Linear prediction: a tutorial review. Proc IEEE 1975;63(4):561–580.
[31] Vijayalakshmi P, Reddy MR. Analysis of hypernasality by synthesis, in proceedings of Int. Conf. on Spoken Language Processing (ICSLP), Jeju, South Korea, 2004;525–528.
[32] Vijayalakshmi P, Nagarajan T, Rav J. Selective pole modification-based technique for the analysis and detection of hypernasality. TENCON-IEEE Region 10 Conference, Singapore, 2009:1–5.
[33] Quatieri TF. Discrete-time speech signal processing: principles and practice, 1st ed. Pearson Education, Delhi, India, 2006.

Plínio A. Barbosa, Zuleica A. Camargo and Sandra Madureira

3 Acoustic-based tools and scripts for the automatic analysis of speech in clinical and non-clinical settings

Abstract: This chapter presents three Praat scripts developed for analyzing prosodic acoustic parameters as an aid for acoustic science on prosody modeling and for determining the correlation of prosody production and perception in normal and pathological speech. The SGdetector script assists in language-mediated, semi-automatic identification of syllable-sized normalized duration peaks for investigating prominence and boundary marking. The ProsodyDescriptor script delivers 14 prosodic factors accompanied with duration, F0 and spectral importance, whereas the ExpressionEvaluator script computes additional descriptors of F0 and adds global intensity and long-term spectral parameters useful for expressive speech research. All three scripts have been applied successfully for the study of rhythm, intonation and voice quality for the analysis of expressive and pathological speech as well as for assessing the vocal profile analysis scheme (VPAS) protocol. All scripts are freely available and the languages tested so far were French, German, Swedish, English, Brazilian Portuguese (BP), and European Portuguese.

Keywords: Prosody, Rhythm, Intonation, Voice quality, SGdetector, F0 descriptors, acoustic tools

3.1 Introduction

Prosody research can greatly benefit from the automatization of procedures for describing prosodic forms in differently sized corpora and for investigating such functions as prominence, boundary and discursive relation marking. For the analysis of large corpora, manual procedures are not feasible. Automatization is advantageous because the same procedures can be applied to analyze the entire corpus. It is also helpful for the purpose of arranging and preparing data for the statistical analysis.

This chapter presents three scripts for speech prosody research running on Praat [1]. They measure acoustic parameters which are relevant to be taken into account in describing speech prosody and in such a way they generate robust prosodic descriptors. Since the phonetic literature on speech prosody has shown that duration is a crucial parameter for signaling stress, prominence and

https://doi.org/10.1515/9781501502415-004

boundary in languages such as English, Portuguese, French, German, and Swedish, the scripts were devised in such a way to be able to detect prosody-related acoustic salience, as well as to generate a 12-parameter vector of duration, intensity and F0 descriptors for prosodic analysis. The usefulness of the scripts is discussed regarding the results obtained from their application in previous speech research works.

3.2 SGdetector script for semi-automatic detection of acoustic salience via duration

The SGdetector script for Praat was implemented in 2004 and updated in 2009 and 2010. It allows the semi-automatic detection of local peaks of normalized syllable-sized durations. That kind of duration detection is crucial in the prosodic investigation of languages, such as Brazilian Portuguese (henceforth BP), Swedish [2], English [3, 4], German [5, 6], and French [7] as well as other languages that use duration to signal both stress and prosodic boundary.

Thoroughly tested since 2004 with BP (cf. [8, 9], inter alia), the script has also been used to carry out prosodic research in the aforementioned languages and has potential to be applied to additional languages, at least those genetically related to the ones which have been already tested. It was also used in studies of speech expressivity [10, 11].

The input files for running the script are a TextGrid file containing a phone- or syllable-sized segmentation and a broad phonetic transcription of the corresponding Sound file. Furthermore, a TableOfReal file containing a table listing the means and standard-deviations in milliseconds of the phone durations of the language under study is provided. This latter file is delivered as part of the script and is available for BP, European Portuguese, British English, German, Swedish and French.

As a first step, syllable-sized segmentation is intended to capture prosodic-relevant duration variation along the utterances [12] and is taken here as an interval between two consecutive vowel onsets. This unit constitutes a phonetic syllable called a VV unit, that is, a unit containing a vowel and all the consonants following it. It extends from the onset of one vowel to the onset of the next vowel. Each vowel followed by one or more consonants is a VV unit.

Besides the crucial importance of vowel onset detection for speech signal processing [13], a clear advantage of a segmentation based on vowel onsets is its potential for automatic detection [9]. Even under moderately noisy conditions, the script performs well, what makes it suitable for forensic applications as well.

Since audios submitted to forensic analysis are usually noisy and distorted due to bad recording conditions, their analysis is challenging, and VV unit duration can be a robust measure to be taken into account [14, 15]. For extracting measures other than duration for forensic purposes, the script ForensicDataTracking (Barbosa, P. A. 2013) can be used to automatically extract the following acoustic parameters: three formant frequencies (F1, F2, and F3), median fundamental frequency, spectral emphasis, fundamental frequency baseline, and F0 inter-peaks duration. Passetti [16] applied the ForensicDataTracking to the analysis of Portuguese vowels in data collected by mobile phones and direct recordings.

Detection of vowel onsets can also be carried out using the Praat script BeatExtractor, which was developed in 2004 [9, 12]. Constantini [17] analyzed speakers' speech samples from seven Brazilian regions, using the BeatExtractor script to segment speech samples into VV units and applying the ProsodicDescriptorExtractor script to extract eight prosodic measures: VV unities per second to evaluate speech rate; mean, standard deviation, and skewness of the normalized z-score; peaks of z-score per second for detecting prominence rate; fundamental frequency median, spectral emphasis and rate of non-prominent VV units.

The BeatExtractor script was repeatedly tested for BP along the years, confirming its usefulness and appropriateness for detecting local peaks of syllable-sized duration for describing potential perceived speech prominence and prosodic boundaries, as shown by the experimental research presented later in this chapter.

In the SGdetector script, the detection of peaks of prosodic-relevant VV duration is carried out by serially applying a normalization technique as well as a smoothing technique, as explained in the following paragraphs.

For normalizing VV duration, the script uses the z-score transformation given in equation (3.1), where *dur* is the VV duration in ms and the pair (μ_i, var_i) is the reference mean and variance in ms of the phones within the corresponding VV unit. The reference descriptors for the aforementioned languages are included in the file TableOfReal delivered with the script.

$$z = \frac{dur - \sum_i \mu_i}{\sqrt{\sum_i var_i}} \qquad (3.1)$$

For smoothing, the script applies a five-point moving average filtering technique given by equation (3.2) to the sequence of z-scores (z_i).

$$z^i_{smoothed} = \frac{5.z^i + 3.z^{i-1} + 3.z^{i+1} + 1.z^{i-2} + 1.z^{i+2}}{13} \qquad (3.2)$$

The two-step procedure which has been just described aims at minimizing the effects of intrinsic duration and number of segments in the VV unit, as well as attenuating the effect of the implementation of lexical stress irrelevant for the prosodic functions of prominence and boundary marking. Local peaks of smoothed *z-scores* are detected by tracking the position of the VV unit for which the discrete first derivative of the corresponding smoothed z-score changes from a positive to a negative value.

The effect of the application of the two-step procedure can be seen in Figure 3.1 from raw duration contour in Figure 3.2. Observe that only five peaks appear in Fig. 1, from which three peaks signaled in the figure are the most relevant ones, corresponding with the perception of prominence and/or boundary. In Figure 3.2, there are 11 local peaks of VV duration: just a few correspond to perceived prominence, as can be seen in Figure 3.1.

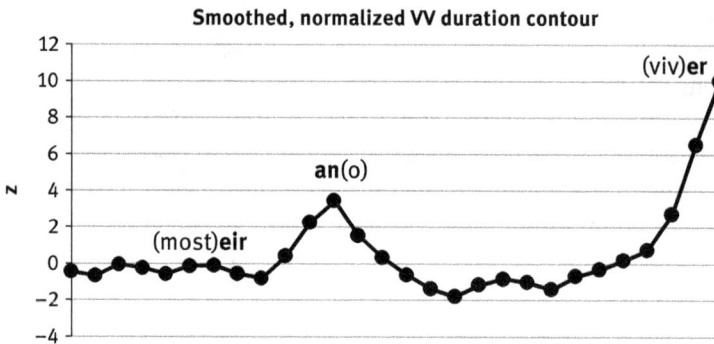

Figure 3.1: Smoothed, normalized VV duration contour of sentence "Manuel tinha entrado para o **mosteiro** há quase um **ano**, mas ainda não se adaptara àquela maneira de **viver**." by a female speaker.

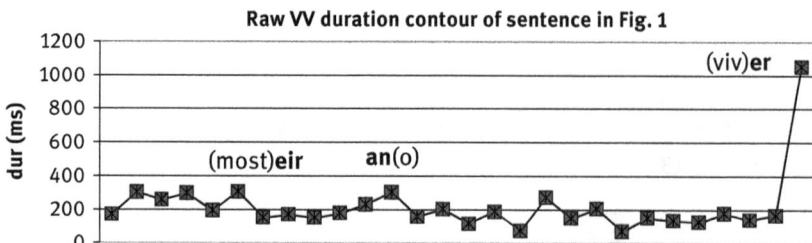

Figure 3.2: Raw VV duration contour (in ms) of sentence depicted in Figure 3.1.

At the output, the script generates two text files, a TextGrid object and an optional plot of the syllable-sized smoothed and normalized duration along the time-course of the Sound file under analysis. The first text file is a five-column table displaying the following values for each VV unit: (a) its given transcription recovered from the TextGrid itself, for example, "eNs," "at" (even for the case where the segmentation is made phonewise), (b) its raw duration in milliseconds, (c) its duration z-score, the result of equation (3.1), (d) its smoothed *z-score*, the result of equation (3.2), and (e) a binary value indicating whether its position corresponds to a local peak of smoothed *z-score* (value 1) or not (value 0).

The second text file is a two-column table containing (1) the raw duration in milliseconds of the acoustically defined stress groups, which are delimited by two consecutive peaks of smoothed *z-scores* and (2) the corresponding number of VV units in these stress groups. These corresponding values were often used to do linear regressions to evaluate the degree of stress-timing of a speech passage, for instance in Barbosa et al. [18].

The TextGrid generated by the script contains an interval tier delimiting the detected stress group boundaries, synchronized with the input TextGrid, which allows, when selected with the corresponding Sound file, to listen to the chunks that end with a duration-related salience. The optional feature, implemented when the option *DrawLines* is chosen in the input parameters window, plots a trace of the smoothed z-scores synchronized with the VV unit sequence: each value of smoothed z-score is plotted in the y-axis in the position of each vowel onset along the plotted original TextGrid. The advantage of this choice for integrating intonation and rhythm descriptions is discussed the next section.

The correspondence between smoothed z-scores peaks and perceived salience, which refers to both prominence and prosodic boundary, is striking. In Barbosa [9], we demonstrated an accuracy range varying from 69 to 82% between

Table 3.1: Precision, recall, and accuracy in percentage (%) for semi-automatically detected salience against perceived salience for the Lobato corpus read by a female (F) and a male (M) speaker at slow (s), normal (n), and fast (f) rates.

Sp/rate	precision	recall	accuracy
F/n	90	74	82
F/f	73	57	69
M/s	88	67	73
M/f	61	70	70

perceived and produced salience, as shown in Table 3.1 for the semi-automatic algorithm described here.

Perceived salience was determined by asking two groups of 10 listeners to evaluate two readings of a passage by two BP speakers (a male and a female) at three distinct rates (normal, slow, and fast). The listeners in both groups were lay undergraduate students in Linguistics. They were free to listen to the four readings as many times as they wanted.

In the first group, each listener was given a handout with the orthographic transcription of the recording and was instructed to circle all the words s/he considered highlighted by the speaker.

The second group was instructed to circle the words that preceded a boundary. In each group, the percentage of listeners that circled each word in the text for each reading was initially used to define three levels of salience, according to a one-tailed z-test of proportion. Since the smallest proportion significantly distinct from zero is about 28% for $\alpha = 0.05$ and N=10, words circled by less than 30% of the listeners were considered non-salient. For $\alpha = 0.01$, the threshold for rejecting the null hypothesis is about 49%. Thus, words circled by 50% the listeners or more were considered strongly salient. Words circled by between 30 and 50% of the listeners were considered weakly salient. For the purpose of computing the performance measures in the table, weakly and strongly salient words were both considered as "salient" *tout court*.

The relatively high correspondence between perceived and produced salience allowed us to evaluate the degree of stress-timing in two different speaking styles for two varieties of Portuguese [18] This work revealed that the speech rhythm of Portuguese speakers differs remarkably from the rhythm of Brazilian speakers when both groups narrate but not when both groups of speakers read. This was possible to demonstrate through the linear correlation on interval durations delimited by smoothed z-score peaks and number of VV units in the same interval. These two series of values were recovered from one of the tables generated by the SGdetector script.

3.2.1 The SGDetector script for describing the relations between F0 trace and syllable-sized duration trace

The smoothed, normalized syllable-sized duration plot obtained with the *DrawLines* option of the SGdetector script was conceived in such a way as to give the value of normalized duration along the vowel onsets of the utterance. This feature allows the possibility of plotting the F0 contour of the utterance against the evolution of normalized duration and examining the VV units for which pitch accents and boundary tones coincide with normalized duration peaks [8].

Table 3.2 presents results of such coincidences in terms of a priori and conditional probabilities for both read paragraphs (two male subjects) and spontaneous speech (a male and a female subject).

Table 3.2: A priori probability of pitch accent p(F0) and duration peak p(dur) in percentage (%) of number of phonological words. Speaker and speaking style are indicated. Stars signal significant differences between a priori and conditional probabilities α = 0.02).

sp (sp.sty)	p(F0)	p(F0/dur)	p(dur)	p(dur/F0)
F (spont.)	63*	79*	49*	63*
M (spont.)	73	80	48	56
AC (read)	54	66	56*	76*
AP (read)	70	83	65	74

A priori probabilities are the proportion of pitch-accents, p (F0), and normalized duration peaks, p (dur), considering the total number of phonological words. Conditional probabilities, on the other hand, consider the co-occurrence between a duration peak with a pitch accent over the total number of duration peaks, p (F0/dur), or the total number of pitch accents, p (dur/F0).

A significant difference, computed from a test of proportions with α = 0.02, between a priori and conditional probabilities signals, a dependence between pitch accent and duration peak.

The table shows that there is dependence between duration peak and pitch accent for the female speaker in spontaneous speech, as well as for speaker AC in read speech: for the latter, a pitch accent implies 76% of chance of a duration peak. For the female speaker both are inter-related.

This inter-relation is confirmed when the analysis is restricted to major prosodic boundaries in read speech (utterance boundaries, clause and subject-predicate boundaries): 98% (for speaker AP) and 100% (for speaker AC) of the time, both pitch accent and duration peak occur in the same lexical item, usually in the pre-stressed or stressed vowel for pitch accents, and in the stressed or pre-pausal VV unit for duration peaks.

Figure 3.3 illustrates how both traces can be visualized. This was possible with the use of the *DrawLines* option of the SGdetector script. In this figure, the labels

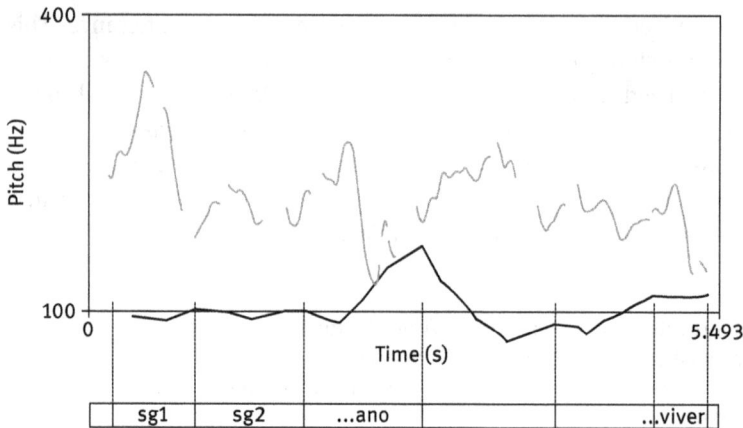

Figure 3.3: F0 contour superposed on the VV smoothed, normalized duration contour of read utterance "Manuel tinha entrado para o mosteiro há quase um ano, mas ainda não se adaptara àquela maneira de viver."

sg1 and *sg2* signal the first two stress groups. The first rising F0 contour during *sg1* signals a melodic salience not accompanied by a duration peak. This salience is perceived by almost all listeners as a prominence in the word "Manuel," the character of the story. The two low boundary tones inside the stress groups ending in *ano* and *viver* occur during a VV unit with a duration peak.

3.3 The ProsodyDescriptor for semi-automatic extraction of global and local prosodic parameters

The ProsodyDescriptor script delivers 14 phonetic-prosodic parameters for whole utterances or chunks of the same utterance to allow research on the link between prosody production and perception.

This script has as input parameters names of the Sound file and corresponding TextGrid file. The TextGrid file must be composed of two interval tiers, one with the labeling and segmentation of the VV units (VV tier), and the other with the delimitation of the chunks of the audio file for analysis (Chunk tier), if this option is chosen. The number of intervals in the Chunk tier can vary from one to any number of units corresponding to any kind of phrasing needed for the intended analysis (e.g., syntactic phrases, prosodic constituents such as stress groups, content-based chunks, among others). F_0 contour is also computed, thus, it is necessary, as for the Pitch buttons in Praat, to inform minimum and maximum pitch range.

For the entire audio file (or for each chunk in the corresponding interval tier), the algorithm generates (a) six duration-related measures computed from the metadata obtained using the algorithm of the previously described SGdetector script, (b) seven descriptors obtained from the Pitch object computed by the script and (c) a measure of spectral emphasis as defined by Traunmüller and Eriksson [19].

The six duration-related measures computed in each chunk are: speech rate in VV units per second (sr), mean, standard deviation and skewness of smoothed VV duration z-score, rate of smoothed VV duration z-score local peaks (pr), and rate of non-salient VV units. The seven F0 descriptors are F0 and first derivative of F0 median, standard deviation and skewness, as well as F0 peak rate. For computing the latter measure, a smoothing function (with cut-off frequency of 1.5 Hz) followed by a quadratic interpolation function are applied before the F0 peak rate computation. The 14th parameter is spectral emphasis, a measure of relative intensity correlated to vocal effort [20].

Speech rate is a classic measure in prosodic research whose change signals aspects such as changes across speakers, speaking style, hesitation, parenthetical constructions, prominence, and boundary marking. Computed for a single audio file, it allows comparison across these audio files only. That is why local measures of duration throughout an audio file are necessary, such as mean, standard deviation, skewness, rate of smoothed VV duration z-score local peaks, and rate of non-salient VV units. These measures reveal local changes in syllabic duration that signals prosodic changes such as prominence and boundary marking. The seven descriptors of F0 are computed for the entire audio files and reveal melodic aspects of prosodic structure related to range, mean, pitch accent rate, and mean and dispersion of rate of F0 change (F0 derivative). Spectral emphasis reveals vocal effort: the greater its value, the higher the effort for uttering a sound or audio file.

These 14 measures can be used both to study the evolution of these prosodic parameters throughout a speech signal as well as to correlate prosody production and perception. As regards the latter, we used the difference of these values between paired utterances as predictors of the degree of discrepancy between perceived manner of speaking [21]. The experimental design consisted in instructing 10 listeners to evaluate two subsets of 44 audio pairs combining three different speakers of BP and two speaking styles, storytelling, and reading. The instruction was "Evaluate each pair of excerpts as to how they differ according to the manner of speaking given a scale from 1 (same manner of speaking) to 5 (very different manner of speaking)." After testing more than 50 models of multiple linear regression, results showed that the best model was the one which explained 71% of the variance of the listeners' responses (lr), as given in equation (3.3) with *p*-value of at least 0.009 for all coefficients ($F_{3,11}$ = 12.4, $p < 0.0008$).

$$lr = -1.5 + 10.4pr + 2.65sr - 10.75pr*sr \qquad (3.3)$$

This reveals that the significant production parameters that explain the listeners' performance are speech rate in VV units/s and normalized duration peak rate, which can be associated with the syllable succession and salient syllable succession.

Recently, this script was used to compare prosodic parameters in professional and non-professional speaking styles (Barbosa, Madureira and Boula de Mareüil, submitted). The professional stimuli were composed of excerpts of broadcast news and political discourses from six subjects in each case. The non-professional stimuli were made up of recordings of 10 subjects who read a long story and narrated it subsequently. All these materials were obtained in four language varieties: Brazilian and European Portuguese, standard French and German. The corpus was balanced for gender. Eight melodic and intensity parameters were retained after extracting them from excerpts of 10 to 20 seconds. We showed that six out of eight parameters partially distinguish professional from non-professional style in the four language varieties. Classification and discrimination tests carried out with 12 Brazilian listeners using delexicalized speech showed that these subjects were able to distinguish professional style from non-professional style with about 2/3 of hits irrespective of language. In comparison, an automatic classification using a Linear Discriminant Analysis (LDA) model performed better in classifying non-professional (96%) against professional styles, but not in classifying professional (42%) against non-professional styles.

3.4 The ExpressionEvaluator script for describing dynamic and vocal quality features

The ExpressionEvaluator script is similar to the Prosodic script. It extracts five classes of acoustic parameters and four statistical descriptors, producing 12 acoustic parameters. The five classes of acoustic parameters comprise the fundamental frequency (F0) with the extraction of the following descriptors: median, inter-quartile semi-amplitude, skewness, and 0.995 quantile, the fundamental frequency first derivative (dF0) with the descriptors mean, standard-deviation and skewness; global intensity skewness, spectral tilt (SpTt), and long-term average spectrum (LTAS) standard-deviation. Spectral tilt is a correlate of vocal effort and was set to the difference of intensity in dB between the bands 0–125 Hz and 1,250–4,000 Hz.

The F0 first derivative was used to detect abrupt changes in the melodic contour. The values of the F0 and dF0 descriptors were z-scored using F0 mean and standard-deviation reference values for adult males (136 Hz, 58 Hz) and females (231 Hz, 120 Hz). Spectral tilt was normalized by dividing its value by the complete-band intensity median, whereas LTAS standard-deviation was normalized by dividing its value by 10.

The ExpressionEvaluator script was applied to analyze voice quality settings in clinical and expressive speech samples [22]. In this line of investigation, the acoustic measures derived by the script were correlated to perceived voice quality settings identified by the application of the vocal profile analysis scheme (VPAS) by Laver et al. [23]. The application of the ExpressionEvaluator script made it possible to distinguish between neutral (modal voice) and non-neutral phonatory settings [24–26]. The identification of the modal voice setting was related to little variation in F0 and to first F0 derivative (df0) values across speech samples of the same speaker. Furthermore, F0 and df0 measures were found to be useful to detect intermittent occurrences of voice quality settings, such as phonatory settings with irregular vocal fold vibration: breathy voice, harsh voice, and creaky voice.

Camargo et al. [27] described, from the perceptual and acoustic (via ExpressionEvaluator script) points of view, the differences in voice quality settings that are related to gender. The corpus was composed by speech samples recorded by 38 subjects, aging from 20 to 58 years old. The data showed the discriminatory capability of F0 and spectral tilt measures in differentiating speaker's gender.

Long-term measures obtained by means of the ExpressionEvaluator script in Camargo et al. [26] were able to predict laryngeal and tension voice qualities. The results showed the discriminant power of long-term acoustic measures to predict neutral (79%) and non-neutral (75%) laryngeal and tension settings. The relevant measures to detect neutral setting (modal voice) were F0 and df0, with high discriminant scores (82%). On the other hand, for the non-neutral settings in laryngeal and tension domains, the combination of spectral tilt and LTAS acoustic measures was influential, with discriminant power of 66%, especially for laryngeal hyper-function and raised larynx settings.

In clinical environment with adult patients, some investigations using the ExpressionEvaluator script have been carried out [28, 29].

Camargo et al.[28] found some correspondences between perceived voice quality and acoustic measures in AIDS patients' speech samples. The relevant measures were F0 (especially for female), spectral tilt, and LTAS measures (especially for male).

Lima-Silva et al. [29] investigated the acoustic and perceptual correlations of voice quality and vocal dynamics in speech samples recorded by teachers with voice complaints and laryngeal disorders. In agglomerative hierarchical cluster-analysis (AHCA), tendencies toward clustering spectral tilt (mean and SD), LTAS in one group, and F0 (median and quantile 0.995) measures in another one group were found. Canonic correlation analysis showed the relevance of spectral tilt and F0 measures in acoustic-perceptual correlations: spectral tilt (skewness) and the following perceptual findings: breathiness (40%), harsh voice (32%), high habitual pitch (288%), and supralaryngeal hyper-function (26 %); spectral tilt (mean) and the following perceptual findings: high habitual loudness (30%), laryngeal hyper-function (30%), and harsh voice (30%); spectral tilt (SD) and the following perceptual findings: pharyngeal constriction (29%) and high habitual loudness (27%); F0 (99.5% quantile) and harsh voice (26%); F0 (median) and inadequate breath support (25%); F0 (interquartile semi-amplitude) and inadequate breath support (21%). Linear regression analysis reinforced the relevance of acoustic measures, F0 (median: 59%), spectral tilt (skewness: 43% and mean: 39%) and perceptual data (harsh voice: 48%, fast speech rate: 47%, retracted tongue body: 41%, breathiness: 40% and pharyngeal constriction: 39%) in relation to laryngeal disorders. These findings reinforce the multidimensional aspect of voice and the importance of acoustic and perceptual profiles to provide a detailed description of teacher vocal behavior.

In clinical studies of children with voice and speech disorders, some explorations were also carried out [30–32]. In a case report, [30]Pessoa et al. [30] applied the ExpressionEvaluator script to speech samples, recorded by a unilateral cochlear implant (UCI) user at the ages of 5 and 6. Data related to F0 measures were influential in discriminating the different speech samples collected in the period of a year.

Pessoa et al. [31] explored the speech characteristics of a hearing impaired child, a three-year and ten-month-old bilaterally implanted user. These findings indicated the influence of laryngeal hyper-function setting and aperiodicity on pitch extension and variability.

In Gomes et al. [32], both the acoustic measures extracted with the ExpressionEvaluator and the voice quality settings described with the VPAS were found to be relevant to segregate speech samples from male and female children with and without respiratory diseases (oral breathing).

The investigation of voice quality based on the measures extracted by means of the ExpressionEvaluator script made it possible to correlate acoustic to perceptual dimensions and to identify instances of co-occurrence of voice quality settings [25]. Those aspects are relevant not only to consider compensatory strategies to voice and speech disturbances in the clinical context (patients with AIDs, voice disorders, including teachers with laryngeal disturbances and children with cochlear implants) but also to foster research on speech expressivity [11, 33].

Madureira [33] discusses specific uses of sound symbolism concerning segmental and prosodic properties in the reading of a poem by a professional actor. The duration values of the VV units in the five repetitions of the stanza chosen for the purpose of analysis were compared by means of Analysis of Variance (ANOVA). No differences were found among repetitions 1, 2 3, and 4. Repetition 5 was found to differ from the others $p = 0.000$. The fifth repetition was also found to differ from the others in relation to F0 (median, 0.995 quantile, skewness, and its first derivate mean, standard deviation, and skewness) and in relation to the LTAS. These differences in LTAS correlate with differences in voice quality identified by means of the VPAS.

In Madureira et al.[34], the ExpressionEvaluator was used in an acoustic and perceptual experiment exploring the characteristics of voice quality and dynamic settings evaluated by means of the VPAS [35]. The objective of the work was investigating whether professional and non-professional speech styles could be differentiated by means of descriptors inserted in a semantic differential questionnaire applied to a group of 80 judges. The corpus was a prose text which was read by eight female subjects aged 21 to 45 years: four of them voice professionals, two university teachers, and two undergraduates. The results indicated that the two styles were differentiated. The quantitative acoustic variables, F0 inter-quartile semi-amplitude (sampquartisf0) and F0 median (mednf0), were found to be significant ($p < 0,05$). These two measures indicate that the varying fundamental frequency and the speed of its variation were relevant to explain the data. Professional speakers more than non-professional speakers tend to vary with fundamental frequency more often and more rapidly assigning prominence to certain words.

Menegon and Madureira [36] investigated voice quality settings in instances of singing following the presentation of metaphors commonly used in the teaching of singing. The ExpressionEvaluator script was applied to extract the acoustic measures. The research subjects were asked to sing a folk song without any instruction given by the teacher and then to sing it again after being presented with the following kinds of metaphors: the prism, the flying saucer, and the cathedral. The results indicated that the configurations of the vocal tract were influenced by the metaphors. From the acoustic point of view, the acoustic measures related to spectral tilt (spectral tilt mean and standard deviation (desvadinclinespec)) were found to be influential in determining these configurations.

In Madureira [37], the ExpressionEvaluator script was applied to stanzas of a poem recited by a professional actor. The objective of the work was to analyze expressive uses of rhotic sounds and prosodic data. Besides the acoustic analysis, perceptual analysis of voice quality settings, voice dynamics by means of the VPAS [35], and the evaluation of the emotional primitive "activation" by a group of judges were carried out. The results indicated that higher degrees of perceived agitation were related to more energy in high frequencies suggesting higher vocal effort involvement on the part of the speaker. Other findings were as follows: more f_0 variability (higher sampquastisf0), higher median values of f_0 (mednf0), a decreased steepness of the overall spectral slope (LTAS and medinclinespec), more extreme values of intensity (assimint), greater number of trill productions, and higher degrees of tenseness, loudness, and pitch. This higher degree of activation and vocal effort was reflected in the choice of trills, since trills were more productive in the speech production of the stanzas perceived as having a higher degree of agitation.

3.5 Summary and availability of the tools

The tools presented here were used to conduct research on speech rhythm analysis and modeling either in a single language or cross-linguistically, on the relation between intonation and rhythm both *stricto sensu* and on the link between speech rhythm production and perception. They were tested in French, German, Brazilian and European Portuguese and less systematically tested in Swedish and English. They proved to be helpful in analyzing expressive speech and clinical speech data, as well as in assessing the VPAS protocol. They are licensed under the terms of the GNU General Public License as published by the Free Software Foundation: version 2 of the License and have been tested in French, German, Brazilian and European Portuguese, Swedish, and English, the latter two less systematically.

Acknowledgments: The authors thank research grants from CNPq: first author, CNPq grant 302657/2015-0), second author, CNPq grant 302602/2016-0, and third author, CNPq grant 306818/2010-8.

References

[1] Boersma p, Weenink D. Praat: doing phonetics by computer [Computer program]. Available at: http://www.praat.org. Version 5.2.44, 2013.
[2] Barbosa PA, Eriksson A, Åkesson J. Cross-linguistic similarities and differences of lexical stress realisation in Swedish and Brazilian Portuguese. In: Asu EL, Lippus [UIP], editors. Nordic prosody. Proceedings from the XIth Conference, Tartu 2012, 97–106. Frankfurt am Main: Peter Lang, 2013.
[3] Wightman CW, Shattuck-Hufnagel S, Ostendorf M, Price PJ. Segmental durations in the vicinity of prosodic boundaries. J Acoust Soc Am 1992;91(3):1707–1717.
[4] Fry DB. Experiments in the perception of stress. Language and Speech, 1958;1:126–152.
[5] Dogil G. Phonetic correlates of word stress and suppress. In: Van der Hulst, editor. Word Prosodic System of European Languages. Berlin: De Gruyter, 1995:371–376.
[6] Sluijter AM. Phonetic correlates of stress and accent. Ph.D. Thesis, Holland Institute of Generative Linguistics, Leiden, 1995.
[7] Barbosa PA. Caractérisation et génération automatique de la structuration rythmique du français. PhD thesis, ICP/Institut National Polytechnique de Grenoble, France, 1994.
[8] Barbosa PA. Prominence- and boundary-related acoustic correlations in Brazilian Portuguese read and spontaneous speech. Proceedings of Speech Prosody 2008, Campinas, 2008:257–260.
[9] Barbosa PA. Automatic duration-related salience detection in Brazilian Portuguese read and spontaneous speech. Proceedings of Speech Prosody 2010, Chicago (100067:1-4), 2010. Available at: http://www.speechprosody2010.illinois.edu/papers/100067.pdf. Accessed June 8th 2018.
[10] Madureira S. Reciting a sonnet: production strategies and perceptual effects. Proceedings of the Speech Prosody 2008 Conference. São Paulo, Editora RG, 2008:1, 697–700.
[11] Madureira S, Camargo Z. Exploring sound symbolism in the investigation of speech expressivity. Proceedings of ISCA Tutorialand Research Workshop on Experimental Linguistics, 2010. Grécia: Universitry of Athens, 2010:1, 105–8.
[12] Barbosa PA. Incursões em torno do ritmo da fala. Campinas: RG/Fapesp, 2006.
[13] Dogil G, Braun G. The PIVOT model of speech parsing, Wien: Verlag, 1988.
[14] Gonçalves CS. Taxa de elocução e de articulação em *corpus* forense do português brasileiro. Unpublished Thesis, 2013.
[15] Machado AP. Uso de técnicas acústicas para verificação de locutor em simulação experimental. Master's thesis. University of Campinas, Brazil, 2014.
[16] Passetti RR. O efeito do telefone celular no sinal da fala: Uma análise fonético-acústica com implicações para a verificação de locutor em português brasileiro. Unpublished Master Dissertation, 2015.
[17] Constantini AC. Caracterização prosódica de sujeitos de diferentes variedades do português brasileiro em diferentes relações sinal-ruído. Brazil: University of Campinas 2014.

[18] Barbosa PA, Viana MC, Trancoso I. Cross-variety rhythm typology in Portuguese. Proceedings of Interspeech 2009– Speech and Intelligence. Brighton, UK. London: Causal Productions, 2009:1011–1014.

[19] Traunmüller H, Eriksson A. The frequency range of the voice fundamental in the speech of male and female adults. Unpublished Manuscript. Available at:: http://www.ling.su.se/staff/hartmut/aktupub.htm.

[20] Eriksson A, Thunberg GC, Traunmüller H. Syllable prominence: a matter of vocal effort, phonetic distinct-ness and top-down processing. Seventh European Conference on Speech Communication and Technology, 2001.

[21] Barbosa PA, R Silva W. A new methodology for comparing speech rhythm structure between utterances: beyond typological approaches. In: Caseli H, et al. editors. PROPOR 2012, LNAI 7243. Springer, Heidelberg, 2012:329–337.

[22] Barbosa PA. Detecting changes in speech expressiveness in participants of a radio program. Proceedings of Interspeech 2009– Speech and Intelligence, 2009, Brighton. Londres: Causal Productions, 2009:2155–2158.

[23] Laver J, Wirs S, Mackenzie J, Hiller SM. A perceptual protocol for the analysis of vocal profiles. Edinburg University Department of Linguistics Work in Progress 1981:14, 139–155.

[24] Camargo Z, Madureira S. The acoustic analysis of speech samples designed for the Voice Profile Analysis Scheme for Brazilian Portuguese (BP-VPAS): long-term F0 and intensity measures. Tutorial and Research Workshop on Experimental Linguistics, 2010, Grécia. University of Athens. Grécia: ISCA International Speech Communication Association, 2010:1, 33–36.

[25] Rusilo LC, Camargo Z, Madureira S. The validity of some acoustic measures to predict voice quality settings: trends between acoustic and perceptual correlates of voice quality. Proceedings of the 4th Isca Tutorial and Research Workshop on Experimental Linguistics, 2011, Paris.. Athens: University of Athens, 2011:1, 115–18.

[26] Camargo Z, Queiroz RM, Rusilo LC, Madureira S. Acoustic and perceptual correlates of voice: trends between short and long-term analysis. Proceedings of 10th Pan-European Voice Conference, 2013, Praga. Praga: Pan European Voice Association, 2013:1, 377–377, 2013.

[27] Camargo Z, Madureira S, Pessoa A, Rusilo LC. Voice quality and gender: some insights on correlation between perceptual and acoustic dimensions. 6th International Conference on Speech Prosody, 2012, Shangai. Abstract Book Speech Prosody 2012. Shangai: Tongji University Press, 2012;1, 115–118.

[28] Camargo Z, Medina V, Rusilo LC, Gorinchteyn JC. Voice quality in Acquired Immunodeficiency Syndrome(AIDS): some perceptual and acoustic findings. Proceedings of 10thPan-European Voice Conference, 2013. Praga: Pan European Voice Association, 2013:1–371.

[29] Lima-Silva MF, Madureira S, Rusilo LC, Camargo Z. Perfil vocal de professores: análise integrada de dados de percepção e acústica. In: Camargo Z, editor. Fonética Clínica. São José dos Campos: Pulso, 2016:100–122.

[30] Pessoa A, Novaes BC, Pereira LC, Camargo Z. Dados de dinâmica e qualidade vocal: correlatos acústicos e perceptivo-auditivos da fala em criança usuária de implante coclear. J Speech Sci 2011;1:17–33.

[31] Pessoa A, Novaes BC, Madureira S, Camargo Z. Perceptual and acoustic correlates of a speech in a bilateral cochlear implant user. In: 6th International Conference on Speech Prosody, 2012, Shangai. Abstract Book Speech Prosody 2012. Shangai: Tongji University Press, 2012:1, 51–54.

[32] Gomes PC, Oliveira LR, Camargo Z. Respiração oral na infância: parâmetros perceptivo-auditivos e acústicos de qualidade vocal. In: Camargo Z, editor. Fonética Clínica. São José dos Campos: Pulso, 2016:86–94.

[33] Madureira S. The investigation of speech expressivity. In: Mello H, Panunzi A, Raso T, editors. Illocution, modality, attitude, information patterning and speech annotation. Firenze: Firenze University Press, 2011:1, 101–118.

[34] Madureira S, Fontes MAS, Fonseca BC. Voice quality and speaking styles. Dialectologia 2016;VI(Special Issue):171–90, 2016.

[35] Laver J, Mackenzie-Beck J. Vocal profile analysis scheme – VPAS. Edinburgh: Queen Margareth University College- QMUC, Speech Science Research Centre, 2007.

[36] Menegon [UIP], Madureira S. Metáforas no ensino do canto e seus efeitos na qualidade vocal: um estudo acústico-perceptivo. In: Madureira S, editor. Sonoridades – Sonorities. São Paulo: Publicação da Pontifícia Universidade Católica de São Paulo, 2016:1, 62–89.

[37] Madureira S. Portuguese rhotics in poem reciting: perceptual, acoustic, and meaning-related issues. In: Gibson M, Gil J, editors. Romance phonetics and phonology. Oxford: Oxford University Press, In the press.

Hemant A. Patil and Tanvina B. Patel

4 Analysis of normal and pathological voices by novel chaotic titration method

Abstract: In most of the current approaches that distinguish between normal and pathological voices, the presence of chaos in the speech production mechanism has been exploited. The goal of the present work is to investigate the potential of a novel chaotic titration-based approach to detect and quantify the amount of chaos that exists in the speech signal. The method determines chaos in the speech signal by titrating the speech signal with noise, which is similar to titrating acid with a base in the chemical titration process. In this chapter, a method based on linear (LP) and nonlinear prediction (NLP) of the speech signal (by the use of Volterra–Wiener (VW) series) is presented. This series works as an indicator during the titration process (such as pH-scale indicator). The amount of chaos measured is related to the noise that is added to titrate the speech signal. This noise value that titrates the speech is known as the noise limit (NL). It is also shown that NLP is better than LP because in NLP, the manner in which the previous samples are combined is also taken into consideration. The experimental results obtained from the NL values for the two classes convey a significant amount of relevant information in terms of the chaotic behavior of the speech, leading to cues for being able to separate normal from pathological voices.

Keywords: novel chaotic titration, vocal folds, speech signals, pathological voices, synthetic speech, noise limit

4.1 Introduction

The speech production system is modeled as a linear system. Linear prediction (LP) analysis has proven to be very effective in speech analysis and speech synthesis applications. Extensive work has been carried out on LP analysis of speech [1, 2]. The LP analysis has an ability to capture implicitly the frequency response of the time-varying vocal tract area function. The assumption in the LP model is that the frequency response of the vocal tract consists of only poles (i.e., all-pole model).

Note: Tanvina B. Patel is now with Cogknit Semantics Pvt Ltd Bangalore, India. The work was done while at DA-IICT Gandhinagar, India, and it does not contain any Cogknit Semantics Pvt Ltd proprietary information.

https://doi.org/10.1515/9781501502415-005

However, such a model is not sufficient to analyze nasal and fricatives sounds. Furthermore, Teagers [3, 4] observed the presence of separated airflow within the vocal tract and the vortices interact with the cavity, forming distributed sources due to a nonlinear exchange of kinetic energy. The nonlinear analysis of the speech signal is also extensively done in [5]. In many applications, LP forms the basis of the source-filter model where the filter is constrained to be an all-pole linear filter. In realistic scenarios, the speech production system has some nonlinearity. The non-linearity exists due to the fact that the human speech produced is the result of a nonlinear system that is excited by the glottal flow waveform. In addition, non-linearity would be present in the coupling (or interaction) of source and system component. The first formant (and higher formants to a certain extent [6]) of the vocal tract system is known to interact nonlinearly with the glottal flow waveform; resulting in sudden drop of acoustic pressure at the lips during the opening phase of the glottis [7]. The vocal fold collision, nonlinear pressure present in the glottis, the nonlinear stress, and strain patterns of the tissues, delayed feedback of the mucosal wave, the turbulence, and the sub-glottal pressure at the glottis; all contributed collectively to the nonlinearity in the speech signal.

In case of abnormal voice (especially those related to the laryngeal pathologies), the nonlinearity present in the speech-production mechanism plays a vital role. Research has been carried out extensively for the development of non-invasive tools for the classification task and to form automated systems to assess voice disorder. These approaches are less expensive and are a convenient solution to the problem of vocal fold disorder analysis and diagnosis. Research has also been directed towards improving the voice therapy effectiveness for various pathologies [8]. The manner of opening and closing of the vocal folds plays a very crucial role to distinguish the natural and pathological classes. The presence of vocal fold pathology can cause significant changes in the vibration patterns of vocal folds. Therefore, it has a significant impact on the resulting quality of speech that is produced. The voice quality depends on the extent and the level of glottal opening or closing. Certain laryngeal pathologies do not allow the vocal folds to close completely during the phenomena of glottal vibration. Following are a few reasons that may lead to incomplete glottal closure [9]:
– Paralysis or injury to either one or both the vocal folds,
– Asymmetry in the vocal folds due to irregular growths,
– Swelling of the vocal folds,
– Difference in muscle tension or length of the vocal folds

Mostly, all pathologies related with the larynx prevent the vocal fold from closing completely during the process of glottal vibration. A few cases of the vocal fold disorder that exists are listed as follows [10],

a) *Nodules*: These are growths developed on or around the vocal folds mainly due to inappropriate use or overuse of vocal apparatus.

b) *Polyps*: These are benign lesions that generally develop on the edge of the vocal folds. They avoid the folds to join at the middle where they meet.

c) *Incompetent larynx*: These include damaged vocal folds movement, that is, it is a condition where either one of the folds or both do not move as required, for example, bilateral or unilateral paralysis.

d) *Laryngeal dysfunction*: It is also known as the spasmodic dysphonia (SD) and occurs due to unstructured and impulsive movements of either one or many muscles in the larynx. There are in turn two types of SD: adductor SD (ASD) and abductor SD (ABSD). ASD have spams which cause sporadic vocal fold closures, resulting in a stressed or choked voice. On the other hand, ABSD has spasms that cause sticky closing of vocal folds and creates sound with disruptions of air.

e) *Presbylaryngis*: It is mainly caused by thinning of the vocal fold muscle and tissues with aging. The folds become thin and less fleshy than a regular larynx due to which midline closure does not occur properly.

f) *Functional disorders:* It includes muscle tension disorders that squeezes the vocal folds and prevents air from moving through the folds, dysphonia plica ventricularis caused by phonation of the ventricular folds, resulting in harsh voice and paradoxical vocal fold dysfunction that occurs due to vocal folds coming close to each other during inspiration.

Figure 4.1(a) and 4.1(b, c) show the normal and pathological vocal folds, respectively. It can be seen that normal vocal folds are smooth with no irregular structure on the surface of the vocal folds. In case of the paralyzed vocal fold (as indicated by an arrow in Figure 4.1(b, c)), the inability of one of vocal folds to move prevents smooth closure of the vocal folds during vibration. There are some techniques available in the medical field for detecting the pathologies. However, these methods require direct inspection of the vocal folds (e.g. laryngoscopy, videoscopy, etc.) due to which the cost and time of diagnosis using such clinical assessment tools increases.

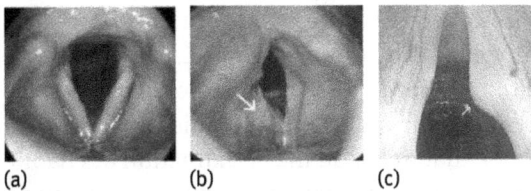

(a)   (b)   (c)

Figure 4.1: Views of the vocal folds: (a) normal vocal fold (b) pathological vocal fold of type paralysis and (c) pathological vocal folds of type cyst. Adopted from [11] and [12].

In case of normal larynx, the glottal flow velocity that forms the source to the system (comprising of the vocal tract and other associated regions) is formed by uniform opening and closing activity of the vocal folds. In case of the pathological vocal folds, the closure of the vocal folds is not always complete. There are regions in the closed phase through which the air passes. The airflow that passes through the vocal folds is different each time the folds close. As a result, *randomness* exists in the pathological voice signals. As chaos in a system is the sensitivity of the system to its initial condition, chaos is expected to be more in pathological voice signals due to more random behavior of the glottal flow waveform. It should be noted that chaos is measurable, however, randomness is not. A nonlinear analysis of time series is, therefore, essential to discriminate between the normal and pathological voices.

Methods of screening laryngeal pathologies [13] included period variability index (PVI), harmonic-to-noise ratio (HNR), stability of pitch generation (STAB), ratio of energy present in the cepstral pitch impulse to that of the total cepstral energy (PECM), etc. In [14] study has been made on clinical values of acoustic jitter, shimmer, and HNR for individuals with and without voice disorders. The disadvantage of these perturbation and noise measures is that they can be applied reliably to only nearly periodic signals or voices as described in the classification by Titze et al. [15], since they require accurate determination of pitch period, which is difficult in case of severely pathological voices. Pathological classification also involves work based on the estimation of acoustic parameters, namely, amplitude and frequency parameters [16], correlation-based features [17], and Mel-frequency cepstral coefficients (MFCC) [18]. However, the nonlinearity in the speech production mechanism cannot be characterized by these methods alone.

The normal voice is known to exhibit periodic and more regular waveform. On the other hand, the pathological voices are found to have a noise-like spectrum with a wider frequency band [19]. The use of entropy-based features is shown in [20–22]. The nonlinear analysis is mainly carried out using two statistics, namely, the largest LE (LLE) and correlation dimension (CD) [20, 22]. The behavior of the trajectories in the state-space plots [22] and the estimation of LE to know the rate of divergence of the trajectories have been very effective in analysis of the two classes [23, 24]. The CD is calculated by the Grassberger Procaccia algorithm (GPA) [25]; however, it has been shown that the Taken's estimator is more computationally efficient [26]. In case of LE, the analysis is based on the fact that with at least one positive LE, the system is said to be chaotic. So far, the application of nonlinear chaotic techniques in speech signal processing is based on either chaotic modeling or extraction of chaotic characteristics. In fact, chaos theory (i.e., the study of behavior of dynamical systems that are highly sensitive to the initial conditions) has been adopted as the new nonlinear approach in the area of speech signal processing [27].

In estimating the sensitive dependence of the system to its initial conditions, the LE is known to be the state-of-the-art approach [5]. The algorithm for calculating LE from a time series was first proposed by [28]. Amongst the many methods to estimate LE, the approach presented by Rosentein et al. [29] and Giovanni et al. [30] is mainly used. In [22], the authors used LLE to differentiate between normal and pathological voices. It was observed that for both the cases, the LLE values were positive, indicating the presence of chaos in both the normal and abnormal speech. Although the LLE and CD showed discrimination properties, such derived nonlinear statistics require the dynamics of speech to be purely deterministic. This assumption is inadequate since randomness due to *time-varying* pressure and turbulence is a natural process in the speech production. In addition, another drawback of using the nonlinear dynamic methods for classification was that they require the time series to be stationary and long, which may not always be the case for the natural speech signal. These parameters can be easily contaminated by noise and hence, other techniques are used for modeling and detecting the system's chaotic behavior [31].

The present work is an extended version of the work carried out in [32], with an attempt to perform nonlinear prediction (NLP) of the speech signals rather than the linear prediction (LP). Attempt to model nonlinearities (and nonlinear dependencies) in speech signal was reported by Thyssen *et. al.* [33] in the framework of speech coding. The work proposed two methods for NLP, namely, second-order Volterra filter and a time-delay neural network. The limitation of this study was that the predictor was applied twice (first for LP model and second for NLP model) [34, 35]. There are attempts to model the global behavior of Volterra–Wiener (VW) series using artificial neural networks [36–38]. The approach in [36] improves an important limitation of computational complexity associated with calculation of Volterra kernel using back propagation training of higher order nonlinear models in the three-layered perceptrons (TLP). However, the approaches do not explain how to compute the Volterra kernels. To address this, an application was presented in [39] to model the nonlinear characteristics of electronic devices. Thereafter, in [40], the instability of VW series NLP filter used for speech coding was studied and then a scheme was proposed that detects those frames for which, after stabilization, including the quadratic predictor is beneficial. Recently, a novel application of Volterra series was presented to analyze the multilayered perceptron (MLP) to estimate the posterior probability of phoneme for automatic speech recognition (ASR) task [41]. In the same study, Volterra kernels are used to capture *spectro-temporal* patterns that are learned from the Mel filterbank log-energies (during training of the system for each phoneme).

Here, we are interested to analyze the normal and pathological voices by estimating the amount of nonlinearity, that is, the chaos in the speech signal through a novel chaotic titration method. The method of chaotic titration is used to estimate or quantify the chaos in the speech signal that exists because of the non-uniform closing of the folds. Further experiments have been carried out to reveal the effectiveness of NLP and variation in the predictor coefficient values estimated by LP and NLP. This work analyzes the LP and NLP coefficients (with respect to their ability to predict samples of speech signal). A fast orthogonal search algorithm [42] is used to determine the nonlinear system coefficients from the VW series. The concept lies in knowing the amount of chaos in the speech by neutralizing the chaos present in the signal via deliberately adding noise in the speech signal [43]. The amount of noise added will give a measure of the chaos in the speech signal. In [44], it has been proved that the noise limit (NL) values give a better reliable estimation about the nonlinear characteristics present in the speech than the other chaos detection methods (such as LE). Several pathological samples are experimented here to study the chaotic nature of pathological voices. The pathological voices (publically available at [10]) are of the following type, namely, abductor SD (ABSD), adductor SD (ASD), muscle tension, dysphonia plica ventricularis (DPV), paradoxial vocalfold dysfunction (PVD), unilateral/bilateral paralysis and presbylaryngis. A vowel\a\extracted from the rainbow passage has been used for analysis purpose. In [23, 24], an analysis of various chaotic-based measures such as phase plane plots, estimating the Lyapunov exponent from the trajectory set along with computation of the Shannon entropy and the permutation entropy, has been carried on these pathological samples. The significance of the work lies in the non-invasive approach to analyze and the feasibility to work with low-cost computation machines.

The rest of the chapter is organized as follows. Section 4.2 discusses the proposed chaotic titration method in detail. This section presents the detailed methodology of LP and NLP. The method of chaotic titration is explained to estimate the chaos in the speech signal. Section 4.3 studies the effectiveness of NLP over the LP. The decrease in the NLP error is highlighted. Experiments conducted on both the normal and pathological speech signals are presented and the results are discussed in detail. Finally, Section 4.4 draws the conclusions and limitations of this study and the future research directions.

4.2 Chaotic titration method

This method was an outcome of the research carried out by Dr Chi-Sang Poon, principal research scientist in the Harvard-MIT Division of Health Sciences and

Technology (HST). Poon and Barahona [44] demonstrated the use of chaotic titration as a technique to quantify the amount of chaos in the signal. In the earlier studies, Poon and Merill [45] discovered that heart disease actually makes the heart beat less chaotic. They proposed the use of analytical methods in nonlinear dynamics to analyze, detect and diagnose congestive heart failure (CHF). These techniques contribute to Poon and Barahona's latest findings, which explain that the intensity of chaos can be measured by titration strength against added noise [44]. As an analysis technique used in chemistry, the titration process determines a reaction's endpoint. Titration also estimates the precise amount or measure of an unknown reagent used in chemical reactions to observe, detect, quantify or produce other substances. Titration is carried out using a standard concentration of a known reagent that reacts with another unknown reagent. Generally, noise is considered as an unwanted signal; however, in this case, it is referred to the random fluctuations present in the signal patterns. Although noise is not a chemical reagent, however, in Poon's work noise is used as a reagent to achieve numerical titration. According to the work in [44], measuring titration strength against added noise is analogous to measuring the strength of an acid by how well it can be titrated against a strong alkaline. The research proves this 'litmus test' analogy and confirms the earlier work that the decrease of heart rate variability in patients with CHF is due to a decrease in the cardiac chaos. It was believed that the numerical titration approach can be applicable to problems in almost any domain, that is, physical, biomedical and socioeconomic systems as well. This may include the identification and control of cardiac arrhythmia, epileptic seizures or other biomedical variables, analysis and forecasting of geological, astrophysical or economic data and also unmasking of chaotically encrypted communication signals [44]. Hence, this work attempts to apply the novel chaotic titration method for the analysis and classification of normal and pathological voices.

4.2.1 Analogy of chemical titration with the chaotic titration

The chaotic titration approach is equivalent to the chemical titration method (i.e., acid-base concept). It is based on the concept of addition of noise to the signal till the noise *neutralizes* the chaos in the signal. To that effect, to estimate the amount of chaos in the signal, noise (with increasing standard deviation (sd)) is added till the chaos present in the signal is neutralized by the added noise. In case of the acid-base titration process, the neutral-level is indicated by the pH indicator scale, that is, if the value of the pH scale is 7 then the solution is considered neutral. In chemical titration process to determine whether the neutral-level is reached, the litmus test is also performed. It is well known that when the blue litmus paper turns red, the solution is acidic and if the red litmus turns blue then the solution is basic. However, if the litmus paper does not show any color change then the solution is neutral. Thus, in case of the chemical titration process, the color change of the litmus paper or the value of the pH scale indicates the neutrality of the solution.

Figure 4.2 shows the chemical titration process analogy with that of the chemical titration process. For example, the acidic nature of the solution can be compared to the amount of chaos in the signal and the noise is compared to an alkaline solution. Just as an acidic solution is neutralized by adding an alkaline solution, to neutralize a chaotic signal, noise is added to it. If a signal is more chaotic then more amount of noise (i.e., noise of more standard deviation) is added to the signal to neutralize the effect of chaos in the signal. The amount of noise is determined by its standard deviation. The value of sd at which the indicator will detect a neutral-level is called the NL. However, the question arises that in case of the chaotic titration process how the neutrality test should be performed? Or as to how the indication of chaotic condition is done? The answer to this is to use the VW series [43]. The VW series serves as an indicator to the chaotic titration process. Thus, it is very important and interesting to know as to how the neutrality is estimated in the chaotic titration. The identification method is described in the next sub-sections.

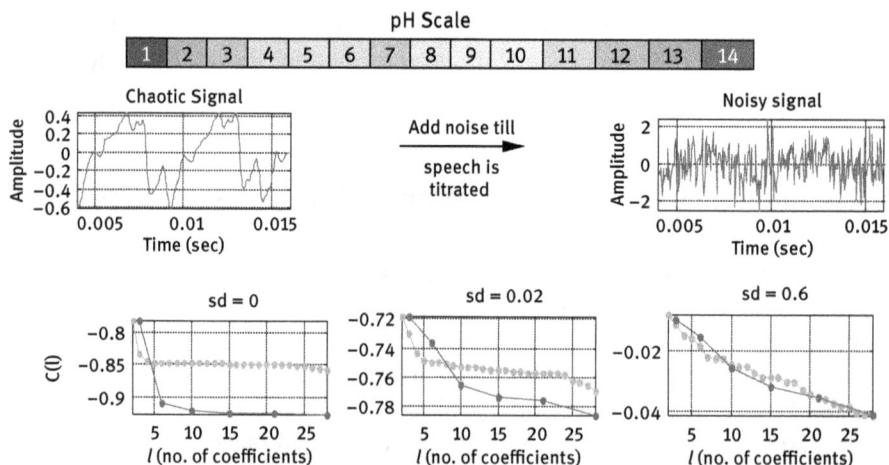

Figure 4.2: Analogy of the chaotic titration process to that of the chemical titration process.

4.2.2 Analogy of pH-scale indicator in chemical titration to the Volterra–Wiener (VW) indicator in the chaotic titration

Fréchet showed that the set of Volterra functionals is *complete* (i.e., every Cauchy sequence converges to a limit point that belongs to the same function space) [46]. Fréchet's theorem means that every continuous functional of a signal $x(t)$ can be approximated with some level of precision as a sum of a finite number of Volterra functions in $x(t)$. This result was again a generalization of the Weierstrass–Stone approximation theorem, that is, it states every continuous function of a variable x to be approximated with arbitrary precision as the sum of finite number of polynomials in x [47]. The VW nonlinear identification method detects chaos by comparing the one-step prediction error of linear model with that of a nonlinear model.

4.2.2.1 The Volterra–Wiener (VW) series

The numerical procedure for design of chaotic titration indicator is as mentioned in [43]. For a time series $y(n)$, (where, $n = 1, 2, 3, ..., N$), a discrete Volterra–Wiener–Korenberg (VWK) series of degree d and memory k is used as a model to estimate the predicted time series $\hat{y}(n)$ as follows:

$$
\begin{aligned}
\hat{y}(n) = {} & a_0 + a_1 y(n-1) + a_2 y(n-2) + a_k y(n-k) + ... \\
& + a_{k+1} y(n-1)^2 + a_{k+2} y(n-1) \times y(n-2) + ... \\
& + a_{M-1} y(n-k)^d = \sum_{m=0}^{M-1} a_m q_m(n),
\end{aligned}
\tag{4.1}
$$

where the functional basis $\{q_m(n)\}$ consists of all the distinct combinations of the *embedding* space coordinates $\{i.e., \ y(n-1), y(n-2), ...y(n-k)\}$ up to degree d, with a total dimension, $M = (k+d)!/(k!d!)$ [43]. Thus, each model is parameterized by d and k, which correspond the degree of nonlinearity and the embedding dimension in the model, respectively. The number of distinct combinations and the nature of combinations are indicated as follows. To estimate the number of combinations, sampling with replacement and without ordering is carried out. Therefore, the number of combinations are ^nC_r, where $n = k-1+d$ and $r = 1, 2, ...,$ d. Let us consider a series $x(n) = (5, 8, 7)$, then for $k = 3$ and $d = 2$, the possible distinct combinations are of $\{5,5\}, \{5,8\}, \{5,7\}, \{8,8\}, \{8,7\}, \{7,7\}$. Thus, the total number of combinations obtained is as follows:

$$
^nC_r = \binom{k-1+d}{d} = \binom{3-1+2}{2} = 6.
$$

Similarly, let us take another series as $x(n) = (1, 6, 3, 9)$, where $k = 4$ and that we assume a degree $d = 3$ polynomial, as the combinations are {1,1,1}, {1,1,6}, {1,1,3}, {1,1,9}, {1,6,6}, {1,6,3}, {1,6,9}, {1,3,3}, {1,3,9}, {1,9,9}, {6,6,6}, {6,6,3}, {6,6,9}, {6,3,3}, {6,3,9}, {6,9,9}, {3,3,3}, {3,3,9}, {3,9,9}, {9,9,9}. Then, the total number of combinations is as follows:

$$^nC_r = \binom{4 - 1 + 3}{3} = 20.$$

Next, the coefficients a_m in the VWK series are estimated by a Gram–Schmidt procedure from linear and nonlinear autocorrelations of the data series [48]. The method of coefficient estimation is described in the next sub-section.

4.2.2.2 Korenberg's fast orthogonal search method

To estimate the coefficients of the VW series, the Korenberg's fast orthogonal search algorithm [42] is used. The method implemented here relies on an orthogonal approach that does not need precise creation of orthogonal functions. The advantage lies in the speed of estimating the coefficients of a nonlinear equation and also the storage requirements are diminished [42]. Consider a second-order finite memory discrete-time Volterra series, that is,

$$y(n) = h_0 + \underbrace{\sum_{i=0}^{R-1} h(i)x(n-i)}_{\text{Linear terms}} + \underbrace{\sum_{i_1=0}^{R-1}\sum_{i_2=0}^{R-1} h(i_1, i_2)x(n-i_1)x(n-i_2)}_{\text{Nonlinear terms}}. \tag{4.2}$$

where, h_0, $h(i)$, $h(i_1, i_2)$ corresponds to the zero-order, first-order and second-order coefficients of a system with input $x(n)$ and output $y(n)$, respectively, and R corresponds to the memory terms. For higher order Volterra series, same algorithm can be applied. The orthogonal technique permits a wide variety of input excitation. The earlier technique used Gram–Schmidt orthogonalization procedure to create a series of orthogonal functions as an intermediate step. The variant [49] of orthogonal estimation used in the current Korenberg's algorithm is associated to an orthogonal technique that identifies the difference equation and functional expansion models by orthogonalizing over the actual data record [42, 50]. The orthogonal search method used over here does not create orthogonal function at any point of the identification process. To understand the orthogonal estimation, let us first consider the earlier techniques in [42, 50]. Let $x(n)$ be an input (where $n = 0$ to $n = N$). The output $y(n)$, that is obtained when the input $x(n)$ passes through a system having coefficients, a_m, is given by,

$$y(n) = \sum_{m=0}^{M} a_m p_m(n),$$ (4.3)

where M is the total number of coefficients, a_m in equation (4.3) corresponds to the kernels $h_0, h(i), h(i_1, i_2)$ in equation (4.2). The $p_m(n)$s are distinct terms of 1, $x(n - i_1)$, $x(n - i_2)$, $x(n - i_1)x(n - i_2)$, where $i_1, i_2 = 0, ..., R - 1$. For $n = 0$ to $n = N$, setting $p_0(n) = 1$, and $p_m(n) = x(n - m + 1)$, gives the x terms, where $m = 1, 2, ..., R$. Similarly, the xx terms can also be generated for combinations of the samples. The algorithm then uses Gram-Schmidt orthogonalization process to create an orthogonal function $w_m(n)$ as a function of $p_m(n)$ as described below. For $n = 0, 1, ..., N$, set $w_0(n) = 1$ and for $m = 1, 2, ...M$,

$$w_m(n) = p_m(n) - \sum_{r=0}^{m-1} \alpha_{mr} w_r(n),$$ (4.4)

where

$$\alpha_{mr} = \frac{\overline{p_m(n)w_r(n)}}{\overline{w^2_r(n)}}, \ r = 0, ..., m - 1.$$ (4.5)

In equation (4.5), the bar denotes the time-average taken from $n = 0$ to $n = N$, that is,

$$\overline{p_m(n)w_r(n)} = \frac{1}{N+1}\sum_{n=0}^{N} p_m(n)w_r(n).$$ (4.6)

Therefore, orthogonal series is,

$$y(n) = \sum_{m=0}^{M} g_m w_m(n),$$ (4.7)

where

$$g_m = \frac{\overline{y(n)w_m(n)}}{\overline{w^2_m(n)}}.$$ (4.8)

Now the a_m in equation (4.3) can be obtained by,

$$a_m = \sum_{i=m}^{M} g_i v_i, \qquad (4.9)$$

$$\text{where } v_m = 1 \text{ and } v_i = -\sum_{r=m}^{i-1} \alpha_{ir} v_r, \quad i = m+1, \dots, M. \qquad (4.10)$$

From (4.10), it is clear that a_ms can be readily obtained once α_{ir} and g_i are known. Both of them can be known using equations (4.5) and (4.8) if certain time-averages involving $w_m(n)$ are available. It does not imply that the $w_m(n)$ need to be created themselves and this is the reason of more efficiency in the algorithm proposed by Korenberg. Thus, to obtain the numerator in equation (4.5) note that for $m = 2, \dots, M$ and for $r = 1, \dots, m-1$, that is,

$$\overline{p_m(n)w_r(n)} = \overline{p_m(n)p_r(n)} - \sum_{i=0}^{r-1} \alpha_{ri} \overline{p_m(n)w_i(n)}. \qquad (4.11)$$

If we define,

$$D(m, r) = \overline{p_m(n)w_i(n)}, \qquad m = 1, \dots, M \qquad r = 0, \dots, m-1, \qquad (4.12)$$

and

$$D(m, 0) = \overline{p_m(n)}, \qquad m = 1, \dots, M \qquad (4.13)$$

because $w_0(n) = 1$. Therefore, from equations (4.11) and (4.12), we get,

$$D(m, r) = \overline{p_m(n)p_r(n)} - \sum_{i=0}^{r-1} \alpha_{ri} D(m, i), \qquad (4.14)$$

for $m = 2, \dots, M$ and $r = 1, \dots, m-1$. Now, to obtain the denominator term in equation (4.5), for $m = 0, \dots, M$,

$$\overline{w^2_m(n)} = \overline{p^2_m(n)} - \sum_{r=0}^{m-1} \alpha^2_{mr} \overline{w^2_r(n)}. \qquad (4.15)$$

Equation (4.15) follows from equations (4.4) and (4.5). Now let us define,

$$E(m) = \overline{w^2(n)}, \qquad m = 0, \dots, M \qquad (4.16)$$

Therefore, from equations (4.14) and (4.15) and as $E(0) = 1$ implies,

$$E(m) = \overline{p^2{}_m(n)} = -\sum_{r=0}^{m-1} \alpha^2{}_{mr} E(r). \tag{4.17}$$

If we know the time-averages $\overline{p_m(n)p_r(n)}$ as from equation (4.6) and α_{mr} then $E(m)$ can be calculated from equations (4.16) and (4.17). Moreover, from equation (4.5), it follows that for $m = 1, \ldots, M$ and $r = 1, \ldots, m-1$, that is,

$$\alpha_{mr} = D(m, r)/E(r). \tag{4.18}$$

From equation (4.18), many equivalent of $D(m, r)$ in equation (4.14) and $E(m)$ in equation (4.17) can be formed. For example,

$$D(m, r) = \overline{p_m(n)p_r(n)} - \sum_{i=0}^{r-1} \frac{D(r, i)D(m, i)}{E(i),} \quad m = 2, \ldots, M \quad r = 1, \ldots, m-1 \tag{4.19}$$

$$E(m) = \overline{p^2{}_m(n)} = -\sum_{r=0}^{m-1} \frac{D^2(m, r)}{E(r),} \quad m = 1, \ldots, M \tag{4.20}$$

To improve the speed and to save memory storage, the time-averages used in equations (4.13), (4.19) and (4.20) can be directly calculated from the mean and autocorrelations of input x [48]. Therefore, after computing α_{mr} and applying in equation (4.10), the coefficients a_ms can be estimated from equation (4.9). After computation the coefficients, the set of series obtained from equation (4.7) will be the predicted series $\hat{y}(n)$ by this fast algorithm. The coefficients obtained by this method are efficient only if the predicted series is more close to the original series $y(n)$ than the series predicted by any LP method. In other words, prediction power of nonlinear method is better than LP. This is illustrated in the next sub-section.

4.2.2.3 Efficiency of nonlinear prediction over linear prediction

Once the coefficients are computed for the LP and NLP, the prediction error can be calculated and the effectiveness of the NLP can be evaluated. The total prediction error is computed for both the predictions and is given by,

$$E = \sum_{n=-\infty}^{\infty} |e(n)|^2, \tag{4.21}$$

where $e(n) = y(n) - \hat{y}(n)$ in (4.21). To visualize the decrease in prediction error by NLP, a vowel \e\ is sampled at *16 kHz* and of size 200 samples is taken. The signal is predicted for different values of degree polynomial d. The number of memory terms required for the prediction are kept constant, that is, $k = 3$. At first, the signal is predicted by $d = 1$ and $k = 3$. The predicted error is calculated to be *0.0806* (Figure 4.3(a)). The same signal is then predicted by $d = 2$ and $k = 3$, the prediction

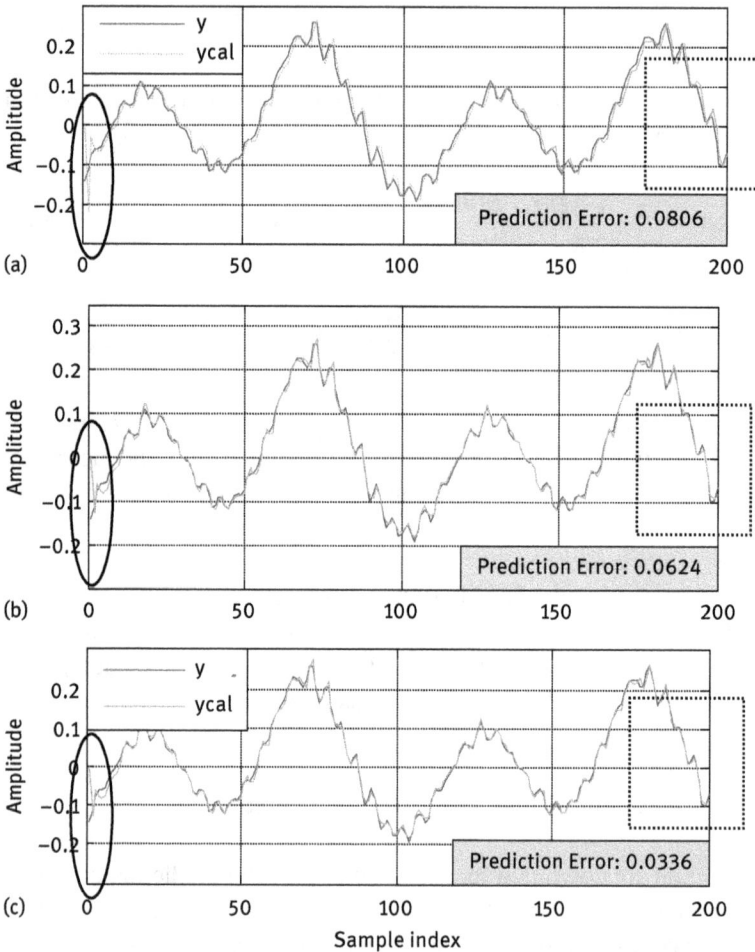

Figure 4.3: The difference between linear and nonlinear prediction by predicting a frame of vowel \e\ of duration 12.5 ms and having sampling frequency *16 kHz:* (a) a frame of vowel \e\ predicted by $k = 3$ and $d = 1$, (b) same frame (as shown in Figure 4.3(a)) of vowel \e\ predicted by $k = 3$ and $d = 2$, (c) same frame (as shown in Figure 4.3(a)) of vowel \e\ predicted by $k = 3$ and $d = 3$. In all the cases, y is the original signal (dark shade curve) and ycal= $\hat{y}(n)$ is the predicted signal (light shade curve).

error decreases to *0.0624* (Figure 4.3(b)). Continuing for $d = 3$ and $k=3$, it can be seen (Figure 4.3(c)) that the prediction error is *0.0336*, which is approximately *58%* less than that of LP [24].

A major difference of LP and NLP by the Korenberg's method lies in the value of initial coefficient, that is, the term a_0. In LP using the autocorrelation method, the value of a_0 is one (i.e., $a_0 = 1$), however, in case of the present method, it is not always so. This eliminates the initial error in the signal. That is, the initial coefficient in NLP is not always *1* (which makes the predicted sample close to that of the actual speech signal), due to which the residual error is less in NLP.

As seen in the Figure 4.3(a) for LP, the manually marked oval region shows that the prediction is not appropriate at the start of the signal (this may be due to poor prediction of samples due to less number of available samples for prediction). The error accumulated at the start is then carried forward in the estimation of the next samples and as a result of which the next samples are not predicted as accurately as the samples predicted with higher degree polynomial d (i.e., the NLP). The other regions in Figure 4.3 (as indicated by manually marked squares) show the improvement in NLP. Therefore, from the above example, it can be seen that the prediction error decreases considerably for NLP without any increase in the memory terms required for the NLP. Therefore, the analysis and prediction done by the NLP method will be relatively more efficient.

Also in [51], the authors have shown that L^1 and L^2 norms of the NLP residual are less as compared to that of the LP residual. This was shown using a LP model ($d = 1, k = 12$) and NLP model ($d = 2, k = 12$) for five instances of voiced segment /aa/ and the unvoiced segment /s/ from *100* speakers. The lesser value of norms of NLP residual indicated that the NLP performed better prediction of the voiced and the unvoiced segments. This was further justified with the help of lower perceptual evaluation of speech quality (PESQ) score of the NLP residual than the LP residual. This relation was also shown using the spectrum of the LP and NLP residuals. The spectrum of the NLP residual was relatively more flat than the LP residual spectrum. Similar analysis was made in [52, 53] showing that the NLP residual has less energy than the LP residual and the peaks around the glottal closure instants (GCI) were less by NLP than LP. This may be due to the fact that the short-term dependencies in the speech signal are captured more effectively via NLP approach and therefore, the intelligibility of the NLP residual is less than the intelligibility of the LP residual. Therefore, the NLP residual capture the higher order statistical relation and the hidden nonlinear dependencies in the sequence of samples of the speech signal.

4.2.2.4 Titration by noise and noise limit (NL) estimation

Barahona and Poon [43] illustrated the use of the short-term prediction to carry out the process of estimating the linear and nonlinear models. In this section, the short-term prediction power of a model is measured by the standard deviation of one-step-ahead prediction error. The use of VW series to estimate or quantify the amount of chaos present in a speech signal is demonstrated here after. The short-term prediction power of a model is measured as follows:

$$\varepsilon^2(k, d) \equiv \frac{\sum\limits_{n=1}^{N} (y_n^{calc}(k, d) - y(n))^2}{\sum_{n=1}^{N} (y(n) - \bar{y})^2}, \tag{4.22}$$

where $y_n^{calc} = \hat{y}(n)$, $\bar{y} = \frac{1}{N} \sum\limits_{n=1}^{N} y_n$ and $\varepsilon^2(k, d)$ are the normalized variances of the prediction error residuals. Next, for each data series, one searches for the optimal model $\{k_{opt}, d_{opt}\}$ that minimizes the following information criterion according to the parsimony principle [54]:

$$C(r) = \log \varepsilon(r) + r/N, \tag{4.23}$$

where for a certain pair $\{k, d\}$, $r \in [1, M]$ is the number of polynomial terms of the truncated Volterra series expansions. Next, the numerical procedure of prediction is carried out as follows. For each of the data series, the best *linear* model is estimated by searching for k^{lin} that minimizes $C(r)$ with $d = 1$. This is repeated with increasing k and $d > 1$, to obtain the best *nonlinear model*. The result is two competing models with standard deviations ε^{lin} (for LP) and ε^{non} (for NLP). The values of r plotted against that of $C(r)$ for NLP and LP will give a $r - C(r)$ curve. Subsequently, to detect the chaos present in the speech signal, it is essential to estimate the NL. The estimated NL indicates as to when the information obtained from the LP and NLP coefficients is almost similar. The indication that the chaos in the speech signal is *neutralized* by the added noise is when the curves of nonlinear and linear $C(r)$ values, (obtained from equations (4.22) and (4.23)) are sufficiently close to each other. That is, the prediction by the linear and nonlinear methods is almost the same (i.e., the chaos present due to nonlinearity in speech production mechanism is nullified by the titration process). The method to obtain this neutral-level is indicated in the next sub-section.

After obtaining the $r - C(r)$ curve, the next step is to obtain the amount of chaos in the system. This is carried out by adding noise (of increasing standard deviation) to the speech signal until a neutral-level is acquired. The neutral-level in this case is achieved when the information obtained by NLP coefficients is same as the information obtained by LP coefficients. As it has been stated that the VW series had been used as an indicator, the indication will be performed when the noise added neutralizes the chaos in the signal, that is, when the $C(r)$ values for NLP and LP techniques are sufficiently close to each other. Therefore, to obtain the neutral value and the corresponding NL at the neutral-level, we add noise of increasing standard deviation (σ) to the speech signal. Each time noise (of increasing standard deviation) is added, both LP and NLP are done and the $r - C(r)$ curve is estimated again to check whether neutral-level is obtained or not. If the differences in nonlinear and linear error values are still large, more noise (i.e., large standard deviation) is again added to the speech signal. The noise of increasing standard deviation (σ) is continuously added till the difference between the $C(r)$ values of LP and NLP is nearly zero (this level is understood as the neutral-level). The value of standard deviation of the noise added when the neutral-level is reached is known as the *NL*, that is, NL = σ. This NL value is represented as the 'noise ceiling' of the speech signal and it corresponds to the amount of chaos. Under the chaotic titration scheme, NL > 0 indicates the presence of chaos, conversely, NL = 0 indicates that the data series is either not chaotic or the chaotic component is already neutralized by the background noise in the original data series. Therefore, the condition NL > 0 is a sufficient test for *chaoticity*. For a speech segment, NL is found frame-by-frame and the final NL *versus* time plot is used to see the amount of chaos in the signal. The complete process of the chaotic titration on the speech signal (carried out frame-by-frame) can be summarized as in Table 4.1.

Poon and Barahona [44] validated the chaotic titration method by a bifurcation diagram of the logistic map to obtain a relation between the largest LE and the NL values obtained from chaotic titration method. They found that there exists a close correlation between the largest LE and NL values. They observed that, over the full bifurcation range, wherever NL had values greater than zero, at the same instant the largest LE also had positive values (i.e., LLE>0). On the other hand, the negative values of LLE mapped to zero NL values. In addition to obtaining a simple and conclusive test for chaos in short and noisy time series, the titration method uses noise itself as a titrant for chaos, as a result of which the NL test is basically robust to the measurement noise. Due to such reliability, the estimation of NL is convenient to determine the chaos in the speech signal. Therefore, in the present work, we use the titration method to determine the chaos in the pathological and normal speech signals for analysis purpose.

Table 4.1: Steps for implementation of the chaotic titration process.

Step 1.	For a frame of speech signal, determine a linear model, that is, for $d = 1$ (find the coefficients of linear predictor).
Step 2.	For the same frame in step 1, determine a nonlinear model, that is, for $d>1$ (find the coefficients of nonlinear predictor).
Step 3.	Plot the $r - C(r)$ curve for both the linear and the nonlinear prediction models, without adding any noise.
Step 4.	Now add noise of certain standard deviation to the speech frame and again obtain the $r - C(r)$ plot.
Step 5.	Repeat the above procedure by adding noise of increasing standard deviation (i.e., σ).
Step 6.	Observe that at a certain standard deviation value, the nonlinearity will not be detected by the indicator and the $r - C(r)$ plots for linear and nonlinear prediction models might overlap with each other (i.e., the given speech frame is titrated).
Step 7.	Note the value of standard deviation at which the indicator does not quantify further the nonlinearity, this standard deviation value is called the noise limit (i.e., NL).
Step 8.	Then, move the window with a shift interval a few points (it may range from *1* to *35* sample shift) and titrate the speech data in the next frame again, till NL is obtained. Estimate NL for the entire utterance.
Step 9.	Plot the curve of NL *vs.* time. Observe that, the more chaotic the signal is, more should be its noise limit.

4.3 Experiments results and discussions

The experiments are performed here on a set of two normal voice signals (one male and one female) along with six pathological voices (i.e., ABSD, muscle tension, DPV, PVD, Bilateral Paralysis and Presbylaryngis). Here, muscle tension and DPV are from male speakers while the remaining pathological samples are from female speakers. For all the experiments, the speech signals are sampled at *25 kHz* and are of *40* ms duration. Before estimating the NL values for the speech signals, the efficiency in NLP for the set of voices is shown in Table 4.2. For a fixed value of predictor memory terms, that is, $k = 6$ and by varying the value of the polynomial degree d, the prediction error of the speech signals are estimated [24].

It can be seen from Table 4.2 that even if the predictor memory term is kept constant, by increasing the polynomial degree d, sufficient reduction in the prediction error can be obtained. Therefore, in NLP (i.e., for $d>1$), the prediction error is less because the number of coefficients value $M = (k + d)!/(k!d!)$ required for predicting the signal will increase with the increase in the degree of the polynomial d. This result indicates that the NLP model best predicts the samples of speech signal than its linear counterpart.

Table 4.2: The residual prediction error for the normal and different pathological voice signals.

Voices	Prediction Error		
	d = 1	d = 2	d = 3
Normal Male	2.19×10^{-4}	1.54×10^{-4}	1.37×10^{-4}
Normal Female	3.92×10^{-2}	3.19×10^{-2}	2.91×10^{-2}
ABSD	0.1123	0.059	0.0566
Muscle Tension	0.0377	0.0358	0.0233
DPV	0.1025	0.0382	0.0375
PVD	0.8204	0.7861	0.6476
Bilateral Paralysis	0.4750	0.4127	0.2846
Presbylaryngis	0.1906	0.1592	0.1395

From the results of Table 4.2, it can be concluded that the prediction (residual) error is relatively very less (for both LP and NLP) for normal voice samples than the pathological speech samples. This may be due to the fact that the pathological voice samples are expected to be more chaotic and nonlinear than the normal signal and hence, will be difficult to predict, thereby resulting in large prediction error.

Figure 4.4 shows the predictor coefficients (i.e., a_ms in (equation 4.1)) obtained by LP for both normal (Figure 4.4(a)) and pathological voices (Figure 4.4(b)). The predictor memory terms, that is, $k = 6$, have been used here. In case of normal voices, the linearly predicted coefficients are more dependent on the initial values. After say five to six coefficients, the rest coefficients are nearly zero indicting that in case of normal voices the speech signal is more dependent on only few previous adjacent or nearby samples [24].

In case of pathological voices at least coefficient index till *20* are necessary for prediction. This means that for LP of pathological voices, more number of speech samples {i.e., $y(n-1), y(n-2), ..., y(n-k)$} are required, that is, the pathological voices are more difficult to predict than that of the normal voices by LP. As a result, if less predictor memory terms are used, then the prediction error will be more for pathological voices. The prediction coefficients estimated by NLP show that in case of both normal voices (Figure 4.5(a)) and pathological voices (Figure 4.5(b)), the coefficients of the terms formed by the combinations of samples (i.e., nonlinear terms in (equation 4.1)) are more effective than the coefficients formed without combinations (i.e., linear terms in (equation 4.1)). Therefore, the NLP is much more effective than that of LP.

The value of $\{a_m\}$ for LP as shown in Figure 4.4 is relatively much lower (almost by a factor of 200) as compared to the $\{a_m\}$ for the nonlinear model. In Figure 4.5(a) and 4.5(b), for $k = 6$ and $d = 2$, after coefficient value a_6 (corresponding to index 7 in

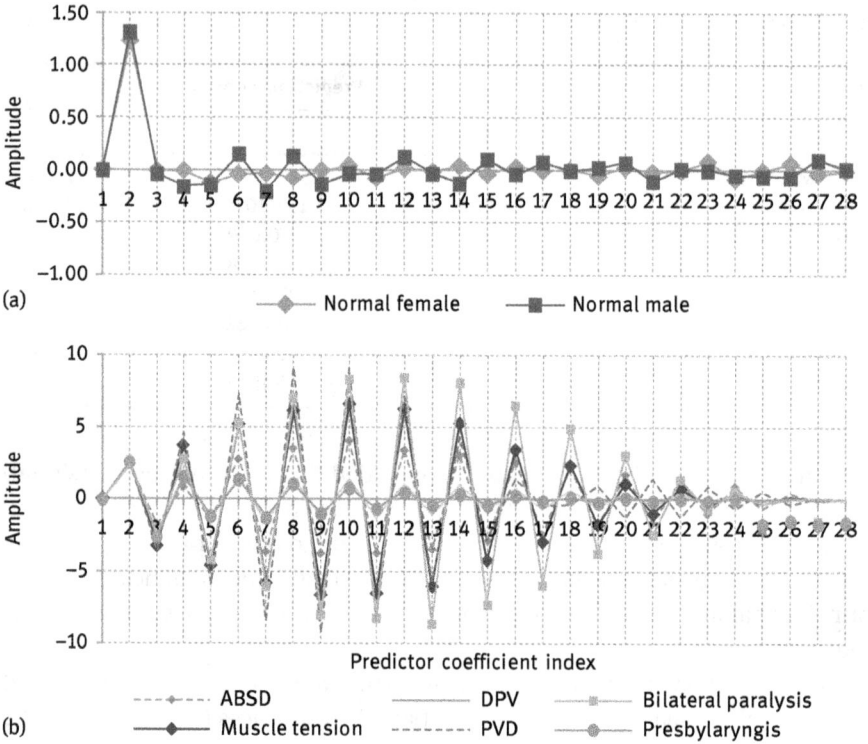

Figure 4.4: The coefficients obtained by linear prediction ($d = 1$). (a) Coefficients for normal voices and (b) coefficients for pathological voices.

the figure), there is a sudden jump in the values of $\{a_m\}$ for the remaining nonlinear portion of the model. This indicates that contribution towards accurate prediction is made by the nonlinear terms {i.e., $y(n-1)^2, y(n-1)y(n-2)$, $y(n-1)y(n-3), ..., y(n-2)^2, y(n-2)y(n-3), ..., y(n-3)^2, ..., y(n-6)^2$}.

This sudden increase in the value of coefficient is further shown in Figure 4.6 (as indicated by the arrows), where the speech signals is predicted ($d = 2$) for different value of predictor memory terms (i.e., $k = 4, k = 5, k = 7$). In all the cases, NLP coefficients are more dominant candidate for prediction than the LP coefficients. Thus, this finding indicates that for the speech signal, prediction of samples only by the linear model is not sufficient. Rather, it is the *manner* in which the previous speech samples are nonlinearly combined, will determine the accuracy of prediction model. These results vary for different pathologies due to the different severity as well as due the fact that the reason of pathology is different. It has been shown in [23, 24] that each of the pathologies discussed

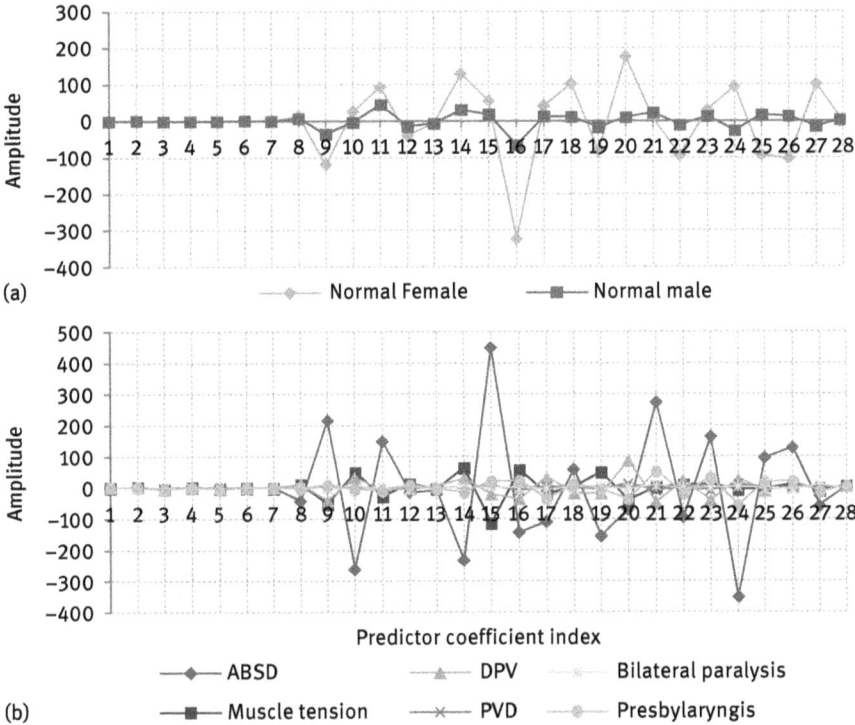

Figure 4.5: The coefficients obtained by nonlinear prediction ($d = 2$). (a) Coefficients for normal voices and (b) coefficients for pathological voices.

has different degrees of randomness (shown by state-space diagrams, entropy and LLE values) and hence, the parameters extracted from these pathological samples are different.

Thereafter, to estimate the chaos in the speech signal, we need to estimate the NL values for the speech signals. For the linear model, we take $d = 1$ and $k = 27$ and for the nonlinear model, the predictor memory terms $k = 6$ and $d = 2$ are taken. Both these values will give total number of coefficients $M = 28$. Figure 4.7 shows a frame of speech of a normal female voice (Figure 4.7(a)) and the corresponding $r - C(r)$ curve in Figure 4.7(b). Pathology of type of abductor SD is shown in Figure 4.7(c) and the $r - C(r)$ curves in Figure 4.7(d). The figures suggest that the difference between $r - C(r)$ curves obtained by NLP and LP is more in case of pathological voice as compared to that of the normal voice. Therefore, to neutralize the chaos in the speech signal, we add noise (of increasing standard deviation (sd)) to the speech signal till the two curves nearly close to each other. Therefore, the NL values will be more for the pathological voice as

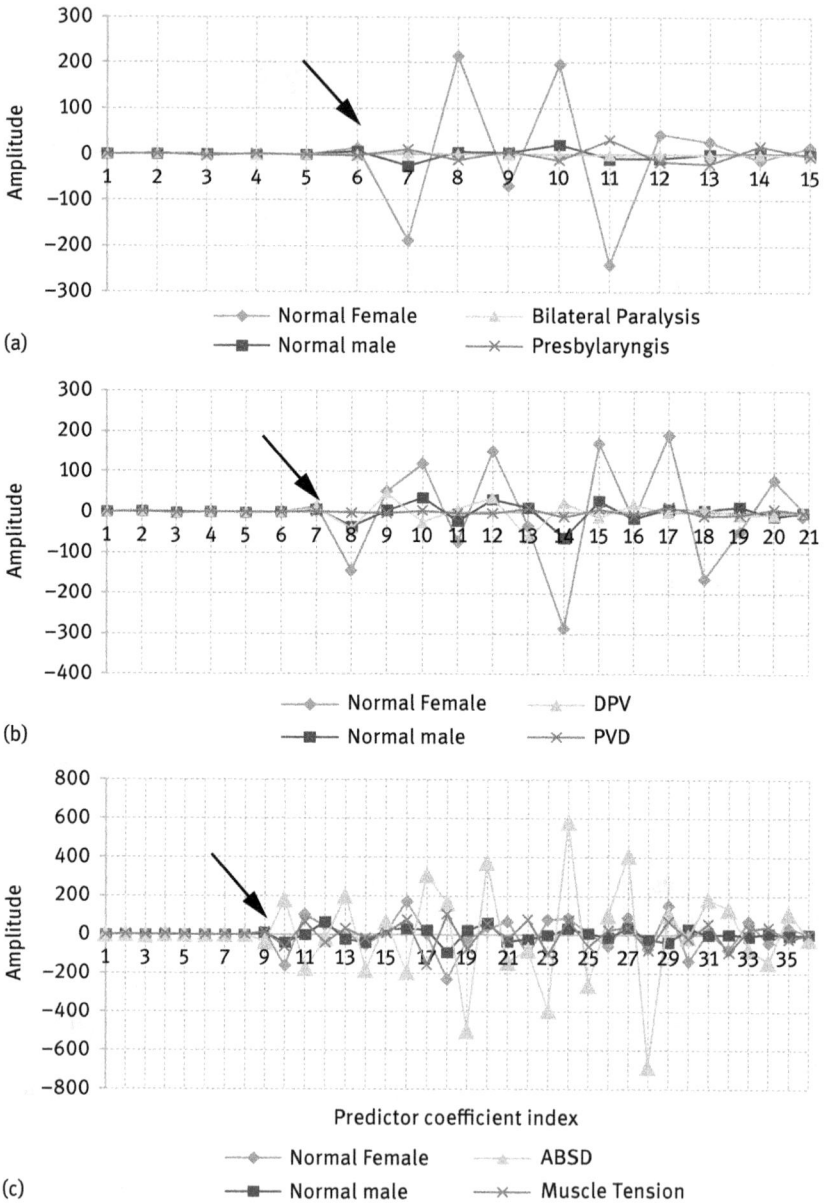

(a)

(b)

(c)

Figure 4.6: The coefficients obtained by nonlinear predictions: (a) for $d = 2$ and $k = 4$, (b) for $d = 2$ and $k = 5$, (c) for $d = 2$ and $k = 7$. The arrows in Figure 4.6 indicate the index of the start of the nonlinear coefficients, that is, a_{k+1}.

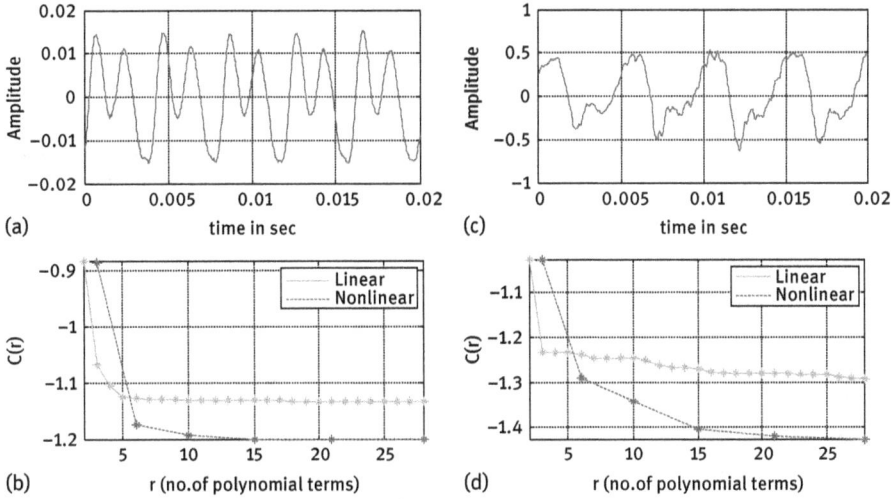

Figure 4.7: Estimating the nonlinear dynamics for analysis purpose: (a) a frame for the normal female voice sampled *at 25 kHz*, (b) the *r- C(r)* curve for the speech signal in (a), (c) a frame of pathological speech signal sampled at *25 kHz* and (d) *r- C(r)* curve for the speech signal in (c).

compared to that of the normal voice. To illustrate this and to understand how the neutralization process takes place, we take a frame of the same speech sample as above and add noise of increasing *sd*. We add noise to the frame of speech signal until the frame gets *titrated* by the added noise. Figure 4.8 shows frames of speech for a normal male voice when noise (of increasing *sd*) is added to it. It is seen that even at a very small *sd* value the linear and nonlinear $C(r)$ curves are sufficiently close to each other. One criterion of measuring the NL is that when the nonlinear $C(r)$ curve crosses the linear $C(r)$ curve, then the *sd* value at that point is assumed to be the NL for that particular frame of speech signal. In Figure 4.8, at *sd = 0.007*, such a condition is met and hence, for the speech frame chosen the NL = *sd = 0.007*. Any further addition of noise to the speech frame will have nearly no effect of the $C(r)$ curves.

If the first criterion is not met, then a second criterion is used to estimate the NL values, that is, if the nonlinear curve does not cross the linear curve then choose the *sd* value at which the curves are sufficiently close to each other and on any further addition of noise (with increasing *sd*) no change in the curves will be observed. Figure 4.9 shows the set of frames of speech for a pathological voice (ABSD) when noise (of increasing *sd*) is added to it. It can be seen that during the addition of noise, a point is reached such that even if more noise is added to the speech signal then there is no variation in the curves. The value of *sd* at which the two curves are close to each other is taken as the NL value for that particular

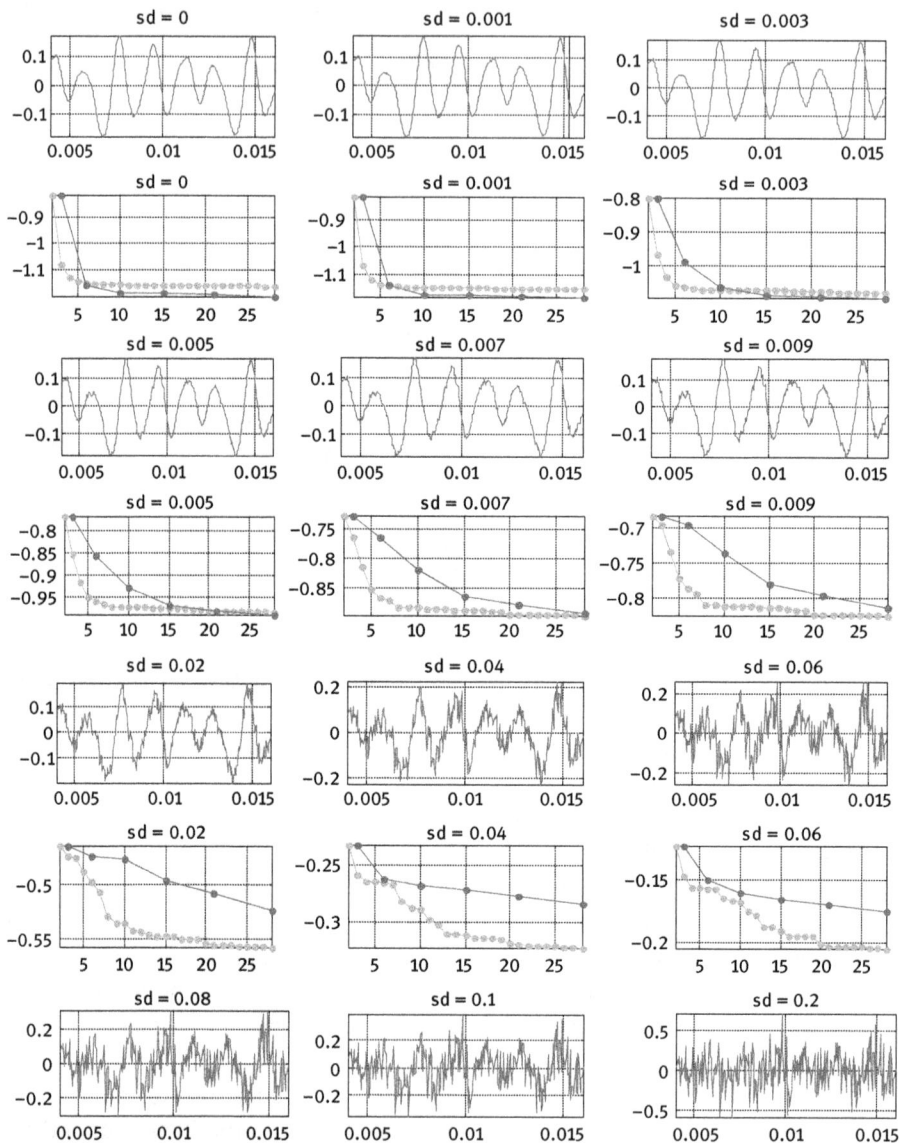

Figure 4.8: A frame of *300* sample points of normal male voice signal when titrated with addition of noise of increasing standard deviation (*sd*). Each sub-figures show two plots: 1) the plot of amplitude *vs.* time (sec) for the frame of normal speech signal sampled at *25 kHz* (top). 2) The r (number of coefficient terms) *vs.* C(r) curve for the speech frame (bottom, i.e., just below the speech signal). The light shade curve indicates the C(r) curve for linear prediction with *d = 1* and *k = 27*. The dark shade curve shows the C(r) curve nonlinear prediction with *d = 2* and *k = 6*. The dots on the line indicate the memory terms.

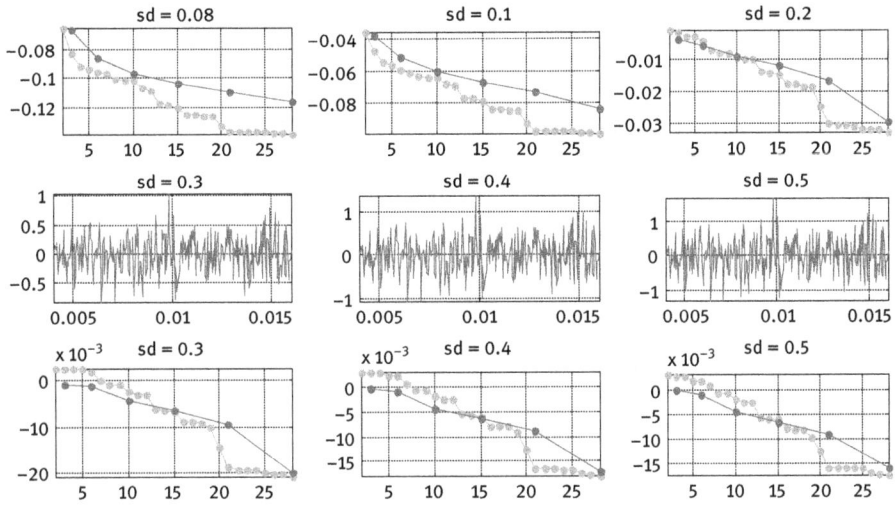

Figure 4.8: continued

frame of speech signal. It can be seen from Figure 4.9 that after an *sd* value of 0.2, not much change is observed in the linear and nonlinear curves. The NL value for the particular speech frame is estimated to be the *sd* value when the difference between the curves is minimum or below a certain value. In the present case, it can be said that the NL value is *sd* = 0.2. Likewise to estimate the NL of the entire speech signal the frame is shifted by certain samples (say *25*) and again the frame of speech is titrated. This is continued till the speech utterance is titrated with noise. The plot of the entire set of NL values *versus* time gives the overall estimate of the speech signal for analysis purpose.

However, prior to the estimation of NL, the amount of frame shift necessary to get the appropriate NL values needs to be estimated. Very less value of shift will be cumbersome, because small shifts will take more time to cover the entire speech utterance. For example, a shift of one sample may prove very effective to determine the chaos in the signal, however, at the same time, the number of NL values will be large. On the other hand, too large value of sample shift does not take into account the NL variations. This is shown in Figure 4.10 by varying the sample shift from *1* to *35* (and the standard deviation is varied from *0* to *1*, with increments of *0.1*). Therefore, an appropriate shift would be between *20 and 30* samples. After fixing a sample shift value such that the time of computation is not too large and also the variation in the NL values are preserved, the NL values for the normal voice and different voices are estimated. Here, the sample shift is taken to be *25* with a window length of *300* speech samples. The speech frame is

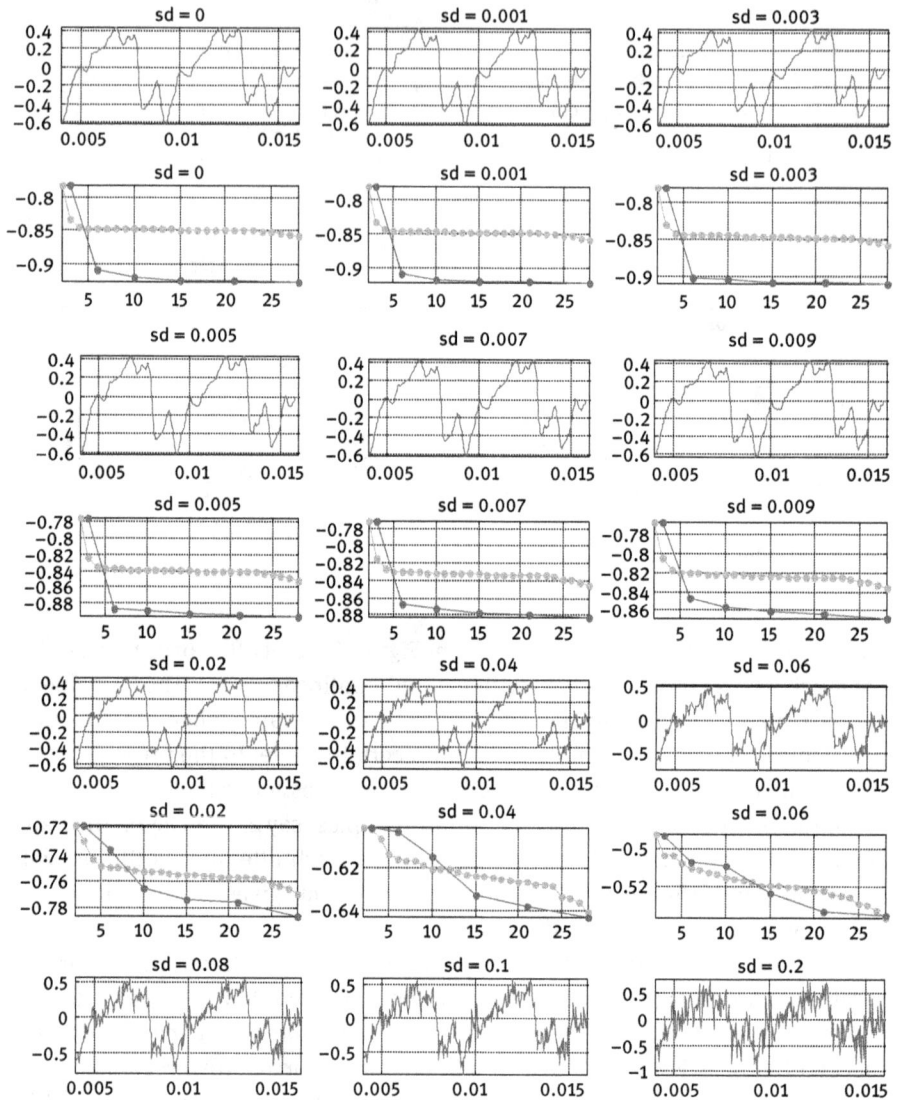

Figure 4.9: A frame of *300* sample points of pathological voice (ABSD) signal when titrated with addition of noise of increasing standard deviation (*sd*). Each sub-figures show two plots: 1) the plot of amplitude *vs.* time (sec) for the frame of pathological speech signal sampled at 25 kHz (top). 2) The r (number of coefficient terms) *vs.* C(r) curve for the speech frame (bottom, i.e., just below the speech signal). The light shade curve indicates the C(r) curve for linear prediction with *d = 1* and *k = 27*. The dark shade curve shows the C(r) curve nonlinear prediction with *d = 2* and *k = 6*. The dots on the line indicate the memory terms.

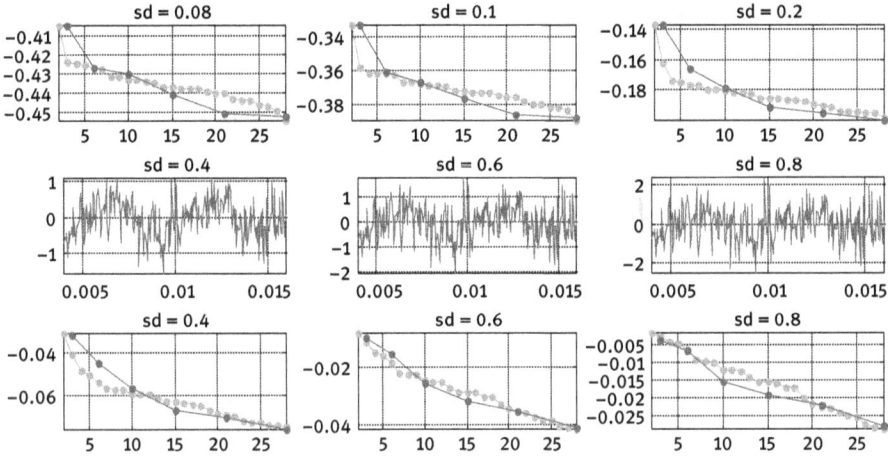

Figure 4.9: continued

titrated to obtain a NL value for the corresponding speech frame. The window is shifted by *25* samples and the next frame is titrated. The titration process is performed frame-by-frame till the entire *40* ms speech utterance is titrated. The titration had been carried out by increasing the standard deviation of noise from *0* to *3*. Therefore, the NL values will range from *0* to *3*. It can be seen from the Figure 4.11 that the NL values of the normal speech signals are relatively much less as compared to that of the NL values obtained for the pathological voice signals [24, 32]. This is due to the fact that the chaos present in the normal speech signal is less due to the smooth closure of the vocal folds. The randomness in movement of vocal folds for the pathological voices being a source for the more chaotic nature of the pathological speech signal is captured in terms of the NL values. Therefore, NL values will be a good test to separate the normal and the pathological voices from each other.

4.3.1 Feature discrimination by J-measure

It should be noted that the classification accuracy may depend on the availability of a large dataset, and it may be dependent on the number of voice samples used in the training and testing set. However, classification can still be carried on different basis, that is, there is a high correlation between separation of class and good classification accuracy. If the classes themselves are large and close to one another or overlapped, clearly the discrimination among them will become poor. The capability of a feature to differentiate between two classes is dependent on

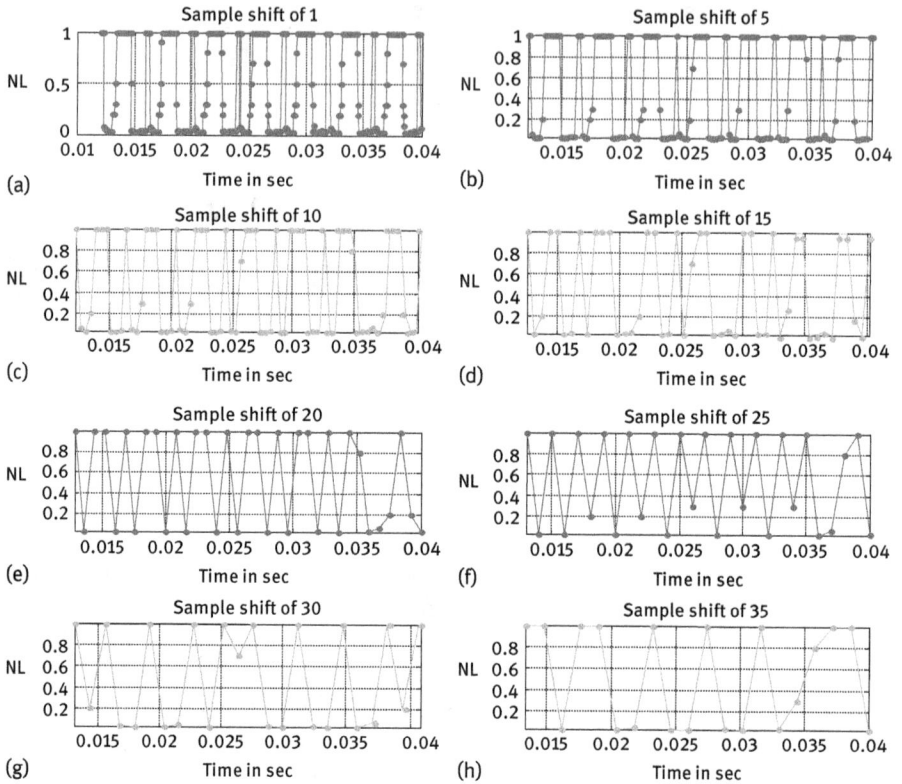

Figure 4.10: The NL values obtained by changing the sample shift parameter starting with (a) with a sample shift of 1 and incrementing in steps of 5 samples (b) to (h) till 35. The sample shift values are stated at the top of each sub-figure.

both the amount of scatter within the classes and the distance between the two classes. Sensible measures of class discrimination takes into consideration both the mean and variance of the classes. Such a measure of the separation between these two classes is well known as Fisher's discriminant or its extended version [55], that is, F-ratio, which is given as,

$$f = \frac{(\mu_1 + \mu_2)^2}{\sigma_1^2 + \sigma_2^2},$$
(4.24)

where μ1 and μ2 represent two means of the classes, and σ1 and σ2 give the standard deviations of the classes. Clearly higher discrimination is measured when the means are further apart and when the spread of the classes is smaller, thereby increasing the overall class separation. Fisher's discriminant is able to measure the separability,

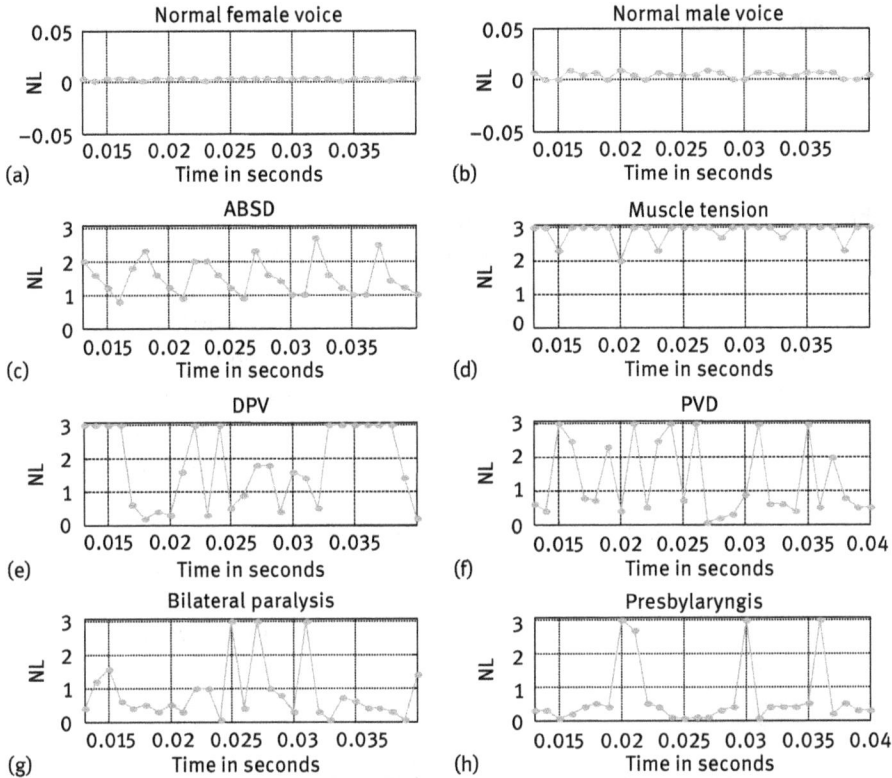

Figure 4.11: The NL *vs.* time plot for the normal and pathological voices computed by taking a frame shift of 25 samples: (a) NL plot for normal female speech signal, (b) the NL plots for the normal male speech signal and (c) to (h) The NL plot for the pathologies: ABSD, muscle tension, DPV, PVD, bilateral paralysis and presbylaryngis, respectively.

which exists between just two classes. For most tasks, there will be considerably more classes than only two classes. The *F*-ratio is an extension of Fisher's discriminant which provides a measure of separability between multiple classes.

$$F-ratio = \frac{\text{variance of mean(between class)}}{\text{mean of variance(within class)}}.$$ (4.25)

If the spread of class means increases or the clusters themselves become narrower, then the separability of the class increases. As these are statistical measures, they form ideal candidates for extracting the between-class and within-class covariance for a given feature space. Therefore, to evaluate the discrimination of an entire feature set, an extension to the F-ratio is needed, that is, J-measures. To compute these measures, let covariance of the class means be matrix B (i.e., between-class covariance) and average of the class covariance be matrix W (i.e., within-class covariance), then,

$$J_1 = trace(W^{-1}B) \text{ and } J_s = \sum_{k=1}^{k=N} \frac{w_{kk}}{b_{kk}}, \tag{4.26}$$

where **b** and **w** are the individual elements of the matrix B and matrix W, respectively [55]. For classification purpose, in addition to the initial six pathological samples two other pathological samples, that is, ASD and unilateral paralysis from [10] (both from female speakers) are used. Further, six samples of normal speech (from equal male and female speakers) were recorded in addition to the earlier two normal samples that are used. Thus, for a population size of *16* speakers (eight normal and eight pathological), the class separation of coefficients and results obtained for J_1 and J_s measures is shown in Table 4.3. Initially, the J-measures for the LP and NLP coefficients for different values of predictor memory *k* and degree *d* are obtained in Table 4.3 [24].

Table 4.3: J-measures for LP and NLP coefficients obtained by varying the polynomial degree *d* and predictor memory terms *k*.

		d = 1 (linear)	d = 2 (Nonlinear)
k = 2	J_1	0.1940	0.3050
	J_s	0.1622	0.3481
k = 3	J_1	0.1963	0.2306
	J_s	0.1281	0.1066
k = 4	J_1	0.1932	0.4460
	J_s	0.1299	0.7998
k = 5	J_1	0.2009	0.8808
	J_s	0.1486	0.7411
k = 6	J_1	0.2438	0.9659
	J_s	0.2100	0.7283

It is very interesting to observe from the results that for NLP, the J-measures are much higher than the LP; indicating that the NLP features have more class discrimination than that for LP. Furthermore, J-measures values increases with increase in degree of Volterra polynomial, which means that the class discrimination is more efficient if the nonlinearities in the sequence of samples of the speech signal is exploited.

4.4 Summary and conclusions

This work discusses a novel chaotic titration approach to study and estimate the chaotic characteristics of the speech signal. We illustrate the effectiveness in NLP of the speech signals than that of LP. The estimation of chaos becomes very useful in the case of pathological signals as they are more sensitive to their initial conditions (i.e., the closure of the vocal folds, which itself is random due to the presence of growths or structures that obstruct the opening and closing phenomena of the vocal folds). In normal voices, the opening and closing of the vocal folds are more certain to occur. The NL values for normal and pathological voices could easily quantify the chaotic nature of the speech signal, therefore, it can be said that the titration process offers a simple yet conclusive test for chaos in short and noisy time series. Further, referring back to the work carried out by Poon and Merill [45], where the electrocardiograms from a set of healthy subjects and those with severe CHF (i.e., a clinical condition associated with a high risk of sudden death) were analyzed, the chaotic dynamics in the CHF data suggested a weaker form of chaos. These findings imply that cardiac chaos is prevailing in healthy heart, and a decrease in such chaos may be a possible indicative of CHF. Methods derived from the field on nonlinear dynamics, or chaos theory, have been useful tools to describe systems from 'life sciences'. It can be applied to wide areas of medicine, namely, cardiology, physiology and neurosciences. The entire analysis has been carried on limited data, however, with sufficient analysis, which can be extended in near future on large databases. Using titration for chaos measures to reveal subtleties between different types of glottal closure would be an important finding, especially if verified with high-speed video of the larynx.

The limitation of the present work is computational load in observing higher degree predictions of speech signal. However, the use of very large degree for prediction model is not necessary in the present case. In addition, Tao et. al. [27] found that chaos not only exists in the speech signal but also in its corresponding residual or prediction error. This has been found by applying the procedure of titrating the LP residual by noise to infer that chaos also exists in the LP residual. This knowledge can also been used in speech synthesis applications where the excitation source, that is, residual is replaced by noise or ideal pitch pulses to synthesize unvoiced and voiced speech signals, respectively. On the similar ground, in [56], the authors synthesize speech using the novel chaotic excitation source (i.e., using noise of known *sd* estimated from chaotic titration method). It was observed that on an average for synthesized voices, the naturalness was more by the chaotic-mixed excitation source. Since nonlinear information of the speech production is contained in the residual, therefore this chaotic characteristic may also be used to improve the quality of synthetic speech.

In [53], the authors have explored the use of LP and NLP residual-based features for detection of natural and synthetic speech. Thus, there is a great possibility of extending the study to quantify the amount chaos in natural and spoofed speech (machine-generated synthetic speech). Thus, this may help in detecting voice forgery, that is, it may assist the forensic scientist to know if the speech was from a genuine speaker or from an impostor.

References

[1] Markhoul J. Linear prediction: a tutorial review. Proc IEEE 1975;63(4):561–580.
[2] Yegnanarayana B, Murthy PS. Enhancement of reverberant speech using LP residual signal. IEEE Trans Speech Audio Process 2000;8(3):267–281.
[3] Teager HM, Some observations on oral air flow during phonation. IEEE Trans Acoust Speech Signal Process 1980;ASSP-28(5):599–601.
[4] Teager HM, Teager SM, Evidence for nonlinear production mechanisms in the vocal tract. Speech Production and Speech Modelling. NATO ASI Series (Series D: Behavioural and Social Sciences). In: Hardcastle WJ, Marchal A, editors. vol 55. Dordrecht: Springer, 1990:241–261.
[5] Kumar A, Mullick SK. Nonlinear dynamical analysis of speech. J Acoust Soc Am 1996;100 (1):615–629.
[6] Ananthapadmanabha TV, Fant G. Calculation of true glottal flow and its components. Speech Commun 1982;1(3–4):167–84.
[7] Quatieri TF. Discrete-time speech signal processing, 2nd ed. Prentice-Hall, Pearson, India 2002.
[8] Van Stan JH, Mehta DD, Petit RJ, Sternad D, Muise J, Burns JA, et al. Integration of motor learning principles into real-time ambulatory voice biofeedback and example implementation via a clinical case study with vocal fold nodules. Am J Speech-Lang Pathol 2017; 26(1):1–10.
[9] Vaziri G, Almasganj F, Behroozmand R. Pathological assessment of patients' speech using nonlinear dynamical analysis. Comput Biol Med 2010;40:54–63.
[10] The pathological voice samples (Texas voice center). Available at: http://www.texasvoicecenter.com/diseases.html. Accessed: 10 Nov. 2017.
[11] Figure of normal vocal folds. Available at: http://www.odec.ca/projects/ 192005/kost5d0/public_html/introduction.html. Accessed: 11 Nov. 2017.
[12] Figure of pathological vocal folds. Available at: http://stanfordhospital.org/clinicsmedServices/clinics/otolaryngology/laryngology/clinicalPicturesMovies.html. Accessed: 03 April 2014.
[13] Boyanov B, Hadjitodorov S. Acoustic analysis of pathological voices: a voice analysis system for screening of laryngeal diseases. IEEE Eng Med Biol Mag 1997;16:74–82.
[14] Brockmann-Bauser M, Bohlender JE, Mehta DD. Acoustic perturbation measures improve with increasing vocal intensity in healthy and pathological voices. Voice Foundation Symposium, Philadelphia, PA, 2016.
[15] Titze IR, Baken RJ, Herzel H. Evidence of chaos in vocal fold vibration. Front Basic Sci 1993;143–188.

[16] Lieberman P. Some acoustic measures of the fundamental periodicity of normal and pathological lLarynges. J Acoust Soc Am 1963;35(3):344–353.

[17] Dubuisson T, Dutoit T, Gosselin B, Remacle M. On the use of the correlation between acoustic descriptors for the normal/pathological voices discrimination. EURASIP J Adv Signal Process 2009;2009:1–19.

[18] Dibazar AA, Narayanan SS. A system for automatic detection of pathological speech. Asilomar Conference on Signal, Systems and Computers, Asilomar, CA, 2002:182–183.

[19] Jiang JJ, Zhang Y. Nonlinear analysis of speech from pathological subjects. Electron Lett 2002;38(6):294–295.

[20] Henríquez P, Alonso JB, Ferrer MA, Travieso MC, Godino-Lorente IJ, Diaz-de-Maria F. Characterization of healthy and pathological voice through measures based on nonlinear dynamics. IEEE Trans Audio Speech Process 2009;17(6):1186–1195.

[21] Maciel CD, Pereira JC, Stewart D. Identifying healthy and pathologically affected voice signals. IEEE Signal Process Mag 2010;27(1):120–123.

[22] Arias-Londoño JD, Godino-Llorente JI, Saenz-Lechón N, Osma-Ruiz V, Castellanos-Domínguez G. Automatic detection of pathological voices using complexity measures, noise parameters, and mel-cepstral coefficients. IEEE Trans Biomed Eng 2011;58(2):370–379.

[23] Patel TB, Patil HA, Acharya KP. Analysis of normal and pathological voices based on nonlinear dynamics. International Conference on Electrical, Electronics and Computer Engineering, Interscience Research Network, Ahmedabad, India, 2012:1–6.

[24] Patel TB. Classification of normal and pathological voices: an approach based on nonlinear dynamics. Master's Thesis, L.D. College of Engineering, Gujarat, India, 2012.

[25] Grassberger P, Procaccia I. Characterization of strange attractors. Phys Rev Lett 1983; 50(5):346–349.

[26] Takens F, Detecting strange attractors in turbulence. Lect Notes Math 1981;898:366–381.

[27] Tao C, Mu J, Du G. Chaotic characteristics of speech signal and its LPC residual. Acoust Lett Acoust Sci Technol 2004;25(1):50–53.

[28] Wolf A, Swift J, Swinney H, Vastano J. Determining lyapunov exponents from a time series. Physica D 1985;16:285–317.

[29] Rosentein MT, Collins JJ, De Luca CJ. A practical method for calculating largest Lyapunov exponent from small data sets. Physica D 1993;65:117–134.

[30] Giovanni A, Ouaknine M, J-M Triglia, Determination of largest lyapunov exponents of vocal signal: application to unilateral laryngeal paralysis. J Voice 1999;13(3):341–354.

[31] Seghaier I, Zaki MH, Tahar S. A statistical approach to probe chaos from noise in analog and mixed signal designs. IEEE Computer Society Annual Symposium on VLSI (ISVLSI), Montpellier, France, 2015: 237–242.

[32] Patil HA, Patel TB. Novel chaotic titration method for analysis of normal and pathological voices. International Conference on Signal Processing and Communication (SPCOM), IISc, Bangalore, 22–25 July, 2012:1–5.

[33] Thyssen J, Nielsen H, Hansen SD. Nonlinear short-term prediction in speech coding. Proceedings of IEEE International Conference on Acoustic, Speech and Signal Process. (ICASSP), Adelaide, South Australia, Australia, 1994:185–188.

[34] Martin S. The Volterra and Wiener theories of nonlinear systems. John Wiley & Sons, New York 1980.

[35] Don RH, Venetsansopoulus AN. Nonlinear digital filters: principles and application. Kluwer Academic Publishers, New York 1990.

[36] Marmarelis VZ, Zhao X. Volterra models and three layers perception. IEEE Trans Neural Networks 1997;8:1421–1433.

[37] Hakim NZ, Kaufman JJ, Cerf G, Meadows HE. Volterra characterization of neural networks. Conference Record of the Twenty-Fifth Asilomar Conference on Signals, Systems and Computers, Pacific Grove, CA, 1991:1128–1132.

[38] Harkouss Y, Rousset J, Chehade H, Ngoya E, Barataud D. Modeling microwave devices and circuits for telecommunications systems design. International Joint Conference on Neural Networks (IJCNN), Anchorage, Alaska, 1998:128–133.

[39] Stegmayer G, Volterra series and neural networks to model an electronic device nonlinear behavior. IEEE Conference on Neural Networks, Budapest, Hungary, 2004:2907–2910.

[40] Savoji MH, Alipoor G. Speech coding using non-linear prediction based on Volterra series expansion. in International Conference on Speech and Computer (SPECOM), St. Petersburg, Russia, 2006:367–370.

[41] Pinto J, Sivaram GV, Hermansky H, Doss MM. Volterra series for analyzing MLP based phoneme posterior probability estimator. IEEE International Conference on Acoustics, Speech and Signal Processing (ICASSP), Taiwan, 2009:1813–1816.

[42] Korenberg MJ. Indentifying nonlinear difference equation and functional expansion representation: the fast orthogonal algorithm. Ann Biomed Eng 1988;16:123–142.

[43] Barahona M, Poon C-S. Detection of nonlinear dynalmics in short, noisy time series. Nature 1996;381:215–217.

[44] Poon C-S, Barahona M. Titration of chaos with added noise. Natl Acad Sci 2001;98:7107–7112.

[45] Poon C-S, Merill CK. Decrease of cardiac chaos in congestive heart failure. Nature 1997;389:492–495.

[46] Frechet M. Surles les fontionelles continues. Annales Scientifiques de L'Ecole Normale Sup 1910;27:193–216.

[47] Mathews VJ, Sicuranza GL. Polynomial Signal Processing. John Wiley & sons, New York 2000.

[48] Korenberg MJ, Bruder SB, McIlroy PJ. Exact orthogonal kernel estimation from finite data records: Extending Weiner's identification of nonlinear systems. Ann Biomed Eng 1988;16:201–214.

[49] Korenberg MJ. Functional expansions, parallel cascades and nonlinear difference equations. Advanced Methods of Physiological System Modeling, Los Angeles, 1987.

[50] Korenberg MJ. Orthogonal identification of nonlinear difference equation models. Midwest Symposium on Circuit and Systems, Louisville, KY, 2985:90–95.

[51] Patil HA, Patel TB. Nonlinear prediction of speech by Volterra-Wiener series. INTERSPEECH, Lyon, France, 2013:1687–1691.

[52] Bhavsar HN. Novel nonlinear prediction based feature for spoof speech detection. M.Tech. Thesis, Dhirubhai Ambani Institute of Information and Communication Technology (DA-IICT), Gandhinagar, Gujarat, India, 2016.

[53] Bhavsar HN, Patel TB, Patil HA. Novel nonlinear prediction based features for spoofed speech detection. INTERSPEECH, San Francisco, 2016:155–159.

[54] Akaike H. A new look at the statistical model identification. IEEE Trans Autom Control 1974;19(6):716–723.

[55] Nicholson S, Milner B, Cox S. Evaluating features set performance using the F-ratio. EUROSPEECH, Rhodes, Greece, 1997;1–4.

[56] Patil HA, Patel TB. Chaotic mixed excitation source for speech synthesis. INTERSPEECH, Singapore, 2014:785–789.

Part II: **Using Acoustic Modeling in the Detection
and Treatment of Cognitive, Affective,
and Developmental Disorders**

Sumanlata Gautam and Latika Singh

5 Speech disorders in children and adults with mild-to-moderate intellectual disability

Abstract: Children and adults with mild-to-moderate intellectual disability (ID) can converse with others; however, they reportedly possess speech and language abnormalities. Language impairments are used as one of the main diagnostic criteria by health professionals to diagnose ID. However, the acoustic nature of these abnormalities and their diagnostic power is currently underestimated, particularly in early detection of these disorders. In this chapter, we quantify speech abnormalities using acoustic parameters including fundamental frequency (F_0), intensity, and spectro-temporal features encoded at different time scales in speech samples of 82 subjects (30 with ID, 52 age-matched controls). Here, the spectro-temporal features are extracted, as these features provide the phonological basis of speech comprehension and production. We find significant differences in these measures between these groups. These differences are used for designing a classification system that can differentiate between speech of ID and control with 97.5% accuracy. The study provided in this chapter is a step toward developing speech-based markers for contributing in early diagnostic of mild-to-moderate ID.

Keywords: Speech disorder, Intellectual disability, Spectro-temporal feature, fundamental frequency, Intensity, Speech production

5.1 Introduction

Speech is spoken and most powerful form of the language. It is a means by which people communicate and share their ideas/thoughts. Developing speech and language skills is one of the main preconditions for successful social life. Acquisition of this skill is one of the most remarkable achievements of life. Within a span of few years, children make the transition from babbling to becoming fluent speakers of the language they are exposed to. Speech and language difficulties are prevalent in children with ID. The ID is a disorder in which a person lacks the basic intelligence essentially required to perform routine activities such as self-help, academic skills, sensory-motor and communication skills. According to DSM-IV [1], there are four levels of intellectual impairments, which reflect four degrees of severity that are mild, moderate, severe, and profound. Whereas it is

https://doi.org/10.1515/9781501502415-006

easy to diagnose severe and profound ID, early detection of mild-to-moderate ID is a challenging task. As per Diagnostic and Statistical Manual of Mental Disorders (DSM-IV), ID is primarily diagnosed by finding out the impairments in two primary areas: intellectual functioning and adaptive behavior. The IQ scores are used to measure disabilities in intellectual functioning. However, these tests cannot be performed during early childhood. Similarly, professionals assess the adaptive behavior by comparing the functional abilities of these special children with age-matched controls. These functional abilities cover social skills, routine living skills, and communication skills. Whereas judgment of behavior in social skills and living skills require certain age criteria, it is easier to examine the communication skills of growing children. It is seen that children with IDs are highly prone to developing speech disabilities. A research [2] shows that it is the primary concern for visits to pediatric clinics and more than 40% of the reported cases have this as a major concern. Similar study has shown that more than 55% of children with IDs have some or the other form of speech and language impairments. Most of the times these impairments are reflected in their speech production skills. Speech production is very well studied using quantitative frameworks that have improved with the advancement of technology. This has led to the belief that these measures can be used as potential bio-markers for understanding intellectual disabilities. However, the exact nature of these abnormalities and their diagnostic power for detecting mild-to-moderate ID is not fully studied.

In the present study, we develop a speech-based system that can differentiate between the subjects with mild-to-moderate IDs and normal subjects. Such a system can contribute to the growing efforts in developing measures for early identification of mild-to-moderate IDs. It also has implications in improving the effectiveness of the therapies. We develop a model by training classifiers using several speech parameters including fundamental frequency(F_0), intensity and spectro-temporal features encoded at different time scales [3]. Spectro-temporal features are the basis of phonological comprehension in the human brain [4–6]. These features can be categorized based on their time scales, which corresponds to different linguistic units [7]. These parameters are used in many studies to provide acoustic milestones of speech development which is explained as follows.

Normally developing children develop the capacity to produce speech-like sounds during the first year of their life. This includes stages of cooing and babbling. Cooing is a stage of pre-linguistic speech that emerges between 6 to 8 weeks and is characterized by the first non-crying verbal behavior [8]. Studies [9, 10] have shown that babbling is a pre-cursor to language development and it contains universal syllabic patterns. During second year of life, children try to imitate sounds and words. They develop a vocabulary of around 50 single words and try to speak short sentences of two to three words [11]. Acoustical studies which investigated the speech production development in children have shown that children start acquiring phrasal stress and boundary cues at the age of 2–3 years [12–14]. Between 3–4 years of age, children start producing sentences with three to six words and possess a mature vocabulary. By the end of 5 years, this increases to six to eight words per sentences [11]. Speech production studies have shown that children start producing adult-like intonation patterns at this age [15, 16]. Also, studies have shown that speech of children exhibit higher pitch, spectral, and temporal variation and longer segmental durations as compared to the adults [17–19]. A similar study [20] conducted on a larger number of subjects showed that the magnitude, temporal and spectral variation reduces with age, and adult-like patterns were observed at 12 years of age.

Children with IDs show delay in speech production and possess many articulatory deficits [21]. Studies [22, 23] have shown impairments in phonological development of children with IDs. Speech of such children exhibit articulatory problems and delay in speech production skills [24]. Limitations in grammar and syntax development are also evident in children with IDs as compared to the age-matched controls [25, 26]. Whereas many studies in past two decades have reported various kinds of deficits in expressive language, very few studies have performed analysis of speech production skills of children with mild-to-moderate IDs using acoustical frameworks. This can be very useful as a measure as it can contribute in development of bio-markers that can help in early diagnosis of such impairments. Also, one can understand the nature of the speech production deficits and can design therapies accordingly for improved rehabilitation of such children. The present study tries to fill this gap partially by analyzing the differences between acoustic parameters of subjects with IDs and age-matched controls. A classification model is also built on the basis of differences observed in these features between the two groups.

The chapter is organized as follows. Section 5.2 describes the speech database and recording setup; Section 5.3 illustrates the speech features and method for their extraction; Section 5.4 presents results and Section 5.5 comprised of discussion and future scope.

5.2 Speech database and recording setup

5.2.1 Speech database

The speech database consists of two groups, Typically Developing (TD) and Intellectually Disabled (ID) with age ranges between 4 and 20 years. The TD group was subdivided into three groups, namely, TD1, TD2, and TD3. The ID group was subdivided into two groups, namely, ID1 and ID2. Table 5.1 shows the detailed description of these groups.

Table 5.1: Details of speech database.

Group		Age	No of Subjects
TD		5–20 years	52
1.	TD1	4.5 years ± 0.5	9
2.	TD2	6.5 years ± 0.5	26
3.	TD3	18.5 years± 0.5	17
ID		6–20 years	30
1.	ID1	6–10 years	9
2.	ID2	14–20 years	21

5.2.2 Experimental settings and procedure

The speech recordings were taken at the sampling rate of 44.1 kHz and 16bit PCM using head-fitted Sony recorder (model ICD-UX533F) kept at an appropriate distance of 5 cm from the mouth of the speaker. The recording procedure included three tasks, namely, picture naming, reading, and story-telling. The first task was picture naming which consisted of naming pictures of common objects, fruits, vegetables, animals, and birds presented before them. The reading task included reading of phonetically rich article. The story-telling task included the recitation of simple stories in English or Hindi language. Young children in TD1 and ID groups could only perform picture naming and story-telling, whereas in TD2 and TD3 groups have performed all the three tasks. The task procedures were explained to all the participants before taking the recordings. The length of each recording was 3 minutes (approximately).

5.3 Acoustic analysis of speech signal

5.3.1 Speech features extraction

Speech is a non-stationary signal that varies with time and frequency. The analysis of speech signal can be carried out effectively by investigating the acoustic parameters. In current study, we have extracted the fundamental frequency (F_0), intensity, and spectro-temporal features that are encoded at two different time scales: the short time scales (25–50 ms) and the long time scales (100–600 ms). Previous studies have shown that significant differences are present in these speech parameters [6, 27]. However, in these studies, the features were taken separately. Moreover, the analysis was performed only using one sampling rate. The maximum class recall for ID group reported in these studies was 91%. In the present study, a larger feature set is constructed by combining the features and performing the analysis using different sampling rates. The design layout is demonstrated in Figure 5.1. The detail procedure of extraction of these features is explained as follows.

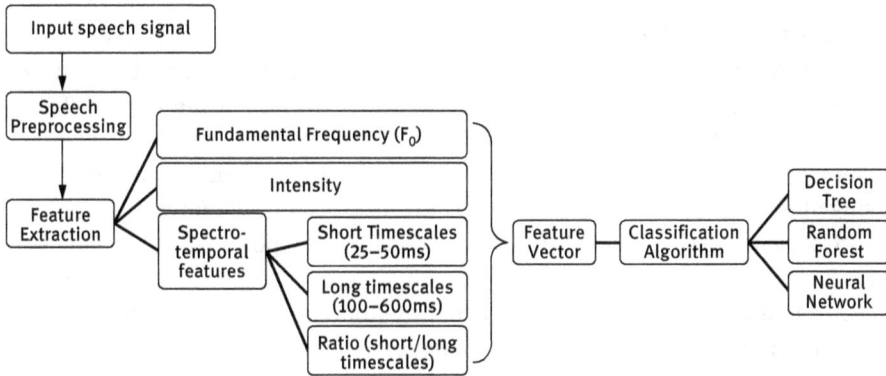

Figure 5.1: Design layout of proposed work.

5.3.1.1 Fundamental frequency analysis

The fundamental frequency values were determined for each speech sample of each group at the time window of 10 ms by interpolation curves with time resolution of 1 ms using autocorrelation method as mentioned in Equation (1) [28, 29].

$$a(z) = \sum_{i=1}^{N-z} y(n)y(n+z) \tag{5.1}$$

where N is total number of sample.

5.3.1.2 Intensity analysis

The intensity values were determined for each speech sample of each group in a window of 10 ms interpolation curves with time resolution of 1 ms using root mean square method [29].

5.3.1.3 Spectro-temporal analysis

Speech signal encodes linguistic and acoustic information at multiple time scales [5, 7, 30]. In this study, spectro-temporal features were characterized into two different time scales: short time scales (25–50 ms), which encode information, such as intonation, voicing, stress, and formant transition and long time scales (100–600 ms), which carry information representing syllabicity, rhythm, and tempo. As shown in Figure 5.1, the speech samples were pre-processed to remove background noise and down-sampled to three different sampling frequencies, namely, 8, 16, and 22 kHz. Entire analysis was performed using three different datasets derived using these three different types of sampling frequencies. To determine spectro-temporal features, the gray-scale spectrogram was generated using 512-point Fast Fourier Transform (FFT) in 22 ms time window. The obtained spectrogram image is then used to extract spectro-temporal features using various filters and applying thresholding to convert the noise-free binary image. The spectro-temporal features were extracted by applying eight connected-component algorithm [31] from these binary images.

5.3.1.4 Classification techniques

All the acoustic features were then combined to construct a feature vector which was used to train different classifiers using 10-fold cross-validation. Three different feature vectors were constructed respective to three different sampling rates, namely, 8, 16, and 22 kHz. However, our classification showed best results with 22 kHz (refer result in Section 5.4). The possible reason for this could be that the short time scale spectro-temporal features in high-frequency energy regions (beyond 5 kHz) play an important role in speech perception [32]. The mean values of the attributes taken for training the classifiers are mentioned in Table 5.2 (for 22 kHz). Three supervised learning algorithms were used for this analysis including Artificial Neural Network (ANN), Decision Tree and Random Forest. The classifier giving the best performance was then selected. These are briefly described as follows:

Table 5.2: Feature set for classification using 22 kHz sampling rate.

S/No.	Attribute	Type	Mean ± SD (TD group)	Mean ± SD (ID group)
1	Fundamental frequency (F_0)	Numeric	267.21 ± 55.49	184.0236 ± 50.45
2	Intensity	Numeric	76.75 ± 2.73	67.40 ± 4.52
3	Number of spectro-temporal encoded at short time scales	Numeric	7,069.19 ± 2,245.36	4,373.56 ± 1,922.46
4	Number of spectro-temporal encoded at long time scales	Numeric	504.69 ± 160.13	342.63 ± 181.21
5	Ratio (short/long time scales)	Numeric	15.31 ± 6.92	12.06 ± 4.44
6	Age	Numeric	10.96 ± 7.12	14.03 ± 4.21

Output Classes: Typically Developing (TD)Intellectually Disable (ID)

Artificial Neural Network (ANN)

Neural network is composed of nodes and connections. In this chapter, feed forward neural networks were trained using the feature set, where the input layer is connected to a hidden layer which in turn is connected to the output layer [33]. The connections have weights which were randomly assigned initially and were changed in process of learning through back-propagation of errors. The nodes determined the output based on the weighted input and activation function. The errors are propagated back and weights are adjusted according to minimize the errors.

Decision Tree

Decision Tree is a tree-like graph with internal nodes as attributes, leaf nodes as class labels, and branches are values that satisfy certain conditions. It is constructed using recursive algorithm in which root of the tree is selected using some splitting criterion like information gain [34].

Random forest

Random forest is an ensemble learning method which is based on decision tree learning. Several decision trees are constructed using subsets of training data and average of these trees is determined. This is done to reduce the variance that is observed in trees [35].

The performances of these models were measured using accuracy, precision, and recall. Accuracy is a measure of how many samples are correctly predicted by the classifier. It is defined as a ratio of number of correctly predicted samples versus total number of samples. Precision refers to the ratio of samples that are actually positive in a group that the model has predicted as positive. On the other hand, recall is defined as the ratio of positive samples that are correctly predicted as positive by the model. For our application, precision is how many speech samples were actually belonging to ID class out of the predicted ones and recall means that out of all belonging to subjects with ID how many were correctly predicted as class ID. Given this context, it is more important to have a model with better recall rather than the precision. The results of the experiments are discussed in the next section.

5.4 Experimental results

In this section, the results of the analysis are provided. Initial exploratory analysis using scatter plots showed differences in attributes across two groups: normal and subjects with ID (Figure 5.4). This was followed by significant testing of individual attributes among various groups which has been discussed as follows.

5.4.1 Fundamental frequency (F_0) analysis

As discussed in Section 5.3, fundamental frequencies for each speech sample were determined using a sliding window of 10 ms. The mean value of F_0 for each sample was then determined by finding the average of this measure over all the windows for that sample. This average is then used as a feature for constructing the feature set. The mean values of fundamental frequencies of subjects in various groups are shown in Figure 5.2(A). Statistically significant differences were observed in fundamental frequencies of TD1 and TD3 supporting the fact that fundamental frequencies of children and adults are different. In addition, significant differences were found in F_0 of children with ID group and with age-matched control (respective TD group){(ID1 and TD1; $p < 0.001$) (ID1 and TD2; $p < 0.001$)}.

5.4.2 Intensity analysis

The mean values of intensity for each sample were determined and are shown in Figure 5.2(B). The average value of intensity for each sample was determined and used as an attribute in feature set. Significant differences were observed

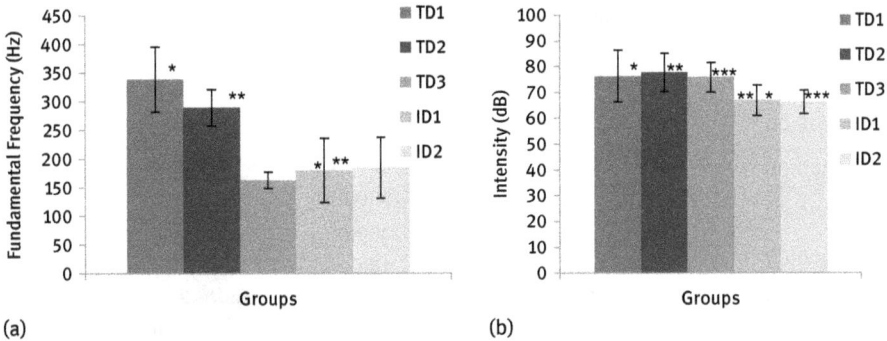

Figure 5.2: Comparative graph representation for Typically Developing (TD) and Intellectually Disabled (ID) groups (A) group-wise mean fundamental frequency (F_0), (B) group-wise mean intensity.
(Note: * and ** symbolizes the significant difference with p<0.001.).

between respective ID and TD groups {(ID1 and TD1; $p < 0.001$) (ID1 and TD2; $p < 0.001$);(ID2 and TD2; $p < 0.001$)}.

5.4.3 Spectro-temporal features

Figure 5.3(A),(B), and (C) show average number of spectro-temporal features encoded at short time scales, long time scales and ratio (short/long time scales), respectively, for each group. This was determined by finding the arithmetic mean of number of these features in each group. The spectro-temporal features encoded at short time scales are found to be significantly different (unpaired t-test: p<0.001 (TD2 and ID1) and p<0.005 (TD3 and ID2)) between age-matched TD and ID groups. Similar patterns of differences were observed for the ratio (short/long time scales), whereas no significant differences were found for long time scales among different groups. Therefore, it can be interpreted that the short time scales are evolving with age in TD groups but very less changes is happening in ID groups. From the above findings, we can conclude that the features encoded at short time scales (25–50 ms) are not matured even in adults with IDs as compared to the features encoded at long time scales. The ratio (short/long time scales) also acts as one of the important differentiating attribute. This differentiation of groups can be utilized to build models that classify speech parameters into two classes, namely, TD and ID. The feature vector for classification consisted of short time scales, long time scales, their ratios, and age.

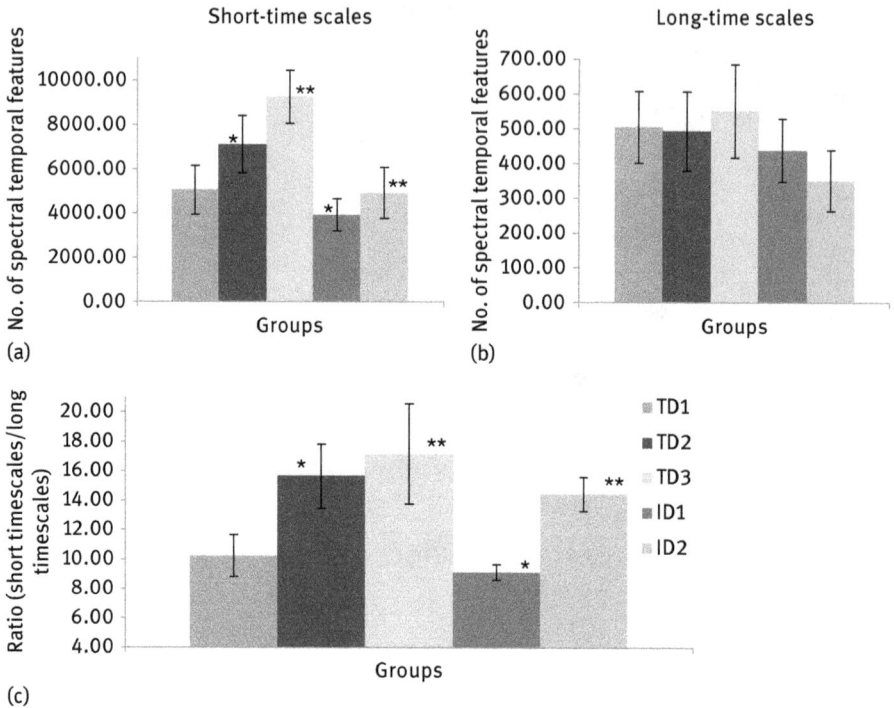

Figure 5.3: Group-wise mean for Typically Developing(TD) and Intellectually Disabled (ID) groups (A) short-time scales, (B) long-time scales, (C) ratio (Short/Long).
* and ** symbolizes the significant difference with $p < 0.001$ and $p < 0.005$ respectively).

5.4.4 Classification results

Tables 5.3, 5.4 and 5.5 show the performance of different classification models, on the obtained datasets with sampling frequency of 22, 16, and 8 kHz, respectively. It can be seen from results that features obtained using 22 kHz sampling rate are giving the best results. Also, it is evident from Table 5.3 that Random Forest has outperformed other classifiers and is giving an accuracy of 97.5% with class recall of 96.6% (for ID). Figure 5.4.

5.5 Summary and discussion

In this study, we report quantitative measures for finding speech abnormalities in mild-to-moderate IDs that are based on spectro-temporal properties

Table 5.3: Performance of classifiers for sampling frequency of 22 kHz.

Classifier	Parameter Setting	Accuracy (%)	Precision (%)	Recall (%)
Decision Tree	Criteria for splitting: gain ratio.	95.00 ± 8.29	90.62	96.67
Random Forest	Criteria for splitting: gain ratio. No. of tree: 200	97.50 ± 5.00	96.67	96.67
Neural Network	Epocs = 700	95.00 ± 8.29	93.33	93.33

Table 5.4: Performance of classifiers for sampling frequency of 16 kHz.

Classifier	Parameter Setting	Accuracy (%)	Precision (%)	Recall (%)
Decision Tree	Criteria for splitting: gain ratio.	93.89% ± 8.29	93.33	90.32
Random Forest	Criteria for splitting: gain ratio. No. of tree: 45	96.25% ± 5.75	93.33	96.55
Neural Network	Epocs = 800	93.89% ± 6.12	93.33	90.32

Table 5.5: Performance of classifiers for sampling frequency of 8 kHz.

Classifier	Parameter Setting	Accuracy (%)	Precision (%)	Recall (%)
Decision Tree	Criteria for splitting: gain ratio.	95.00 ± 8.29	96.67	90.62
Random Forest	Criteria for splitting: gain ratio. No. of tree: 45	93.89 ± 5.12	93.33	90.32
Neural Network	Epocs=200	96.25% ± 5.73%	93.33	96.55

of speech signal. We test these measures on a sample of 30 subjects with IDs and 52 age-matched controls. Our results indicate that fun damental frequency (F_0), intensity, and spectro-temporal features encoded at different time scales in speech of ID groups (children and adults) differed significantly from those of control groups. The values of pitch and intensity are significantly lower in subjects belonging to ID groups. Similarly, ID subjects are producing less number of sounds corresponding to shorter time scales. This is also evident by the differences observed in ratio of short and long time-scales associated with spectro-temporal features. In addition, we use these measures to classify mild-to-moderate ID in the samples with 97.5% success. It is also interesting to see that difference in short time scales and ratio of short-to-long time scales is more evident with sampling frequency of 22 kHz. This indicates that the regions of high frequency contribute equally to short time scale features. Emerging evidence in literature shows that

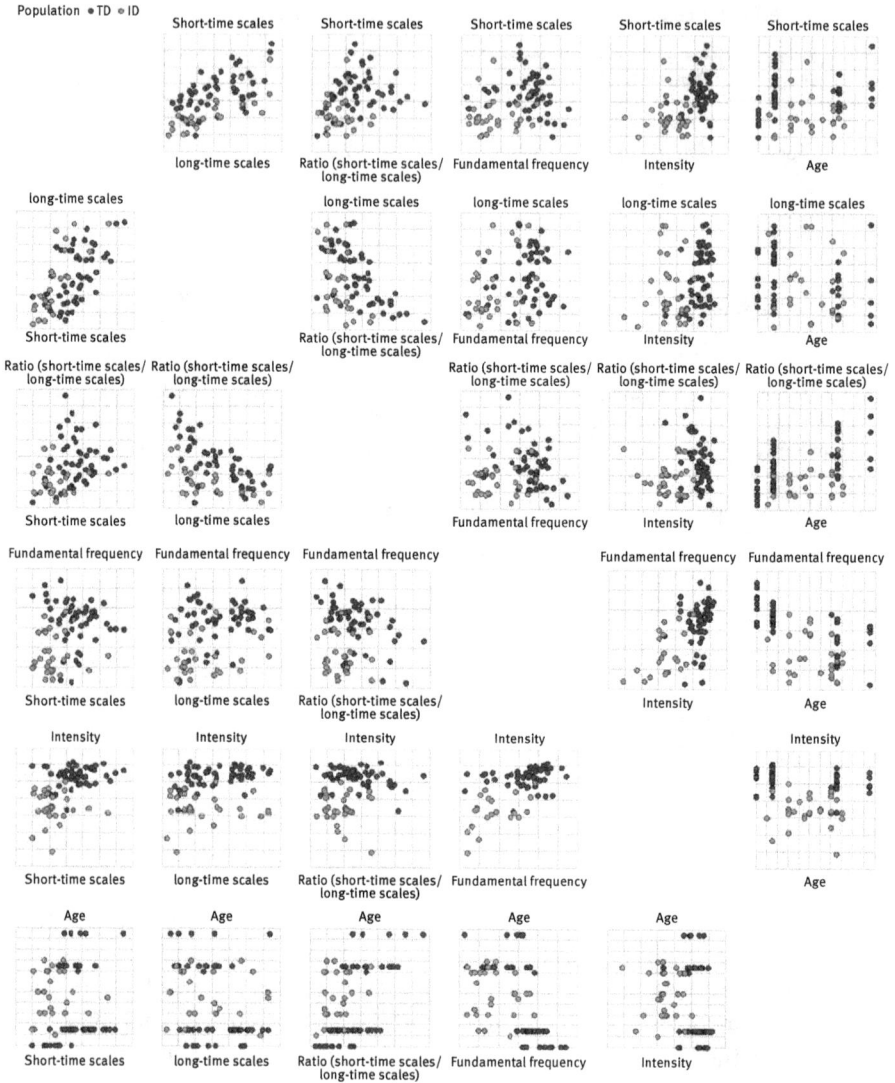

Figure 5.4: Scatter matrix plots for all the attributes used in classification models (sampling frequency 22 kHz).

these high-frequency regions consist of important features that are crucial for speech perception [32].

The results of the present study can be compared with studies carried out on speech production skills and phonological development in ID [21]. In a study [22, 23], the authors investigated the speech of 167 children with mild-to-moderate ID and found that prevalence of speech and language disorders (SLD) in the group were as high as 71.3%. The assessments of SLD in the study were carried out by speech and language therapists; however, the acoustic nature of these disorders was not mentioned. In our study, we have moved a step further by examining the nature of impairments using acoustical framework. Another study [24] has shown that children with ID are slow to acquire the phonological system. This is also evident from our study where deficit in spectro-temporal features is reported. We further add to these results by demonstrating that deficits are more prominent in features of shorter time scales that correspond to intonation, voicing, and formant transition as compared to the features at longer time scales.

These impairments in ID can emerge due to fault in speech perception or production or both. It is difficult to say that the speech production is delayed in children as we have observed deficits in spectro-temporal features encoded at short time scales in speech of adults with ID as compared to their age-matched control. However, not much difference was observed in fundamental frequencies of normal and intellectually disabled adults. This acoustic feature was not able to capture the finer differences in speech production skills of the two groups. An explanation for improper development of speech production skills could be a flaw in the motor control mechanism as speech production is a fine-motor skill. There is a growing body of evidence that sensory impairments (such as hearing, auditory processing, etc) prevalent in ID has detrimental impact on the speech and language skills [36]. Another reason for these impairments can be difficult in association between perception and production, which could arise because of some structure or genetic impairment [37].

This study can be taken as a first step that can be further expanded. We propose that the acoustic parameters in ID can contribute in developing markers for early diagnosis. It can be used in combination with other methods/markers as a potential tool for detection of IDs.

References

[1]   American Psychiatric Association. Diagnostic and statistical manual of mental disorders, 4th ed., 1994.
[2]   Harel S, Greenstein Y, Kramer U, Yifat R, Samuel E, Nevo Y, et al. Clinical characteristics of children referred to a child development center for evaluation of speech, language, and communication disorders. Pediatr Neurol 1996;15(4):305–311. https://doi.org/10.1016/S0887-8994(96)00222-6
[3]   Gautam S, Singh L. Development of spectro-temporal features of speech in children. International J Speech Technol 2017;20(3):543–551. https://doi.org/10.1007/s10772-017-9424-2

[4] Goswami U, Thomson J, Richardson U, Stainthorp R, Hughes D, Rosen S, Scott SK. Amplitude envelope onsets and developmental dyslexia: A new hypothesis. Proc Natl Acad Sci 2002;99(16):10911–10916. https://doi.org/10.1073/pnas.122368599

[5] Leong V, Goswami U. Acoustic-emergent phonology in the amplitude envelope of child-directed speech. PLoS ONE 2015;10(12). https://doi.org/10.1371/journal.pone.0144411

[6] Gautam S, Singh L. Speech impairments in intellectual disability: an acoustic study. Int J Adv Comput Sci Appl 2016b;7(1):259–264.

[7] Rosen S. Temporal information in speech: acoustic, auditory and linguistic aspects. Philos Trans R Soc London 1992. https://doi.org/10.1098/rstb.1992.0070

[8] Semb GB. An introduction to child behavior and development, 7th ed. Kansas: University of Kansas, 2004.

[9] Oller DK. The emergence of the sounds of speech in infancy. Child Phonol 1980;1:93–112. https://doi.org/10.1016/B978-0-12-770601-6.50011-5

[10] Stoel-Gammon C. Prelinguistic vocal development: measurements and predictions. Phonological Developments: Models, Research, Implications, 1992:439–456.

[11] Schwartz RG. Handbook of child language disorders. New York: Psychology Press, 2009.

[12] Clark EV, Gelman SA, Lane NM. Compound nouns and category structure in young children. Child Dev 1985;56(1):84–94. https://doi.org/10.2307/1130176

[13] Kaplan E. Inntonation and language acquistion. Papers and Reports on Child Language Development, 1970:1–21.

[14] Snow D. Phrase-final syllable lengthening and intonation in early child speech. J Speech Hear Res 1994;37(4):831–840. https://doi.org/10.1044/jshr.3704.831

[15] Koike KJ, Asp CW. Tennessee test of rhythm and intonation patterns. J Speech Hear Disord 1981;46(1):81–87.

[16] Loeb DF, Allen GD. Preschoolers' imitation of intonation contours. J Speech Hear Res 1993;36(1):4–13. https://doi.org/10.1044/jshr.3601.04

[17] Hillenbrand JM, Getty LA, Clark MJ, Wheeler K. Acoustic characteristics of American English vowels. J Acoust Soc Am 1995;97(5):3099–3111. https://doi.org/10.1121/1.411872

[18] Kent RD, Forner LL. Speech segment durations in sentence recitations by children and adults. J Phonetics 1980;8:157–168.

[19] Smith BL. Relationships between duration and temporal variability in childrens speech. J Acoust Soc Am 1992;91(4):2165–2174. https://doi.org/10.1121/1.403675

[20] Lee S, Potamianos A, Narayanan S. Acoustics of children's speech: developmental changes of temporal and spectral parameters. J Acoust Soc Am 1999;105(3):1455–1468. https://doi.org/10.1121/1.426686

[21] Memisevic H, Hadzic S. Speech and language disorders in children with Intellectual Disability in Bosnia and Herzegovina. Disability, CBR Inclusive Dev 2013;24. https://doi.org/10.5463/DCID.v24i2.214

[22] Mervis CB. Early conceptual development of children with down syndrome. Children with down syndrome a developmental perspective. 1990:252–301, ST–Early conceptual development of chil).

[23] Mervis CB, Becerra AM. Language and communicative development in Williams syndrome. Mental retardation and developmental disabilities research reviews. 2007. https://doi.org/10.1002/mrdd.20140

[24] Stoel-Gammon C. Down syndrome phonology: developmental patterns and intervention strategies. Down's Syndrome, Research and Practice, 2001;7(3):93–100. https://doi.org/10.3104/reviews.118

[25] Singer Harris NG, Bellugi U, Bates E, Jones W, Rossen M. (1997). Contrasting profiles of language development in children with williams and down syndromes. Dev Neuropsychol 1997; 13(Special Issue: "Origins of language disorders"):345–70. https://doi.org/10.1080/87565649709540683

[26] Tager-Flusberg H, Calkins S, Nolin T, Baumberger T, Anderson M, Chadwick-Dias A. A longitudinal study of language acquisition in autistic and Down syndrome children. J Autism and Dev Disord 1990;20(1):1–21. https://doi.org/10.1007/BF02206853

[27] Gautam S, Singh L. Classification of the speech of normally developing and Intellectually disabled children. Int J Data Min Emerging Technol 2016a;6(1):28–37. https://doi.org/10.5958/2249-3220.2016.00005.7

[28] Boersma P. Accurate short-term analysis of the fundamental frequency and the harmonics-to-noise ratio of a sampled sound. Proc Inst Phonetic Sci 1993;17: 97–110. https://doi.org/10.1371/journal.pone.0069107

[29] Rabiner L, Juang B.-H. Fundamentals of speech recognition. Prentice Hall, 1993. https://doi.org/10.1002/ev.1647

[30] Elhilali M, Chi T, Shamma SA. A spectro-temporal modulation index (STMI) for assessment of speech intelligibility. Speech Commun 2003;41(2–3):331–348. https://doi.org/10.1016/S0167-6393(02)00134-6

[31] Di Stefano L, Bulgarelli A. A simple and efficient connected components labeling algorithm. Proceedings – International Conference on Image Analysis and Processing, ICIAP 1999, 1999:322–327. https://doi.org/10.1109/ICIAP.1999.797615

[32] Monson BB, Hunter EJ, Lotto AJ, Story BH.The perceptual significance of high-frequency energy in the human voice. Front Psychol 2014;5(JUN). https://doi.org/10.3389/fpsyg.2014.00587

[33] Pang-Ning T, Steinbach M, Kumar V. (2006). Introduction to data mining. Lib Congr 2006;796. https://doi.org/10.1016/0022-4405(81)90007-8

[34] Quinlan, J. R. (1986). Induction of decision trees. *Machine Learning*, 1(1), 81–106. https://doi.org/10.1023/A:1022643204877

[35] Breiman L. Random forests. Mach Learn 2001;45(1):5–32. https://doi.org/10.1023/A:1010933404324

[36] Kiani R, Miller H. Sensory impairment and intellectual disability. Adv Psychiatr Treat 2010;16(3):228–235. https://doi.org/10.1192/apt.bp.108.005736

[37] Bathelt J, Astle D, Barnes J, Raymond FL, Baker K. Structural brain abnormalities in a single gene disorder associated with epilepsy, language impairment and intellectual disability. NeuroImage: Clin 2016;12:655–665. https://doi.org/10.1016/j.nicl.2016.07.016

Erik Marchi, Yue Zhang, Florian Eyben, Fabien Ringeval
and Björn Schuller

6 Autism and speech, language, and emotion – a survey

Abstract: Individuals with Autism Spectrum Conditions (ASC) show difficulties in social interaction, communication and tend toward restricted interests and repetitive behavior. They also may experience difficulties in interpreting, modulating, and enhancing spoken content through expressiveness at different communication level – in particular considering emotional and social aspects. This chapter summarizes peculiarities of ASC manifestations in speech and language and as related to emotion. It further explores the interests and challenges of using speech technology for individuals with ASC, by examining these different aspects of communication.

Keywords: Autism Spectrum Conditions, speech technology, affect recognition, atypical speech

6.1 Introduction

The autism spectrum, as defined by DSM-5 criteria [1], is a range of conditions classified as neurodevelopmental disorders. Autism Spectrum Conditions (ASC) are characterized by social communication and interaction difficulties, stereotyped or repetitive behavior and interest, and in some cases, cognitive delays. Individuals with ASC show major difficulties in the acquisition of language, ranging from the almost complete absence of functional communication to adequate use of linguistic knowledge. Such difficulties in language acquisition lead to an inappropriate use of verbal and non-verbal communications, which are yet required for engaging social interactions.

In particular, the Autism Psychiatric Association defined ASC symptoms in three general categories: difficulty in relating to others, speech and language impairments, and restricted, repetitive patterns of behavior [2]. Severity levels are then further defined based on the degree of support needed by the child; level

Note: Erik Marchi is now with Apple Siri. The work was done while at Technische Universität München, Munich, Germany and University of Passau, Passau, Germany, and it does not contain Apple proprietary information.

https://doi.org/10.1515/9781501502415-007

1: requiring support; level 2: requiring substantial support; and level 3: requiring very substantial support.

Individuals with ASC demonstrate several characteristics that affect social interaction skills, such as significant difficulties in the use of multiple non-verbal behaviors, such as eye-to-eye gaze, facial expression, body postures, and gestures to regulate social interaction; failure to develop peer relationships due to delays in the developmental level; a lack of spontaneous seeking to share enjoyment, interests, or achievements with other people (e.g., by a lack of showing, bringing, or pointing out objects of interest); and lack of social or emotional reciprocity [1]. Three decades of research have also shown that individuals (i.e., both children and adults) with ASC experience significant difficulties at recognizing and expressing emotions and more generally, mental states [3, 4].

Difficulties for expressing mental states are related to those met in speech and language production and understanding; children with ASC are often non-verbal when initially diagnosed [5, 6] and any present speech is usually highly deviant and of limited communicative function. Speech usually sounds atypical and is often described as machine-like, "monotonic," or "sing-song". Indeed, individuals with ASC may show atypical use of pitch and control of loudness, as well as use of aberrant stress patterns [7]. Earlier studies on atypical speech patterns are focused on prosody or atypical supra-segmental aspects of speech production [7]. More recent studies have used tools based on speech technology to quantify speech disfluencies in autism through objective measures, such as the long-term average spectrum [8]. Such studies have permitted to show that abnormal speech patterns in autism are mostly reflected in pitch variability and spectral content. This variability may indeed be an indication of abnormal processing of auditory feedback or instability in the mechanisms that control pitch production [27]. Further difficulties are documented in the grammatical and morphological aspects of speech, related to their reduced abilities in the meaningful use of language for social communication [9, 30]. They include, for example, echolalia – "automatic" repetition of vocalizations of others –, pronoun reversal – such as speaking of themselves by their names, you, or (s)he – or poor grammatical structure [10]. In particular, they are known to be challenged by non-literal language, including deception, humor, irony, sarcasm, and figurative language such as metaphors. Individuals diagnosed with autism normally use idiosyncratic speech that makes little sense to those who are not familiar with them. A third main aspect that characterizes ASC symptoms is the tendency to show repetitive behaviors [30]. This applies also to speech and language, where individuals with ASC tend to repeat certain words and phrases over and over [11].

In the following section, we discuss the impact of ASC on speech production and potential implications for automatic speech recognition systems. Section 3 describes the impact of ASC on language and it links to metaphorical language and grammatical structure. Section 4 discusses the difficulties that individuals with ASC have when they attempt to recognize and express emotions. Section 5 concludes this chapter.

6.2 Autism and speech

ASC affects the social and mental development of children. In particular for speech, studies suggest that the perception and filtering of sounds differs between ASC and non-ASC infants and children [12–14]. Especially, accurate abilities to distinguish similar pitch and sounding phonemes, at the cost of a higher abstraction level has been reported in the literature [14, 15]. The loss of such ability for abstraction was also reported in studies showing that ASC children's phoneme recognition rates are significantly lower than those obtained by typically developing (TD) children in noisy acoustic conditions [16]. Further, the attention priorities to various speech and non-speech sounds have been found significantly different between ASC and non-ASC children [17], for example, some ASC children attend more to analytic, non-speech sounds, than to human speech sounds from close relatives or carers.

The perception of speech sounds and the type and amount of attention given to auditory inputs are inherently linked to the childhood language-learning process [18, 19]. Thus, the way a child perceives speech sounds directly influences the learning process of the child's speech production abilities, since the heard sounds serve as reference examples for cognitive processing [18]. Therefore, we might assume that speech produced by ASC children differs in several ways from that of TD children, especially in phonation, prosody, and fluency. To date, few studies, yet, exist to prove this hypothesis from a phonetic production point of view [20]. The majority of existing studies investigated the language acquisition process of children with ASC from a speech perception perspective. Thereby, the behavior and responses of ASC and non-ASC children are compared in various controlled experiments. Techniques such as functional magnetic resonance imaging (fMRI) [21] or event-related potentials (ERP) measured from an electroencephalograph (EEG) [22] are used to monitor the children's responses to stimuli with objective measurements. This is essential, as young children cannot be simply given questionnaires on what type of sounds they have perceived, for example. Studies on the speech production of ASC children exist, though focused on a higher level than the phonetics, namely, disfluencies at the word and phrase levels. Findings suggest that ASC children show a significantly higher amount of disfluencies than usually present in TD children [23, 24].

The importance of speech prosody, that is, rhythm, stress, intonation, and expressivity, with respect to several aspects of voice and language impairment in ASC, has been investigated with growing interest over the last two decades [25–29]. Indeed, atypical prosody has been identified as a core feature of individuals with ASC [30]. The observed differences with TD children include monotonic or machine-like intonation, aberrant stress patterns, deficits in pitch and intensity control, and a "concerned" voice quality. In particular as prosodic deficits contribute to language, communication, and social interaction difficulties which may lead to social isolation, the atypical prosody in individuals with communication difficulties became increasingly a research topic. It appears that prosodic awareness underpins language skills, and a deficiency in prosody may affect both language development and social interaction. It has been, however, very difficult to characterize prosodic production difference between ASC and TD children, using manual procedures [31, 32]. Some recent studies have thus proposed automatic systems to assess prosody production [33], speech atypicalities [34], or even early literacy [35] in children.

It is important to know about the properties of speech production of ASC children and adults, and how they differ from TD children and adults for many technical applications, especially for the analysis of speech, for example, automatic speech recognition (ASR), recognition of affect, and – more general – paralinguistics [36]. Differences in phonation, that is, unclear or incomplete phonation, and especially speech disfluencies severely degrade the performance of ASR systems [37, 38]. One could, however, ask the question why these ASR technologies are required to work for ASC children. The answers are nevertheless quite obvious: such technologies will be widely spread in our society during the next coming decades, and thus must work reliably for all groups of individuals in order not to exclude minorities. Major efforts are spent at present to make speech technologies, in particular ASR and speech synthesis, work reliably for many diverse languages [39], including "sparse" languages where very few training resources are available for automatic systems [40, 41]. Moreover, such technologies can be used explicitly to train ASC children in a possibly playful and intuitive way to improve their phonation and social awareness [42, 43]. They could also be very helpful to help clinicians in the diagnosis of ASC, by providing them useful information measured in an objective way, for example, automatic analysis of atypical production of speech sounds.

Phonation and low-level acoustics is, however, the only one issue among others. Another major one met in ASC concerns the linguistic level, which will be discussed in the next section.

6.3 Autism and language

Language impairment is an important criterion used for the diagnosis of ASC [44]. Yet, the language skills observed across individuals with autism are marked by an outspread heterogeneity, ranging from (selective) mutism – an anxiety resulting in partial inability to speak in specific social situations or to specific people – and low functional communication to (over) complex syntactic capabilities and high functional speech. The variability of language profiles met in ASC requires a differentiated investigation of the individual language features, but also a general consideration of the systematicity behind the specific patterns of language skills and impairments.

For the purpose of autism diagnosis, the oral language can be regarded as the interplay of four major linguistic components: pragmatics, semantics, phonology, and syntax [45]. Pragmatics reflects social conventions of language use within social interactions. These include specific behaviors, such as the use of eye contact, gestures, or social smiling as well as constraints of verbal conversation, for example, turn-taking, measures of formality of speech, topic selection, and relevance of contributions to conversations [45]. Semantics refer to the word meanings and concepts. It impacts on our ability to acquire new words and their meanings, to organize concepts in memory and to produce or respond to those words during meaningful communication with a partner [45]. Phonology refers to the rules governing the perception and pronunciation or articulation of speech sounds (cf. Section 2). Finally, syntax refers to the structural aspects of language and, thus, relates to the rules governing the structure of sentences. To deal with all these different components of linguistics, an approach of "language profiling" has been developed for assessing language skills and comparing those between TD children and children with ASC [46]. In the following, we describe the prominent language characteristics in autism emerging in pragmatics, semantics, and syntax by reflecting a systematic dissociation of form (language structure) and function (language use).

6.3.1 Language use (Pragmatics)

Pragmatic deficits are common to all individuals with autism, regardless of their actual language level since this domain involves both verbal and non-verbal communication [45]. The salient characteristic governing the non-verbal behaviors in autism is the deficit in coordinated attention between a partner and environmental circumstances [47–50]. As an example, eye gaze or gesture patterns remain relatively intact for instrumental or purely social communication, but show selective impairment when the social context requires sharing information within "joint attention" [45]. Frequently cited verbal limitations in the pragmatic domain include turn-taking, persistent questioning as well as immediate and delayed repetition of words or phrases, a phenomenon called echolalia (cf. section 1) [51].

6.3.2 Symbolic behavior (Semantics)

Semantic development is often delayed in autism and often involves unusual lexical patterns such as made-up words, that is, private neologisms [45, 52]. Such delays and abnormalities have been reported for other developmental disorders as well and thus cannot be considered as syndrome-specific. However, they are distinctive in autism for their heightened frequency and persistence [45]. In the review work [45], it is noted that individuals with autism do not show principle deficits in relating words to concepts or in organizing the concepts in memory, but in the application of conceptual and symbolic knowledge to functional (often social) tasks. Particularly, individuals with autism are described as having difficulties with figurative language, despite a normal or even erudite vocabulary. Stylistic devices of language such as humor, irony, simile, and metaphor generally cannot be comprehended due to overliteral interpretations [53].

6.3.3 Syntax and morphology

In the syntactic domain, individuals with autism show no specific deficits or delays relative to other language domains, or relative to other peers with developmental disabilities [45]. A syntactic hallmark of autism is the reversal of pronouns which has been reported almost exclusively for autism since Kanner's (1943) first description of the syndrome [30]. However, a study explicitly designed to explore understanding and production of personal pronouns led to the assumption that the problem may not lie in the ability of individuals with autism to identify referents for personal pronouns, but in the application of deictic terms during conversation in social context [54]. Further, Bartolucci (1980) found that children with autism were inclined to omit certain morphemes, particularly articles ("a", "the"), auxiliary and copula verbs, past tense, third-person present tense, and present progressive [10]. All these peculiarities represent evidences that underpin the systematic pattern of form/function dissociation.

6.3.4 Borderlands of ASC and SLI

ASC is characterized by lack of general delays in language and cognition but marked by social deficits [52]. Specific language impairment (SLI) refers to a case where a child fails to develop spoken language on the normal schedule in selective aspects [55]. According to conventional diagnostic frameworks, SLI and ASC are mutually exclusive diagnoses despite their frequent co-occurrence [56, 57]. Kjelgaard and Tager-Flusberg [58] performed a wide-ranging battery of language tests commonly used to diagnose SLI in a group of 89 children with autism. The main findings were a significant variation in language abilities and, particularly, similarities between the profile of performance for the language-impaired children with ASC and the profile that defines SLI. Subsequently, Tager-Flusberg and Joseph [59] have noted that children with autism are impaired on nonsense word repetition, which is a deficit considered to be a psycholinguistic marker of the SLI [60–62]. These studies led to the suggestion that there is a subtype of children with autism who show the same neurocognitive phenotype as that seen in children with SLI, indicating the possibility of an etiological overlap at a deeper level between autism and SLI [58, 59]. So far, this proposal has remained controversial. Whitehouse suggested that poor nonsense word repetition in autism is related to the presence of substantial deficit in multiple autistic domains [60].

6.3.5 Longitudinal language development in autism

Often, parents of children with autism first begin to notice that something is different in their child's development because of delays or regressions in the development of speech, sometime during the second year, when the majority of peers already have acquired vocabularies of numerous words [63]. Generally, language regression is a gradual process involving deceleration of the rate of learning new words, or loss of already learnt words. It has been suggested that regression of vocabulary occurs early in development in about one-third of children with autism [64]. A large-scale systematic longitudinal study of children by Lord, Shulman, and DiLavore found that language regression after a pattern of normal language onset was unique to autism and not found among children with other developmental delays [6, 52, 65].

Prognosis studies in autism have shown that functional language use by school age entails better long-term outcomes in autism [66, 67]. Besides, production of speech before the age of five years has been related to later advanced development in language and other intellectual domains [52, 68]. Further, it has been noted that better joint attention skills are a positive prognosis for later language development [69]. Moreover, Paul and Cohen [67] found that both receptive and expressive abilities continue to improve through adolescence and adulthood. In another series of follow-up studies, almost all of the participants with autism showed substantial improvements in formal aspects of language into adulthood [70]. In contrast, once spoken language is acquired, atypical prosody remains evident throughout the lifespan [71]. It has also been observed that individuals with autism, who had serious receptive language deficits in early childhood, remained more severely language delayed as a whole [72].

The study of language in autism is a complex endeavor due to several methodological problems including 1) diversity of language profiles in the autism population, 2) the difficulty in early diagnosis and in predicting developmental change with age, 3) the concomitant phenomenon of mental retardation in most of the individuals with autism diagnosis, and 4) sample size and ascertainment [73]. As result of our investigation, it can be summarized that specific features of skill and difficulties have been reported in each of the language domains. The profiling approach brings the apparently unrelated deviances in correlation by demonstrating a systematic syndrome-specific pattern involving a dissociation of form (language structure) and function (language use) [74].

Language is, however, only a further issue. The other major area which is affected is the emotional expression and recognition. This will be discussed in the next section.

6.4 Autism and emotion

Individuals with ASC lack the sense of social reciprocity and fail to develop and maintain age appropriate peer relationships [44, 75]. Several studies have documented that adolescents and adults with ASC show significant difficulties recognizing and expressing emotions [3, 4]. These difficulties are apparent when individuals with ASC attempt to recognize emotions from facial expressions [76–79], from vocal intonation [80, 81], from gestures and body language [82, 83], and from the integration of multimodal emotional information in context [84–86]. Limited emotional expressiveness in non-verbal communication is also characteristic in ASC, and studies have demonstrated that individuals with ASC have difficulties directing appropriate facial expressions to others [87, 88], modulating their vocal intonation appropriately when expressing emotion [27, 89–91] and using appropriate gestures and body language [92]. Integration of these non-verbal communicative cues with speech is also hampered [93].

Recognition and analysis of human emotions have attracted a great deal of interest in the past two decades and have been studied extensively in computer sciences. As the human face is our preeminent means of communicating and understanding affective states and intentions [94], automatic analysis of facial expressions has attracted the interest of many researchers quite early. A bit more recently, the analysis of effect from vocal signals has also gained attention [95–97] as the voice is our primary mean of communication with other people. Our vocal utterances implicitly carry information about ourselves, our current state, and our attitude toward others in a dialogue. Individuals with ASC have limited abilities in understanding and interpreting such cues, and more generally affective states of others, and in controlling their tone of voice and their non-verbal utterances [27].

6.4.1 Automatic emotion recognition in atypical voice

Most of the past research in machine analysis of affect has focused on recognition of prototypic expressions of rather basic emotions based on data that was often posed/acted on demand by adults and acquired in laboratory settings [95, 98, 99]. Still, mounting evidence suggests that deliberate or posed behavior systematically differs in appearance and timing from that which occurs in daily life [100]. Hence, due to the availability of long proposed more naturalistic databases [101], more recently, there has been a shift toward recognition of affective displays recorded in naturalistic settings as driven by real-world applications [96, 102,103]. Many recent studies dealing with naturalistic emotions, however, still deal only with adult typical speech. The main reason is likely that many applications of emotion recognition technology, such as monitoring in call centers, in-car safety, and advanced computer gaming, are primarily intended for typically developed adults.

In comparison, very little work exists that deals with children's vocal emotion [104] and its automatic recognition [80, 104] or such of ASC individuals, or the combination (i.e., children with ASC) [105–108, 126, 127]. In [80], Boucher et al. indicated that autistic children show differences in control of articulation and intonation when compared to regular children.

A relevant aspect in automatic emotion recognition focuses on the turn or sentence fragment level as basic analysis units. This has given good results for prototypical emotions and adult speech, where these fragments are well-defined. Under naturalistic conditions, the identification of sentence fragment boundaries is a non-trivial and error-prone task. Batliner et al. investigate various segmentation unit lengths [109]. For children and adults with ASC, which might show serious deviations in their grammar and/or pronunciation, the proper segmentation is likely an even more important aspect, which so far has not been studied computationally. A further aspect of speech, closely linked to affective states, is the presence of non-linguistic vocalizations such as laughter or sighs. Hudenko et al. [110] found that more voiced laughter is produced by autistic children while almost no unvoiced laughter occurs. Methods exist to automatically detect laughter in child [111, 112] and adult speech [113–115]. Applying these methods to the speech of individuals with ASC seems feasible, although no reports exists that this has ever been done.

The speech features used for state-of-the-art automatic emotion recognition systems heavily depend on the applied unit of segmentation [108, 116, 117] and the type of modeling chosen: for frame-wise, dynamic modeling, usually prosodic, spectral, and voice-quality low-level descriptors such as energy, pitch, and critical band spectra or cepstra [118, 119] are used. As an alternative to dynamic modeling, one finds frame-wise analysis and static modeling of full speech segments that relies on statistical functionals applied to low-level descriptors over the whole speech segment [95, 120–122]. These statistics typically include mean values, statistical moments, extreme values, ranges, percentiles, and regression coefficients, for example. A real-time speech feature extractor [123] was used in [106, 124–126] to analyze relevant audio features in the recognition of emotional vocal expressions of children with ASC, to investigate the usefulness of simple prosodic features against large sets of features that include a vast number of acoustic, spectral, and cepstral features. In the result based on binary arousal grouping, binary valence grouping, and a nine-class emotion task, the authors report that ASC children seem to use prosodic information to encode emotion, albeit in a different way than TD children do.

6.4.2 Linguistic content

Besides analyzing "how" something is said, the analysis of "what" is said also reveals vital information about a person's emotional state. Various attempts to integrate linguistic information into the emotion recognition process have been studied and have been able to improve speech-based emotion recognition performance [127, 128]. This of course requires reliable and potentially self-improving automatic speech recognition or keyword detection [129], which is known to be problematic for (possibly emotional) children's speech [130] and even more of a challenge for autistic individuals' speech due to additional differences in phonation, fluency, and grammar (cf. Section 2 and Section 3). To the authors' best knowledge, however, studies more or less lack that report on experience with ASC individuals' language alteration as related to (automatic) linguistic emotion recognition.

6.5 Assistive speech technologies for the autistic population

Early intervention is very important, and several technologies and approaches have been developed recently. Such assistive technologies aim at enhancing specific communication skills ranging from language development to emotion expression and recognition [131, 132].

6.5.1 Assistive technologies dealing with language impairment

At present, there are a number of alternative and augmentative communication (AAC) approaches and technologies developed to enhance, expand, and develop communication skills. Depending on the sophistication, the technologies are categorized into three levels, that is, low tech, mid tech, and high tech.

Low tech refers to any communication system that does not require a power source. Low-tech products include: communication books, picture exchange communication systems, topic boards, picture communication symbols, and pragmatic organization dynamic display (PODD) communication books.

Mid tech refers to any communication system that requires a source of power and is "very easy" to program. However, it may require proper training to adequately program and maintain an according device. There are many products available on the market such as StepByStep™, TechTalk™, and GoTalk™. Step-by-step features three message levels that support four minutes of recording time and can be used for pre-recording sequential messages to be used at specific times of the day, or for recording and storing sequential messages that are used on a regular basis. TechTalk features high-quality speech playback and provides multiple recording levels and message cells. GoTalk is a small device which stores recording of 10–30 seconds and has a play button and a picture sticker; it helps people who cannot speak to communicate with a few most important phrases or sentences, for example, for emergency situations. These products generally feature sequential recording, speech playback, reading a story, conducting a class report, participating in a school play, and so on.

High tech refers to any communication system that requires a power source and extensive training to competently program and maintain the device. Such devices incorporate sophisticated electronics or computers with keyboard and screen. They generally feature functionalities including quick and accurate input methods, language representations, speech synthesis, and communication modalities/methods. Some of the well-known high-tech products on the market include: Accent™ and ECO2™ produced by Prentke Romich. Depending on the advance and complexity of their hardware and software configurations, their series can facilitate different levels of functionalities and features that help ASC children communicating.

6.5.2 Assistive technologies dealing with emotion recognition and expression

Several programs aim to teach socio-emotional communication and emotion recognition from pictures or facial expression such as *FEFFA* [133], *Emotion Trainer* [134], and *Let's Face It* [135]. Further programs enable individuals with ASC to learn emotions in facial expressions *and* tone of voice such as the *Mind Reading DVD* [136] and the *Transporters* [137]. Embodied conversational agents (ECA) were also proposed to facilitate the collection of socio-emotional data from autistic children, allowing further automatic analysis of these data. The Rachel ECA was, for example, proposed to encourage children with ASC to produce effective and social behaviors [138].

A recent technological solution, developed within the European Union funded ASC-Inclusion project [42, 43, 139], deals with children's vocal emotion recognition. The project has proposed an internet-based serious game platform that can help assist children with ASC, to improve their socio-emotional communication skills, attending to the recognition and expression of socio-emotional cues, and to the understanding and practice of conversational skills.

Another interesting assistive technology is currently being developed under the also European Union–funded DE-ENIGMA project [140]. DE-ENIGMA realizes a robust, context-sensitive, multimodal, and naturalistic human-robot interaction aimed at enhancing the social imagination skills of children with autism. To measure in particular the engagement of the children in such a context, efforts of automatic measurement in ASC child and robot interaction are currently made in the European Union–funded EngageME project [141].

These programs can be seen as a medium to enable interests for social and effective behaviors for children and adults having ASC. They can further provide a mean to collect data from those individuals and quantify the relevance of particular tasks designed to improve their skills on different aspects of language and communication. A number of further similar efforts exist.

6.6 Summary and conclusions

In this chapter, we discussed the impact of ASC and its implications on speech technology by examining three different aspects: acoustic, linguistic, and emotional cues. We first gave a description of the impact of ASC on the acoustic speech level and potential implications for automatic speech recognition systems. Then, we analyzed the language level and its link to metaphorical language and grammatical structure. Finally, we highlighted the difficulties that individuals with ASC have when they attempt to recognize and express emotions in relation to automatic emotion recognition.

The more we are able to understand the way that autism affects speech, the better we are able to create speech analysis technologies that can understand autistic individuals and include them in our societies, and even help them to train their speaking abilities to be able to communicate more easily with others. On that avenue, one will at the same time to master a range of ethical challenges when it comes to data privacy and the protection of a user group with specific needs that ultimately may largely benefit from effective, yet responsible artificially emotionally and socially intelligent tools.

Acknowledgments: This work was supported by the European Union's Seventh Framework and Horizon 2020 Programs under grant agreements No. 289021 (ASC-Inclusion), No. 688835 (RIA DE-ENIGMA), and No. 338164 (ERC StG iHEARu). The responsibility lies with the authors.

References

[1]   American Psychiatric Association, DSM 5. American Psychiatric Association. 2013.
[2]   Wing L, Gould J. Severe impairments of social interaction and associated abnormalities in children: Epidemiology and classification. J Autism Dev Disord 1979;9(1):11–29.
[3]   Baron-Cohen S. Mindblindness: an essay on autism and theory of mind. Boston: MIT Press/Bradford Books, 1995.
[4]   RP Hobson: Autism and the development of mind. Hove: Lawrence Erlbaum Associates, 1993.
[5]   Bauman ML, Kemper TL. The neurobiology of autism. Baltimore, MD, US: JHU Press, 2005.
[6]   Kurita H. Infantile autism with speech loss before the age of thirty months. J Am Acad Child Psychiatry 1985;24(2):191–196.
[7]   Bonneh YS, Levanon Y, Dean-Pardo O, Lossos L, Adini Y. Abnormal speech spectrum and increased pitch variability in young autistic children. Front Hum Neurosci 2011;4:237.
[8]   Löfqvist A, Mandersson B. Long-time average spectrum of speech and voice analysis. Folia Phoniatrica Logopaedica 1987;39(5):221–229.

[9]   Landa R. Social Language Use in Asperger Syndrome and High-functioning Autism. A. Kin, F. R. Volkmar, S. S. Sparrow (eds.), Asperger Syndrome, New York, NY, US: Guilford Press, 125–155, 2000.

[10]   Bartolucci G, Pierce SJ, Streiner D. Cross-sectional studies of grammatical morphemes in autistic and mentally retarded children. J Autism Dev Disord 1980;10(1):39–50.

[11]   South M, Ozonoff S, McMahon WM: Repetitive behavior profiles in Asperger syndrome and high-functioning autism. J Autism Dev Disord 2005;35(2):145–158.

[12]   Constantino JN, Yang D, Gray TL, Gross MM, Abbacchi AM, Smith SC, Kohn CE, Kuhl PK: Clarifying the associations between language and social development in autism: a study of non-native phoneme recognition. J Autism Dev Disord 2007;37:1256–1263.

[13]   Boddaert N, Chabane N, Belin P, Bourgeois M, Royer V, Barthelemy C, Mouren-Simeoni MC, Philippe A, Brunelle F, Samson Y, Zilbovicius M. Perception of complex sounds in autism: abnormal auditory cortical processing children. Am J Psychiatry 2004;161(11):2117–2120.

[14]   Bishop DV, Maybery M, Wong D, Maley A, Hill W, Hallmayer J. Are phonological processing deficits part of the broad autism phenotype? Am J Med Genet 2004;128B(1): 54–60.

[15]   Lepistö T, Kajander M, Vanhala R, Alku P, Huotilainen M, Näätänen R, Kujala T. The perception of invariant speech features in children with autism. Biol Psychol. 2008; 2007;77(1):25–31.

[16]   Alcantara JI, Weisblatt EJ, Moore BC, Bolton PF. Speech-in-noise perception in high-functioning individuals with autism or Asperger's syndrome. J Child Psychol Psychiatry 2004;45(6):1107–1114.

[17]   Ceponiene R, Lepisto T, Shestakova A, Vanhala R, Alku P, Naatanen R, Yaguchi K. Speech-soundselective auditory impairment in children with autism: they can perceive but do not attend. Proc Natl Acad USA 2003;100:5567–5572.

[18]   Kuhl PK: A new view of language acquisition. Proc Natl Acad Sci USA 2000;97(22):11850–11857.

[19]   Kuhl PK, Tsao FM, Liu HM: Foreign-language experience in infancy: Effects of short-term exposure and social interaction on phonetic learning. Proc Natl Acad Sci USA 2003;100 (15):9096–9101.

[20]   Shriberg LD, Paul R, McSweeny JL, Klin A, Cohen DJ, Volkmar FR: Speech and prosody characteristics of adolescents and adults with high-functioning autism and Asperger syndrome. J Speech Lang Hear Res 2001;44(5):1097–1115.

[21]   Just MA, Cherkassky VL, Keller TA, Minshew NJ: Cortical activation and synchronization during sentence comprehension in high-functioning autism: evidence of underconnectivity. Brain 2004;127:1811–1821.

[22]   Kuhl PK, Coffey-Corina S, Padden D, Dawson G. Links between social and linguistic processing of speech in preschool children with autism: behavioral and electrophysiological measures. Dev Sci 2005;8:F1–F12.

[23]   Scott KS, Tetnowski JA, Flaitz JR, Yaruss JS: Preliminary study of disfluency in school-aged children with autism. Int J Lang Commun Disord 2014;49(1):75–89.

[24]   Wetherby AM, Prutting CA: Profiles of communicative and cognitive-social abilities in autistic children. J Speech Hear Research 1984;27(3):364.

[25]   Demouy J, Plaza M, Xavier J, Ringeval F, Chetouani M, Perisse D, Chauvin D, Viaux S, Golse B, Cohen D, Robel L. Differential language markers of pathology in autism, pervasive developmental disorder not otherwise specified and specific language impairment. Res Autism Spectr Disord ELSEVIER, 2011;5(4):1402–1412.

[26] Bonneh YS, Levanon Y, Dean-Pardo O, Lossos L, Adini Y. Abnormal speech spectrum and increased pitch variability in young autistic children. Front Hum Neurosci 2011;4(237):1–7.

[27] McCann J, Peppé S. Prosody in autism spectrum disorders: a critical review. Int J Lang Commun Disord 2003;38(4):325–350.

[28] Russo N, Larson C, Kraus N. Audio-vocal system regulation in children with autism spectrum disorders, Exp Brain Res Springer, 2008;188(1):111–124.

[29] Van Lancker D, Cornelius C, Kreiman J. Recognition of emotional prosodic meanings in speech by autistic, schizophrenic, and normal children. Dev Neuropsychol Taylor & Francis Group, 1989;5(2–3):207–226.

[30] Kanner L. Autistic Disturbances of affective contact. Nerv Child. 1943;2:217–250.

[31] Martínez-Castilla P, Peppé S. Developing a test of prosodic ability for speakers of Iberian-Spanish. Speech Commun (SPECOM), ELSEVIER, 2008;50(11–12):900–915.

[32] Diehl JJ, Paul R. Acoustic Differences in the imitation of prosodic patterns in children with autism spectrum disorders. Res Autism Spectr Disord ELSEVIER, 2012;6(1):123–134.

[33] van Santen JPH, Prud'hommeaux ET, Black LM: Automated assessment of prosody production. Speech Commun (SPECOM), ELSEVIER, 2009;51(11):1082–1097.

[34] Maier A, Haderlein T, Eysholdt U, Rosanowski F, Batliner A, Schuster M, Nöth E. PEAKS – a system for the automatic evaluation of voice and speech disorder. Speech Commun (SPECOM), ELSEVIER, 2009;51(5):425–437.

[35] Black M, Tepperman J, Kazemzadeh A, Lee S, Narayanan S. Automatic pronunciation verification of english letter-names for early literacy assessment of preliterate children. Proc. of ICASSP, Taipei, Taiwan, pp. 4861–4864, April 2009.

[36] Schuller B, Steidl S, Batliner A, Vinciarelli A, Scherer K, Ringeval F, Chetouani M, Weninger F, Eyben F, Marchi E, Salamin H, Polychroniou A, Valente F, Kim S. The INTERSPEECH 2013 computational paralinguistics challenge: social signals, conflict, emotion, autism. Proc. of INTERSPEECH, ISCA, Lyon, France, pp. 148–152, August 2013.

[37] Green P, Carmichael J, Hatzis A, Enderby P, Hawley MS, Parker M. Automatic speech recognition with sparse training data for dysarthric speakers. In INTERSPEECH, Geneva, Switzerland, September 2003.

[38] Yildirim S, Narayanan S. Automatic detection of disfluency boundaries in spontaneous speech of children using audio–visual information. IEEE Trans Audio Speech Lang Process (TASLP), 2009;17(1):2–12.

[39] Ghoshal A, Swietojanski P, Renals S. Multilingual training of deep neural networks. Proc. of ICASSP, Hong Kong, China, April 2013.

[40] Swietojanski P, Ghoshal A, Renals S. Unsupervised cross-lingual knowledge transfer for DNN-based LVCSR. Proc. IEEE Speech Language Technology (SLT), Miami, FL, USA, December 2012.

[41] Thomas S, Hermansky H. Cross-lingual and multistream posterior features for low resource LVCSR systems. Proc. of INTERSPEECH, Makuhari, Chiba, Japan, pp. 877–880, September 2010.

[42] Schuller B, Marchi E, Baron-Cohen S, O'Reilly H, Robinson P, Davies I, Golan O, Friedenson S, Tal S, Newman S, Meir N, Shillo R, Camurri A, Piana S, Bölte S, Lundqvist D, Berggren S, Baranger A, Sullings N. ASC-inclusion: interactive emotion games for social inclusion of children with autism spectrum conditions. Proc. of International Workshop on Intelligent Digital Games for Empowerment and Inclusion (IDGEI 2013) held in conjunction with the 8th Foundations of Digital Games 2013 (FDG), ACM, SASDG Digital Library, Crete, Greece, May 2013.

[43]   Schuller B, Marchi E, Baron-Cohen S, O'Reilly H, Pigat D, Robinson P, Davies I, Golan O, Fridenson S, Tal S, Newman S, Meir N, Shillo R, Camurri A, Piana S, Staglianò Al, Bölte S, Lundqvist D, Berggren S, Baranger A, Sullings N. The state of play of ASC-Inclusion: integrated internet-based environment for social inclusion of children with autism spectrum conditions. Proc. of International Workshop on Digital Games for Empowerment and Inclusion (IDGEI 2014) held in conjunction with the International Conference on Intelligent User Interfaces (IUI 2014), ACM, Haifa, Israel, February 2014.

[44]   American Psychiatric Association: diagnostic and statistical manual of mental disorders, 4th ed. (DSM-IV). American Psychiatric Association: Washington, DC, 1994.

[45]   Wilkinson KM: Profiles of language and communication skills in autism. Mental Retardation Dev Disabilities Res Rev 1998;4(2):73–79.

[46]   Wetherby AM, Prizant BM: Communication and symbolic behavior scales: CSBS. Chicago, IL: Riverside Publ., 1993.

[47]   Lewy AL, Dawson G. Social stimulation and joint attention in young autistic children. Journal of Abnormal Child Psychology 1992;20(6):555–566.

[48]   McArthur D, Adamson LB: Joint attention in preverbal children: Autism and developmental language disorder. J Autism Dev Disord 1996;26(5):481–496.

[49]   Mundy P, Sigman M, Ungerer J, Sherman T. Defining the social deficits of autism: the contribution of non-verbal communication measures. J Child Psychol Psychiatry 1986; 27(5):657–669.

[50]   Wetherby AM: Ontogeny of communicative functions in autism. J Autism Dev Disord 1986;16(3):295–316.

[51]   Prizant BM, Rydell PJ: Assessment and intervention considerations for unconventional verbal behavior. Communicative alternatives to challenging behavior: Integrating functional assessment and intervention strategies. 1993:263–297.

[52]   Tager-Flusberg H, Paul R, Lord C. Language and communication in autism. Handbook of autism and pervasive developmental disorders. 2005;1:335–364.

[53]   Happé F. Understanding minds and metaphors: insights from the study of figurative language in autism. Metaphor Symbol 1995;10(4):275–295.

[54]   Lee A, Hobson RP, Chiat S. I, you, me, and autism: An experimental study. J Autism Dev Disord, 1994;24(2):155–176.

[55]   Bishop DV, Norbury CF: Speech and language disorders. Rutter's child and adolescent psychiatry, 5th ed. 2008:782–801.

[56]   Bishop DVM. Overlaps between autism and language impairment: phenomimicry or shared etiology?. Behav Genet 2010;40(5):618–629.

[57]   Bishop DVM. Pragmatic language impairment: A correlate of SLI, a distinct subgroup, or part of the autistic continuum. Speech and language impairments in children: causes, characteristics, intervention and outcome, 2000:99–113.

[58]   Kjelgaard MM, Tager-Flusberg H. An investigation of language impairment in autism: Implications for genetic subgroups. Lang Cogn Process 2001;16(2–3):287–308.

[59]   Tager-Flusberg H, Joseph RM: Identifying neurocognitive phenotypes in autism. Philos Trans R Soc London. Series B: Biol Sci 2003;358(1430):303–314.

[60]   Whitehouse AJ, Barry JG, Bishop DV. Further defining the language impairment of autism: Is there a specific language impairment subtype? J Commun Disord 2008;41(4):319–336.

[61]   Bishop DV, North T, Donlan C. Nonword repetition as a behavioural marker for inherited language impairment: Evidence from a twin study. J Child Psychol Psychiatry 1996; 37(4):391–403.

[62]   Conti-Ramsden G, Botting N, Faragher B. Psycholinguistic markers for specific language impairment (SLI). J Child Psychol Psychiatry 2001;42(6):741–748.

[63]   Short A, Schopler E. Factors relating to age of onset in autism. J Autism Dev Disord 1988;18 (2):207–216.

[64]   Brown J, Prelock P. Brief report: The impact of regression on language development in autism. J Autism Dev Disord 1995;25(3):305–309.

[65]   Lord C, Shulman C, DiLavore P. Regression and word loss in autistic spectrum disorders. J Child Psychol Psychiatry 2004;45(5):936–955.

[66]   DeMyer M, Barton S, DeMyer W, Norton J, Allen J, Steele R. Prognosis in autism: A follow-up study. J Autism Childhood Schizophr 1973;3(3):199–246.

[67]   Paul R, Cohen D. Outcomes of severe disorders of language acquisition. J Autism Dev Disord, 1984;14(4):405–421.

[68]   Venter A, Lord C, Schopler E A follow-up study of high-functioning autistic children. J Child Psychol Psychiatry, 1992;33(3):489–597.

[69]   Mundy P, Sigman M, Kasari C. A longitudinal study of joint attention and language development in autistic children. J Autism Dev Disord, 1990;20(1):115–128.

[70]   Cantwell D, Baker L, Rutter M, Mawhood L. Infantile autism and developmental receptive dysphasia: A comparative follow-up into middle childhood. J Autism Dev Disord 1989; 19(1):19–31.

[71]   Baltaxe C, Simmons J III: Prosodic development in normal and autistic children. Communication Problems in Autism. Springer US, 1985:95–125.

[72]   Rutter M, Mawhood L, Howlin P. Language delay and social development. Specific Speech Lang Disord Children 1992:63–78.

[73]   Tager-Flusberg H. Strategies for conducting research on language in autism. J Autism Dev Disord 2004;34(1):75–80.

[74]   Tager-Flusberg H. A psycholinguistic perspective on language development in the autistic child. Autism: Nature Diagn Treat 1989:92–115.

[75]   World-Health-Organization. ICD-10 – International classification of diseases. 10th ed. Geneva, Switzerland: World Health Organisation; 1994.

[76]   Celani G, Battacchi M, Arcidiacono L. The understanding of the emotional meaning of facial expressions in people with autism. J Autism Dev Disord. 1999;29(1):57–66.

[77]   Deruelle C, Rondan C, Gepner B, Tardif C. Spatial frequency and face processing in children with autism and Asperger syndrome. J Autism Dev Disord. 2004;34(2):199–210.

[78]   Golan O, Baron-Cohen S, Hill J. The Cambridge Mindreading (CAM) Face-Voice Battery: testing complex emotion recognition in adults with and without Asperger Syndrome. J Autism Dev Disord. 2006;36(2):169–183.

[79]   Hobson R. The autistic child's appraisal of expressions of emotion. J Child Psychol Psychiatry. 1986;27:321–342.

[80]   Boucher J, Lewis V, Collis G. Voice processing abilities in children with autism, children with specific language impairments, and young typically developing children. J Child Psychol Psychiatry All Discip 2000;41(7):847–857.

[81]   Golan O, Baron-Cohen S, Hill J, Rutherford M. The 'Reading the Mind in the Voice' test – Revised: A study of complex emotion recognition in adults with and without Autism Spectrum Conditions. J Autism Dev Disord. 2007;37(6):1096–1106.

[82]   Grezes J, Wicker B, Berthoz S, de Gelder B. A failure to grasp the affective meaning of actions in autism spectrum disorder subjects. Neuropsychologia 2009;47(8–9): 1816–1825.

[83]   Philip R, Whalley H, Stanfield A, Sprengelmeyer R, Santos I, Young A. Deficits in facial, body movement and vocal emotional processing in autism spectrum disorders. Psychol Med 2010;40(11):1919–1929.

[84]   Golan O, Baron-Cohen S, Golan Y. The 'Reading the Mind in Films' Task [child version]: complex emotion and mental state recognition in children with and without autism spectrum conditions. J Autism Dev Disord. 2008;38(8):1534–1541.

[85]   Silverman L, Bennetto L, Campana E, Tanenhaus M. Speech-and-gesture integration in high functioning autism. Cognition 2010;115(3):380–393.

[86]   Yirmiya N, Sigman MD, Kasari C, Mundy P. Empathy and cognition in high-functioning children with autism. Child Dev 1992;63:150–160.

[87]   Kasari C, Sigman M, Mundy P, Yirmiya N. Affective sharing in the context of joint attention interactions of normal, autistic, and mentally retarded children. J Autism Dev Disord. 1990;20(1):87–100.

[88]   Kasari C, Sigman M, Yirmiya N, Mundy P. Affective development and communication in young children with autism. Enhancing Children's Communication: Research Foundation for Early Language Interventions. New York: Paul H. Brooks; 1993:201–222.

[89]   Kasari C, Chamberlain B, Bauminger N. Social emotions and social relationships: Can children with autism compensate? The Development of Autism: Perspectives from Theory and Research. Mahwah, NJ: Lawrence Erlbaum, 2001:309–323.

[90]   H Macdonald, M Rutter, P Howlin, P Rios, A Le Conteur, C Evered: Recognition and expression of emotional cues by autistic and normal adults. J Child Psychol Psychiatry 1989;30(6):865–877.

[91]   Paul R, Augustyn A, Klin A, Volkmar F. Perception and production of prosody by speakers with autism spectrum disorders. J Autism Dev Disord 2005;35(2):205–220.

[92]   Attwood T. Asperger's syndrome: a guide for parents and professionals. London: Jessica Kingsley, 1998.

[93]   de Marchena A, Eigsti I. Conversational gestures in autism spectrum disorders: asynchrony but not decreased frequency. Autism Res 2010;3(6):311–322.

[94]   Keltner D, Ekman P. Facial expression of emotion. In: Lewis M, Haviland-Jones JM, editors. Handbook of Emotions.New York: Guilford Press, 2000:236–249.

[95]   Ververidis D, Kotropoulos C. Emotional speech recognition: resources, features, and methods. Speech Commun 2006;48(9):1162–1181.

[96]   Schuller B, Steidl S, Batliner A. The INTERSPEECH 2009 emotion challenge. Proc. of INTERSPEECH, ISCA, Brighton, UK, ISSN 1990-9772, 2009:312–315.

[97]   Schuller B, Steidl S, Batliner A, Burkhardt F, Devillers L, Müller C, Narayanan S. The INTERSPEECH 2010 paralinguistic challenge. Proc. of INTERSPEECH, ISCA, Makuhari, Japan, pp. 2794–2797, 26–30.09.2010.

[98]   Burkhardt F, Paeschke A, Rolfes M, Sendlmeier W, Weiss B. A database of German emotional speech. Proc. of INTERSPEECH, Lissabon, Portugal, pp 1517–1520. 2005.

[99]   Zeng Z, Pantic M, Roisman GI, Huang TS. A Survey of affect recognition methods: audio, visual, and spontaneous expressions. IEEE Trans Pattern Anal Mach Intell 2009;31(1):39–58.

[100] Schmidt K, Bhattacharya S, Denlinger R. Comparison of deliberate and spontaneous facial movement in smiles and eyebrow raises. J Nonverbal Behav 2009;33:35–45.

[101] Douglas-Cowie E, Campbell N, Cowie R, Roach P. Emotional speech: Towards a new generation of databases. Speech Commun 2003;4(1–2):33–60.

[102] Cowie R, Gunes H, McKeown G, Vaclavu-Schneider L, Armstrong J, Douglas-Cowie E. The emotional and communicative significance of head nods and shakes in a naturalistic

database. Proc. of the Workshop on Corpora for research on Emotion and Affect, LREC 2010 pp. 42–46, 2010.

[103] Devillers L, Cowie R, Martin J-C, Douglas-Cowie E, Abrilian S, McRorie M,: Real life emotions in French and English TV video clips: an integrated annotation protocol combining continuous and discrete approaches. Proc. of International Conference on Language Resources and Evaluation (LREC), Genoa, Italy, 2006.

[104] Loveland KA, Tunali-Kotoski B, Chen YR, Ortegon J, Pearson DA, Brelsford KA, Gibbs MC. Emotion recognition in autism: verbal and nonverbal information. Dev Psychopathol 1997;9:579–593. Cambridge University Press.

[105] Marchi E, Schuller B, Baron-Cohen S, Golan O, Bölte S, Arora P, Häb-Umbach R. Typicality and emotion in the voice of children with autism spectrum condition: evidence across three languages. Proc. of INTERSPEECH, Dresden, Germany, pp. 115–119, ISCA, September 2015.

[106] Ringeval F, Marchi E, Grossard C, Xavier J, Chetouani M, Cohen D, Schuller B. Automatic analysis of typical and atypical encoding of spontaneous emotion in the voice of children. Proc. of INTERSPEECH, San Francisco, CA, pp. 1210–1214, ISCA, September 2016.

[107] Schmitt M, Marchi E, Ringeval F, Schuller B. Towards cross-lingual automatic diagnosis of autism spectrum condition in children's voices. Proc. of ITG Conference on Speech Communication, vol. 267 of ITG-Fachbericht, Paderborn, Germany, pp. 264–268, ITG/VDE, IEEE/VDE, October 2016

[108] Marchi E, Frühholz S, Schuller B. The Effect of narrowband transmission on recognition of paralinguistic information from human vocalizations. IEEE Access 2016;4:6059–6072.

[109] Batliner A, Seppi D, Steidl S, Schuller B. Segmenting into adequate units for automatic recognition of emotion-related episodes: a speech-based approach, Advances in Human Computer Interaction (AHCI), Special Issue on Emotion-Aware Natural Interaction, Hindawi Publishing Corporation, vol. 2010, Article ID 782802, 15 pages, 2010.

[110] Hudenko WJ, Stone W, Bachorowski J. Laughter Differs in Children with Autism: An Acoustic Analysis of Laughs Produced by Children With and Without the Disorder, J Autism Dev Disord 2009;39(10):1392–1400.

[111] Batliner A, Steidl S, Eyben F, Schuller B. Laughter in child-robot interaction. Proc. of Interdisciplinary Workshop on Laughter and other Interactional Vocalisations in Speech (Laughter 2009), Berlin, Germany, 27.-28.02.2009.

[112] Batliner A, Steidl S, Eyben F, Schuller B. On Laughter and Speech Laugh, Based on Observations of Child-Robot Interaction, to appear in The Phonetics of Laughing, Jürgen Trouvain, Nick Campbell (eds.), Trends in Linguistics, Mouton de Gruyter, Berlin and New York, 23 pages, 2010.

[113] Eyben F, Petridis S, Schuller B, Tzimiropoulos G, Zafiriou S, Pantic M. Audiovisual classification of vocal outbursts in human conversation using long-short-term memory networks. Proc. of ICASSP, Special Session on Audio/Visual Detection of Non-Linguistic Vocal Outbursts, IEEE, Prague, Czech Republic, May 2011.

[114] Schuller B, Eyben F, Rigoll G. Static and dynamic modelling for the recognition of nonverbal vocalisations in conversational speech, in perception in multimodal dialogue systems. Proc. of IEEE Tutorial and Research Workshop on Perception and Interactive Technologies for Speech-based Systems (PIT 2008), Springer LNCS Volume 5078/2008, ISBN 978-3-540-69368-0, Springer Berlin/ Heidelberg,pp. 99–110, Kloster Irsee, Germany, 16.-18.06.2008.

[115] Weninger F, Schuller B, Wöllmer M, Rigoll G. Localization of non-linguistic events in spontaneous speech by non-negative matrix factorization and long short-term memory. Proc. of ICASSP, Special Session on Audio/Visual Detection of Non-Linguistic Vocal Outbursts, IEEE, Prague, Czech Republic, May 2011.

[116] Eyben F, Woellmer M, Graves A, Schuller B, Douglas-Cowie E, Cowie R. On-line emotion recognition in a 3-D activation-valence-time continuum using acoustic and linguistic cues. J Multimodal User Interfaces 2010; 3 (1-2): 7–19.

[117] Schuller B, Rigoll G. Timing levels in segment-based speech emotion recognition. Proc. of INTERSPEECH, Pittsburgh, pp. 1818–1821, 2006.

[118] Batliner A, Steidl S, Schuller B, Seppi D, Laskowski K, Vogt T, Devillers L, Vidrascu L, Amir N, Kessous L, Aharonson V. Combining efforts for improving automatic classification of emotional user states, in Language Technologies, IS-LTC 2006, Ljubljana, Slovenia, pp. 240–245, Infornacijska Druzba (Information Society), 2006.

[119] Fernandez R, Picard RW: Classical and novel discriminant features for affect recognition from speech. Proc. of INTERSPEECH, Lisbon, Portugal, pp. 473–476, ISCA, 2005.

[120] Pachet F, Roy P. Analytical Features: A Knowledge-based approach to audio feature generation. J Audio Speech Music Process EURASIP, pp. 1–23, 2009.

[121] Schuller B, Batliner A, Seppi D, Steidl S, Vogt T, Wagner J, Devillers L, Vidrascu L, Amir N, Kessous L, Aharonson V. The Relevance of feature type for the automatic classification of emotional user states: low level descriptors and functionals. Proc. of INTERSPEECH, pp. 2253–2256, 2007.

[122] Schuller B, Wimmer M, Mösenlechner L, Kern C, Arsic D, Rigoll G. Brute-forcing hierarchical functionals for paralinguistics: a waste of feature space?. Proc. of ICASSP, pp. 4501–4504, 2008.

[123] Eyben F, Woellmer M, Schuller B. openEAR – introducing the munich open-source emotion and affect recognition toolkit2. Proc. of ACII, Amsterdam, The Netherlands, pp. 576–581, 2009.

[124] Marchi E, Batliner A, Schuller B, Fridenzon S, Tal S, Golan O. Speech, emotion, age, language, task and typicality: trying to disentangle performance and feature relevance. Proc. of International Workshop on Wide Spectrum Social Signal Processing (WS3P), Satellite Event of the International Conference on Social Computing (SocialCom), Amsterdam, Netherlands, pp. 961–968, September 2012.

[125] Marchi E, Schuller B, Batliner A, Fridenzon S, Tal S, Golan O. Emotion in the speech of children with autism spectrum conditions: prosody and everything else. Proc. of Workshop on Child, Computer and Interaction (WOCCI), Satellite Event of INTERSPEECH, Portland, ISCA, OR, September 2012.

[126] Marchi E, Schuller B, Baron-Cohen S, Lassalle A, O'Reilly H, Pigat D, Golan O, Friedenson S, Tal S, Bölte S, Berggren S, Lundqvist D, Elfström MS. Voice emotion games: language and emotion in the voice of children with autism spectrum condition. Proc. of International Workshop on Intelligent Digital Games for Empowerment and Inclusion (IDGEI 2015) as part of the ACM International Conference on Intelligent User Interfaces, Atlanta, GA, ACM, March 2015. 9 pages.

[127] Schuller B, Rigoll G, Lang M. Speech emotion recognition combining acoustic features and linguistic information in a hybrid support vector machine – belief network architecture. Proc. of ICASSP, Montreal, Quebec, Canada, pp. 577–580, IEEE, 2004.

[128] Wöllmer M, Schuller B, Eyben F, Rigoll G. Combining long short-term memory and dynamic bayesian networks for incremental emotion-sensitive artificial listening. IEEE Journal of

Selected Topics in Signal Processing (J-STSP), Special Issue on Speech Processing for Natural Interaction with Intelligent Environments, 2010, vol. 4, no. 5, IEEE.

[129] Wöllmer M, Eyben F, Graves A, Schuller B, Rigoll G. Bidirectional LSTM networks for context-sensitive keyword detection in a virtual agent framework, cognitive computation. Special Issue on Non-Linear Non-Conventional Speech Process 2010;2(3):Springer.

[130] Steidl S, Batliner A, Seppi D, Schuller B. On the impact of children's emotional speech on acoustic and language models. EURASIP J Audio Speech Music Process (JASMP), Special Issue on Atypical Speech, Hindawi Publishing Corporation, 2010;2010(783954):14.

[131] Marchi E, Ringeval F, Schuller B. Voice-enabled assistive robots for handling autism spectrum conditions: an examination of the role of prosody, Speech and Automata in Health Care (Speech Technology and Text Mining in Medicine and Healthcare), De Gruyter, 2014, pp. 207–236.

[132] Sabouret N, Schuller B, Paletta L, Marchi E, Jones H, Youssef AB. Intelligent user interfaces in digital games for empowerment and inclusion. Proc. of International Conference on Advancement in Computer Entertainment Technology, ACE 2015, Iskandar, Malaysia, ACM, November 2015. 8 pages,

[133] Bölte S, Hubl D, Feineis-Matthews S, Prvulovic D, Dierks T, Poustka F, Facial affect recognition training in autism: can we animate the fusiform gyrus? Behav Neurosci 2006;120(1):211.

[134] Silver M, Oakes P, Evaluation of a new computer intervention to teach people with autism or Asperger syndrome to recognize and predict emotions in others. Autism 5 2001;3:299–316.

[135] Tanaka JW, Wolf JM, Klaiman C, Koenig K, Cockburn J, Herlihy L, Brown C, Stahl S, Kaiser MD, Schultz RT, Using computerized games to teach face recognition skills to children with autism spectrum disorder: the let's face it! program, J Child Psychol Psychiatry 51 2010;8:944–952.

[136] Baron-Cohen S, Golan O, Wheelwright S, Hill JJ. Mind reading: The interactive guide to emotions. London: Jessica Kingsley, 2004.

[137] Baron-Cohen S, Golan O, Chapman E, Granader Y. Transported to a world of emotion. Psychol 2007;20(2):76–77.

[138] Mower E, Black M, Flores E, Flores E, Williams M, Narayanan S. Rachel: design of an emotionally targeted interactive agent for children with autism. Proc. of International Conference on Multimedia & Expo (ICME), Barcelona, Spain, pp. 1–6, July 2011.

[139] Schuller B, Marchi E, Baron-Cohen S, Lassalle A, O'Reilly H, Pigat D, Robinson P, Davies I, Baltrusaitis T, Mahmoud M, Golan O, Friedenson S, Tal S, Newman S, Meir N, Shillo R, Camurri A, Piana S, Stagliano A, Bölte S, Lundqvist D, Berggren S, Baranger A, Sullings N, Sezgin M, Alyuz N, Rynkiewicz A, Ptaszek K, Ligmann K. Recent developments and results of ASC-Inclusion: An integrated internet-based environment for social inclusion of children with autism spectrum conditions. Proc. of International Workshop on Intelligent Digital Games for Empowerment and Inclusion (IDGEI 2015) as part of the ACM International Conference on Intelligent User Interfaces, IUI 2015, Atlanta, GA, ACM, March 2015, 9 pages.

[140] Rudovic O, Evers V, Pantic M, Schuller B, Petrovic S. DE-ENIGMA robots: playfully empowering children with autism. Proc. of XI Autism-Europe International Congress, Edinburgh, Scotland, Autism Europe, The National Autistic Society, September 2016. 1 page.

[141] Rudovic O, Lee J, Mascarell-Maricic L, Schuller BW, Picard R. Measuring engagement in autism therapy with social robots: a cross-cultural study, frontiers in robotics and AI, section humanoid robotics. Special Issue on Affective Soc Signals HRI 2017;4(36):1–17.

Joshua John Diehl

7 Clinical applications of speech technology for Autism Spectrum Disorder

Abstract: Individuals with Autism Spectrum Disorder (ASD) show considerable variability in their speech deficits, but some aspects of the speech signal are considered some of the most identifying features of the disorder. Research on speech performance in individuals with ASD has noted that differences from peers are the norm, but the differences range from deficits in the functional linguistic/ affective uses of prosody to more subtle differences in the manner in which prosody is used in communication. In this chapter, we discuss recently how technological developments show promise for early identification of vocal deficits in ASD and the potential for speech technology to improve treatment of the disorder. We will discuss the clinical characteristics of ASD, the early diagnosis of ASD,and the latest discoveries in terms of the use of speech technology for the early identification and diagnosis of ASD, an area which has received an explosion of cutting edge research in the past decade. We will then explore the applications of speech technology to clinical therapy, where theoretical applications such as voice modeling hold a lot of promise. Throughout the chapter, we will highlight the importance of interdisciplinary collaboration between speech and clinical scientists, and we will identify the most pressing areas in need of research.

Keywords: Autism Spectrum Disorder (ASD), communication, Language, speech technology, psycholinguistics, prosody

7.1 Clinical applications of speech technology for autism spectrum disorder

Autism Spectrum Disorder (ASD) is a neurodevelopmental disorder that affects approximately 1 in 68 individuals [1].[1] ASD is characterized by deficits in social-communication and restricted, repetitive behavior patterns/interests [2]. It is important to note that it is defined by a set of behaviors, rather than an etiology, which makes accurate behavioral measurement and characterization crucial for

---

[1] Estimates of incidence/prevalence of ASD vary. Estimates have been both slightly higher and slightly lower, but for the purposes of this chapter, we are referencing the number used by the Centers for Disease Control and Prevention.

https://doi.org/10.1515/9781501502415-008

diagnosis and early identification. Unfortunately, many of the distinguishing features of ASD, such as pragmatic and prosodic deficits, are difficult to measure using available tools. Moreover, many of the core criteria used to diagnose ASD fully emerge after the first two years of life, making early identification/diagnosis challenging. Even after appropriate diagnosis and treatment, many individuals with ASD who develop fluent spoken language (sometimes called "high-functioning autism," [3]) have persistent difficulties in aspects of pragmatics and vocal communication, despite years of empirically supported intervention targeting expressive and receptive language and communication.

In this chapter, we discuss recently how a number of technological developments show promise for early identification of vocal deficits in ASD and how voice modeling has the potential to do for speech what video modeling has done for behavior in the treatment of the disorder. First, we discuss the clinical characteristics of ASD, focusing on aspects that are directly related to vocal communication. Next, we examine the early diagnosis of ASD and focus on specific aspects of vocal communication that show promise for early detection. Finally, we investigate the latest discoveries in terms of the use of speech technology for the early identification and diagnosis of ASD, an area which has received an explosion of cutting edge research in the past decade. Throughout the chapter, we will highlight the importance of interdisciplinary collaboration between speech and clinical scientists, and we will identify the most pressing areas in need of research.

7.2 Clinical characteristics of communication in ASD

One of the two main diagnostic criteria for ASD (refer Table 7.1) is the presence of deficits in social communication and social interaction [2]. This broad diagnostic criterion represents the combination of previously separate criteria (social inter-action, communication) in the previous version of the diagnostic criteria [4]. This category encompasses deficits in social reciprocity, non-verbal communication, and maintaining relationships, all of which represent broad sub-categories that contain a diverse number of behaviors. For example, deficits in "non-verbal" communication could be represented by differences in gesture, facial expression, prosody, and/or body language, or even poorly integrated verbal and non-verbal communication. Importantly, there is no concrete behavioral manifestation of the deficits, and there is considerable individual variability in how the deficits appear in the ASD population [5].

Table 7.1: DSM-5 Autism spectrum disorder diagnostic criteria (American Psychiatric Association, 2013).

A.	Deficits in social communication and social interaction (currently or historically), including: a. Deficits in social-emotional reciprocity (e.g., conversation, social interactions) b. Deficits in non-verbal communicative behaviors used for social interaction (e.g., verbal and non-verbal communication) c. Deficits in developing and maintaining, and understanding relationships (e.g., difficulties with play or making friends)
B.	Restricted, repetitive patterns of behavior, interests, or activities (currently or historically), including at least two of the following: a. Stereotyped or repetitive motor movements, speech, or use of objects b. Insistence on sameness, inflexible adherence to routines, or ritualized patterns of behavior c. Highly restricted, fixated, or circumscribed interests d. Hyper- or hyporeactivity to sensory input or unusual interest in sensory aspects of the environment
C.	Symptoms must be present in early developmental period
D.	Symptoms cause clinically significant impairment in social, occupational, or other areas of current functioning
E.	Disturbances are not better explained by intellectual disability or global developmental delay

Generally speaking, deficits in the pragmatics of communication are pervasive throughout the autism spectrum, whereas speech and language deficits are more variable [6, 7]. Still, certain aspects of vocal communication have been consistently discussed as features of the disorder through all of the diagnostic changes and are often some of the most identifying characteristics of individuals with ASD. Even in the earliest characterizations of the disorder, both Leo Kanner and Hans Asperger described differences in the manner in which their patients communicated [8–10]. Asperger noted:

> one can invariably pick up these kinds of abnormalities in the language of autistic individuals, and their recognition is, therefore, of particular diagnostic importance... [8]; as translated by [11]).

Asperger also described the considerable variability that he perceived in the speech of his patients. He said that the individuals could sound soft, shrill, or have intonation that had a singsong quality or did not fall at the end of a declarative statement. Asperger emphasized that "we do not intellectually understand many of these qualities and can only feel them intuitively" (p. 70).

Beyond these original descriptions, there has been considerable variability in the descriptions of the speech patterns of individuals with ASD, and the one unifying characteristic among the different descriptions is the fact that individuals with ASD display differences in speech production (especially in prosody performance) in ways that distinguish them from their peers. For example, clinical and research descriptions of prosodic patterns in individuals with ASD have ranged from flat or monotonous to variable, pedantic, and/or having a singsong quality [12–16]. These prosodic differences often persist even when other areas of language improve after intervention [17] and can be seen as a stigmatizing barrier to social acceptance [18]. Prosodic differences have been found to be significantly related to general ratings of social and communicative functioning as well, which emphasizes their close relationship to the diagnostic criteria [19, 20]. Based on clinical observations and descriptive research, it is clear that understanding prosodic differences in ASD is both important and difficult [21–23]. As such, prosody performance has been the major focus of research relating to the speech signal in individuals with ASD [23, 24].

There have been numerous attempts to measure and quantify the speech characteristics of individuals with ASD, with a particular focus on aspects of prosody. Initially, there were a number of studies that examined putative prosody processing deficits that could underlie (and possibly explain) production differences. This was an important step in understanding prosody and its relationship to speech functioning in ASD. Several aspects of language comprehension precede production in early development [25, 26]. Prosody processing has been shown to facilitate other aspects of early language development [27]. Perception of prosodic features is present during the first year of life. Infants with 7–10 months of age have been shown to prefer filtered speech (with no consonant information; containing only vowels and intonation contours) that matches the prosodic patterns of the language they are learning [28]. Filtered speech with "motherese" prosody (marked by higher pitch and wider pitch excursions, [29]) is preferred by infants as early as one month of age over speech with adult-directed characteristics [30, 31]. Infants in the first year of life have been shown to be sensitive to both pauses as signals to syntactic units within sentences [32] and to stress patterns within and across words [33].

Many of the early studies focused on understanding emotion in the voice, given the rich literature on the difficulties of individuals with ASD with emotional understanding (see [34, 35], for reviews). This research had deep roots in the theory that individuals with ASD had primary deficits in understanding Theory of Mind. A large number of studies found differences in processing emotion in the voice of individuals with ASD (e.g., [20, 36–41], although these findings were not

universal [42–44]. As a result, studies looked at comprehension of both pragmatic (e.g., [20, 37, 45–47] and grammatical [45–51] aspects of prosody in individuals with ASD. Even with extensive research in this area, there still does not
seem to be a clear consensus in the pattern of prosody processing in individuals
with ASD.

There is a similar amount of inconsistency found in research on productive
aspects of prosody. Moreover, it would be important to consider production
differences even in the absence of comprehension deficits, because there is
evidence that production deficits persist, even with receptive abilities intact
[52]. Initial studies in the area focused on clinical judgments/ratings and simple
forced choice behavioral tasks to examine prosodic production (e.g., [20, 47]). As
would be expected, these findings were mixed. Many times, tasks were either too
simple or too difficult for the participants and were not sensitive to subtle
differences that were picked up in clinical evaluations ([17, 20, 21, 53].
Moreover, there were considerable individual differences, with one study noting
that there were not consistent patterns of differences in any particular area of
prosodic functioning across the entire group and that the only major consistency
was that the majority of individuals with ASD struggled in one or more areas of
prosodic functioning [47].

Given these trends, a number of research groups started focusing on the
speech signal as a way to examine subtle differences in prosody production in
individuals with ASD. Acoustic analysis of speech afforded a number of benefits that have greatly enhanced the research conducted in this area [54].
Acoustic analyses are more objective in that they rely on data, rather than
subjective judgments of behavior. Additionally, acoustic analyses might be
more sensitive to subtle differences in the "manner" of speaking, which allows
us to shift focus away from the correct application of a linguistic concept (e.g.,
stress marking, discourse structure) and more toward stylistic components of
speech (e.g., is prosody more variable than expected?). Perhaps most importantly, the identification of acoustic markers might enable the use of automated analyses to identify and distinguish the speech of individuals with ASD
(and possibly other groups with speech-related deficits) from their typically
developing peers.

A number of studies indicated the potential for increased variability in the
fundamental frequency (f0) in the speech of individuals with ASD of varying
age ranges. These differences were found during speech that was echolalic
[55–62] in nature. For example, Diehl et al. [59] increased f0 during narrative
retelling of highly verbal individuals with ASD in two different samples (children and adolescents), and these differences were found to be related
to diagnostic measures. Studies have also found notable differences in the

duration of utterances ([50, 57, 58, 63]. Importantly, research has shown that these differences are present both for correct and incorrect examples of the functional use of prosody [54], indicating that prosodic production differences might be most accurately linked to the manner of speaking, rather than necessarily to its application to linguistic or affective concepts [61]. Moreover, in almost all of these studies, there was considerable overlap between the groups, and although acoustic differences often differentiated ASD groups from typically developing peers, they did not always differentiate individuals with ASD from other clinical groups [54, 57], and did not always map onto subjective clinical ratings of behavior [64]. These latter two findings highlight the challenges that individual differences present for using acoustic measures for clinical purposes [23, 53].

More and more, researchers are focusing on the extent to which ASD can be diagnosed in the first two years of life. Early diagnosis is crucial because early diagnosis leads to early intervention, which is predictive of positive outcomes for individuals with the disorder [65]. As such, there is an urgent search for early diagnostic characteristics of the disorder. Unfortunately, many of the diagnostic criteria emerge later in development, and the focus has shifted from these diagnostic cues to their precursors.

Aspects of vocal communication have shown some promise as identifying characteristics of ASD. As part of a longitudinal study, Wetherby et al. [66] identified unusual prosody and difficulty coordinating vocal communication with non-verbal communication as two of the nine early diagnostic markers for infants and toddlers with ASD. Paul et al. [67] tracked vocal production in the younger siblings of individuals born with ASD at 6, 9, and 12 months. Because of the strong contribution of genetics to the etiology of ASD, these individuals are considered to be at higher risk for developing an ASD. Paul and colleagues compared vocal communication in these infants to that of infants who did not have an older sibling with an ASD (i.e., low-risk infants). Infant siblings produced fewer "speech-like" vocalizations, and an increased number of non-speech vocalizations (sounds without characteristics of native language speech). This finding included fewer babbling sounds that resembled consonants and canonical syllable shapes. Patten et al. [68] also found differences in canonical babbling and vocalizations in individuals later diagnosed with ASD in a retrospective video study. In contrast, a study by Schoen et al. [69] did not find phonological differences in the speech of toddlers with ASD in comparison with age- and language-matched peers. However, Schoen and colleagues did replicate a finding that toddlers with ASD produce a larger number of atypical vocalizations (such as squeals and other non-linguistic sounds) in their speech [66, 69, 70].

A compelling series of studies by Esposito and colleagues examined the acoustic characteristics of cries made by infants (refer [71], for a review). In an initial study, Esposito and Venuti [72] found that the cries of 3- to 5-year olds with ASD were acoustically different than those of their typically developing peers and peers with an intellectual disability. Moreover, it was harder for parents to ascribe a communicative intent to the cries (e.g., hungry, tired, etc.). A subsequent study [73] examined interactions between mothers and infants/toddlers with ASD (approximately 1 year old) and found that the cries of the infants with ASD had less waveform modulation and greater dysphonation. Similar to the previous study, it appeared that mothers of individuals with ASD also had trouble interpreting these cries. Esposito and Venuti [74] used retrospective videos to examine the fundamental frequency of cries by individuals with ASD compared with typically developing peers and peers with developmental disabilities. The researchers found that individuals with ASD on average had a higher fundamental frequency to their cries, which is thought to be a more distressed and aversive cry. Moreover, the authors subsequently found that vocal cries were more atypical indicators of distress in 18-month olds with ASD (in comparison with typically developing peers and peers with developmental disabilities) than were other distress cues such as facial and body cues [75]. These acoustic cues (in particular high fundamental frequency and shorter pause duration) were then found to be cross-culturally significant, different, and atypical indicators of distress in infants with ASD [76].

Findings from the Esposito group on cry acoustics were replicated and extended by a separate group of researchers [77]. Sheinkopf and colleagues looked at cry acoustics of infant siblings of individuals with ASD (high-risk group) in comparison with infants without a sibling with ASD at 6 months of age. The authors found a higher and more variable fundamental frequency in the cries of infant siblings of individuals with ASD. Moreover, of those infant siblings who were later diagnosed with ASD at 36 months, their fundamental frequency was the highest and most variable of all participants.

In sum, it is clear that aspects of vocal communication have the potential to be used as clinical indicators of ASD. Additionally, aspects of vocal communication have been isolated as some of the main targets for the early diagnosis of ASD. Still, both in early development and later in life, it appears that even in the most studied characteristics of vocal communication (e.g., prosody), there is considerable variability in vocal performance of individuals with ASD. Moreover, there is meaningful overlap between individuals with ASD and comparison groups, such as peers with intellectual and developmental disabilities and typically developing peers. These behavioral profiles present numerous challenges for clinical applications of speech technology.

7.3 Role of speech technology in ASD diagnosis

ASD is defined and diagnosed based on a set of behaviors, which differentiates it from diagnoses such as Down syndrome (Trisomy 21) or Williams–Beuren syndrome (chromosome 7 q11.23 deletion), which have a known etiological pathway. There is no biological or medical test that can easily identify the disorder, and categorically differentiate it from other conditions. Therefore, the current tests used to diagnosis rely on behavioral observations and parent report. The idea of using the speech signal and prosody in, particular, clinical diagnosis is not novel to the field; in fact, in early stages of ASD research, it was proposed that prosodic differences were a key to differential diagnosis between previous diagnostic categories, such as Autistic Disorder and Asperger Syndrome [78]. In this section, we will review current diagnostic tools for ASD, discuss the potential role of speech technology, and then review research on available tools.

The current gold-standard diagnostic tools for ASD are the Autism Diagnostic Observation Schedule, 2nd Edition (ADOS-2, [79]) and the Autism Diagnostic Interview-Revised (ADI-R, [80]). The ADOS-2 is a semi-structured interview that attempts to elicit social behaviors with age-appropriate tasks and conversational topics. It has different modules that make it appropriate to a wide range of individuals with ASD (toddlers through adulthood). In essence, diagnostic characteristics (including deficits in vocal communication) are subjectively rated by the examiner based on clinical observation during the session. The ADI-R is a detailed diagnostic and developmental interview that relies on parent report of a child's current level of functioning and historical performance in social-communication including vocal communication. There are a number of other checklists that can be used, most of which involve parent report. None of these instruments are sufficient for a diagnosis; clinical judgment using the DSM diagnostic criteria is still the primary mode of diagnosis. Still, these instruments often help provide tangible examples of social performance in individuals with ASD that are quite useful in making diagnoses.

There are currently very few options available clinicians when assessing prosodic performance, and those that are available, such as the Profiling Elements of Prosody in Speech-Communication (PEPS-C, [81]), and the Prosody Voice Screening Profile (PVSP, [82]) are time-consuming and lack standardization. In terms of assessing prosody, Diehl and Paul [21] outlined a number of important areas of consideration, both for behavioral measures and for automated measures of acoustic characteristics of the speech signal if the assessment will be used for clinical evaluation/diagnosis. Any test of prosodic performance should have: (1) a representative (normative) comparison sample,

(2) sensitivity to developmental changes, (3) the ability to examine different functions of prosody such as affect and discourse structure, (4) tasks with ecological validity, and (5) practicality for evaluations, including ease of administration.

It is most likely that automated measures of the speech signal will serve as a similar function to the behavioral and parent-report ASD diagnostic tests (ADOS-2, ADI-R), although the range of behaviors they would describe would be much smaller than these tests. It should be noted that automated analysis of speech would likely be most useful for the early identification of speech/language delays to identify infants at high-risk for developing ASD and other language/communication disorders. For example, programs that can analyze vocal communication characteristics could be useful to a clinician in that they could provide early indicators that an infant or toddler was displaying atypical cry or vocal acoustics (e.g.,[73, 83]). It is unlikely that they would be used for a definitive diagnosis, given that there are so many behavioral factors that go into a diagnosis beyond the speech signal. An additional obstacle would be that there is considerable individual variability and overlap between individuals with ASD and comparison groups with and without language impairments. In essence, there are not clear known categorical boundaries that differentiate individuals with ASD from other populations on these measures as of right now. As such, it is probably important to consider these tools as one component in a diagnostic process.

Another potential clinical benefit to automated tools would be a measurement of behavioral improvement, which has been a serious challenge in the ASD field [84]. At this current stage, most clinical measurements of speech and prosodic improvement are based on subjective measures [81, 82]. In theory, automated measures of vocal performance would give objective, quantifiable measures of improvement in vocal performance. Still, the challenge continues to be identifying the vocal characteristics that would be useful to target in therapy, and what change would look like in these measures.

Even when considering these obstacles, there are a number of research groups who have started to examine automated measurement and analysis of speech patterns as potential diagnostic measures and tools to measure behavioral change. One tool that has been used in a number of studies is the Language Environment Analysis (LENA) system [85–87]. The LENA system is worn by the child, collects naturalistic speech/sound data from the environment and can record up to 16 h of continuous data. It provides automatic reports of data such as child/adult vocalizations, conversational turns, and general audio environment. Additionally, it allows for fine-grained analysis of morphology and phonology, although these analyses are not automated. Oller et al. [86] used the LENA system to examine vocal characteristics of individuals with ASD and both language delayed and typically developing peers (ages range from 10 months to 4 years). In particular, the researchers created an algorithm within the LENA system to examine acoustic aspects of speech, including articulation (or "syllabification"), pitch, and duration. The researchers found that the LENA system differentiated the two clinical groups from the typically developing group with high sensitivity and specificity. They also found differences between the ASD and language-delayed group, although sensitivity and specificity was much lower. Surprisingly, articulation (or "syllabification") appeared to best differentiate the three groups, although it appears that the ASD group might have been more language-impaired. Even though the groups were matched on language level, the ASD group showed the largest discrepancy between chronological age and estimated age based on language level, which might explain differences in basic speech functions more than diagnostic category. The authors argue that speech parameters might need to be refined in LENA to make distinctions between clinical groups, because there was less sensitivity and specificity for these groups. Still, on a functional level, the idea of LENA as a way to identify early characteristics of communication delays is promising, regardless of its ability to identify clinical subgroups.

Importantly, Oller et al. [86] also found that the LENA system was sensitive to developmental changes (particularly in articulation), a finding which is promising for studies of behavioral change and improvement in clinical groups. Subsequent studies have indicated that only a single-day recording of vocalizations is needed to achieve an accurate measure of the stage of vocal development [87]. Other studies have found that the basic automated measurements produced by the LENA system (including number of child vocalizations) are moderately correlated with standardized measures of expressive communication, although they are not correlated with ADOS scores [85]. LENA and other technology under development have been found to produce reliable measures of language for individuals with ASD, although the predictive validity of the instruments for predicting future vocabulary performance was less consistent [88]. These preliminary data suggest that LENA has more utility for the evaluation of the stage of language development than for diagnostic or predictive purposes. Still, even when used in its simplest terms, the LENA system could provide a detailed measure of the number of conversational turns and length of utterances used by individuals with ASD (refer [89], which would also be useful as measures of behavioral change. In sum, LENA shows some promise in identifying individuals with language impairments at an early age, and also for identifying markers of developmental/behavioral change, but its utility as a diagnostic tool for ASD is a matter in need of greater investigation.

Van Santen and colleagues have also investigated automated analysis of the speech signal in individuals with ASD for markers of prosodic performance [63], for measures of repetitive speech [90], and for patterns of disfluency [91]. In contrast to previous studies of prosodic performance in ASD which examined specific aspects of prosody (e.g., fundamental frequency, duration), Van Santen and colleagues argued that the major differences between individuals with ASD and their peers in prosodic performance was the balance among fundamental frequency, amplitude, and duration [63]. More specifically, Van Santen and colleagues created an algorithm to measure stress patterns (e.g., the temporal alignment of stress patterns with speech) in speech during the PEPS-C (described above). The researchers found quantifiable group differences, but interestingly these differences (mostly in duration) were different than what clinicians are required to use for judgments (fundamental frequency) during the PEPS-C. Therefore, the PEPS-C and Van Santen's algorithm might be measuring different things; the PEPS-C is picking up on linguistic errors and Van Santen's algorithm is picking up on the more stylistic aspects of prosodic use related to manner of speaking [53].

Van Santen and colleagues have also applied automatic speech algorithms to measuring repetitive speech [90], which is one of the major diagnostic criteria for ASD [2]. In particular, Van Santen and colleagues focused on echolalia (repeating what someone else says) and self-repetitions. Although the algorithm was used to test research questions related to echolalia, the authors were able to use it to distinguish between individuals with ASD having a comorbid language impairment, individuals with ASD (and no language impairment), and typically developing peers in terms of the amount of echolalia used. The important finding from a diagnostic standpoint is that the authors have a fully automated algorithm that can measure these differences. However, without further development, it only measures one aspect of the diagnostic criteria (refer Table 1 for other aspects of repetitive behaviors) and could not in itself be a diagnostic tool for that criterion. Still, it has potential to provide a clinician with data that would be useful when pulling together information to make an overall diagnosis.

In sum, the majority of research on diagnostic utility of automatic measures of the speech signal comes from the publicly available LENA system, although there is considerable work that needs to be done to determine its diagnostic utility. Minimally, it appears to be a potentially good measure of developmental changes in speech production. There also has been some research on automated analysis of prosody production and repetitive speech, but these areas of inquiry are in their infancy and need a substantial amount of research to be useful in a clinical setting. Ideally, an automated system for measuring vocal development would open source and would allow the development and integration of multiple algorithms [92] to measure multiple aspects of the diagnostic criteria spanning vocal aspects of social-communication and vocal repetitive behaviors.

7.4 Role of speech technology in ASD treatment

At this point, the use of speech technology related to the speech signal to improve speech and communication in ASD is predominantly theoretical in nature. Broadly speaking, early research has indicated that the use of technology is promising for social skills development (refer [93], for a review), but the research on improving speech is limited. Speech–language pathologists are most likely to be the primary professionals working with individuals with ASD on speech issues, and they typically use traditional speech behavior methods. It is important to note, however, that prosody is not typically a targeted behavior in speech–language pathology interventions [23], and there is great potential for speech technology to fill a need in clinical speech therapy. One intriguing possibility would be the use of voice modeling to work with difficulty with non-linguistic aspects of prosodic performance (or "manner") that has been found in a number studies [54, 63]. Voice modeling could build off an existing approach called video modeling, which is typically used for modeling appropriate behavior [92, 94]. For example, in the video-modeling approach, individuals with ASD watch interactions that model appropriate social behavior. Another example of video modeling is to record an interaction between an individual with ASD and their peer and allow the individual with ASD to observe their own behavior. This has been a very successful approach for addressing complex social skill development [92], such as the appropriate use of compliments [95]. It is possible that applications could be built to provide a similar setup for voice modeling, with the difference being that individuals with ASD could listen to their own vocalizations [96, 97]. Speech technology could also give the individual with ASD the opportunity to visualize their own speech and prosodic patterns through a visual spectrograph, which could then be compared with a normative example [96, 97]. For example, Simmons et al. [96] piloted a mobile application in which a speech–language pathologist would have the application to generate a visual representation of a prosodic contour, and then they would show it to the client for them to replicate the pattern. Their pilot study found that participants with prosodic disorders (with and without ASD) showed improvements in prosodic performance in the brief intervention. To our knowledge, however, at the time of this report this was the only investigation of clinical applications of speech tools for use with ASD published in peer-reviewed clinical journals. Therefore, clinical applications of speech technology are promising, but have yet to be sufficiently investigated to have useful clinical applications.

7.5 Summary and future directions

Individuals with ASD show considerable variability in their speech deficits, but some aspects of the speech signal (e.g., prosody) are considered as some of the most identifying features of the disorder. Research on prosody performance in individuals with ASD has noted that differences from peers are the norm, but the differences range from deficits in the functional linguistic/affective uses of prosody to more subtle differences in the manner in which prosody is used in communication. One of the most exciting areas of research is the examination of early markers for ASD diagnosis through the speech signal; differences in the acoustics of cries and in babbling are promising areas that could lead to earlier identification of high-risk infants for ASD and other language impairments. Research on the automated analysis of speech differences for diagnosis is in its infancy, but a number of groups have started to develop algorithms related to diagnostic criteria and examine the sensitivity and specificity of these measures. Moreover, the LENA system, which is publicly available for purchase, has shown promise for tracking aspects of language development in clinical and typically developing populations. There is almost no research on the applications of speech technology to clinical therapy, although theoretical applications such as voice modeling hold a lot of promise.

In sum, this chapter should serve as a call for interdisciplinary collaboration to improve clinical applications of speech technology for use with individuals with ASD and other speech/language impairments. To answer the important questions posed in this chapter, it will take the clinical expertise of clinicians (speech–language pathologists and clinical psychologists) in combination with the experts from the areas of linguistics/psycholinguistics and computer science/technology to adapt speech technology in ways that will have meaningful clinical utility. Speech technology has the potential to improve the diagnosis of ASD and also to target areas such as prosody that previously have not been the focus of speech treatments.

References

[1]   Christensen DL, Baio J, Braun K, Bilder D, Charles J, Constantino JN, Daniels J, Durkin MS, Fitzgerald RT, Kurzius-Spencer M, Lee L, Pettygrove S, Robinson C, Schulz E, Wells C, Wingate MS, Zahorodny W, Yeargin-Allsopp, M. Prevalence and characteristics of autism spectrum disorder among children aged 8 Years – autism and developmental disabilities monitoring network, 11 Sites, United States, 2012. MMWR Surveillance Summary, 2016;65 (No. SS-3):1–23. DOI: 10.15585/mmwr.ss6503a1.
[2]   American Psychiatric Association. Diagnostic and statistical manual of mental disorders, 5th ed. Arlington, VA: American Psychiatric Publishing, 2013.
[3]   Diehl JJ, Tang K, Thomas B. High-functioning autism (HFA). In: Volkmar F, Paul R, Pelphrey K, Powers MD, editors. Encyclopedia of autism spectrum disorders New York: Springer, 2013:1504–1507.
[4]   American Psychiatric Association. Diagnostic and statistical manual of mental disorders, text revision, 4th ed. Washington, DC: American Psychiatric Association, 2000.
[5]   Magiati I, Tay XW, Howlin P. Cognitive, language, social and behavioural outcomes in adults with autism spectrum disorders: a systematic review of longitudinal follow-up studies in adulthood. Clin Psychol Rev 2014;34(1):73–86.
[6]   Tager-Flusberg H, Paul R, Lord C. Language and communication in autism. In: Volkmar FR, Paul R, Klin A, Cohen DJ, editors. Handbook of autism and pervasive developmental disorders: Diagnosis, development, neurobiology, and behavior, 3rd ed. Hoboken, NJ: John Wiley & Sons, Inc, 2005:335–364.
[7]   Young EC, Diehl JJ, Morris D, Hyman SL, Bennetto L. The use of two language tests to identify pragmatic language problems in children with autism spectrum disorders. Lang Speech Hear Serv Schools 2005:36(1):62–72. doi:10.1044/0161-1461 (2005/006).
[8]   Asperger H. Die 'autistischen psychopathen' im kindesalter. Archive Fur Psychiatrie Und Nervenkrankheiten, 1944;117:76–136. doi:10.1007/BF01837709
[9]   Kanner, L. Irrelevant and metaphorical language in early infantile autism. Am J Psychiatry 1946;103:242–246.
[10]   Kanner L. Autistic disturbances of affective contact. Nerv Child 1943;2(3):217–250.
[11]   Frith U. Autism and asperger syndrome. Cambridge: Cambridge University Press, 1991.
[12]   Amoroso H. Disorders of vocal signaling in children. In: Papousek H, Jurgens U, Papousek M, editors. Nonverbal vocal communication: comparative and developmental approaches. Cambridge: Cambridge University Press, 1992:192–204.
[13]   Baltaxe CA. Use of contrastive stress in normal, aphasic, and autistic children. J Speech Hear Res 1984;27(1):97–105.
[14]   Fay W, Schuler AL. Emerging language in autistic children. Baltimore: University Park Press, 1980.
[15]   Goldfarb W, Braunstein P, Lorge I. A study of speech patterns in a group of schizophrenic children. Am J Orthopsychiatry 1956;26:544–555.
[16]   Provonost W, Wakstein M, Wakstein D. A longitudinal study of speech behaviors and language comprehension in fourteen children diagnosed as atypical or autistic. Exceptional Children 1966;33:19–26.
[17]   McCann J, Peppé S. Prosody in autism spectrum disorders: a critical review. Int Journal of Lang Commun Disord 2003;38(4):325–350. doi:10.1080/1368282031000154204.

[18] Shriberg LD, Paul R, McSweeny JL, Klin A, Cohen DJ, Volkmar FR. Speech and prosody characteristics of adolescents and adults with high-functioning autism and asperger syndrome. J Speech Lang Hear Res 2001;44(5):1097–1115. doi:10.1044/1092-4388 (2001/087).

[19] McCann J, Peppé S, Gibbon FE, O'Hare A, Rutherford MD. Prosody and its relationship to language in school-aged children with high-functioning autism. J Lang Commun Disord 2007;42(6):682–702. doi:10.1080/13682820601170102.

[20] Paul R, Augustyn A, Klin A, Volkmar F. Perception and production of prosody by speakers with autism spectrum disorders. J Autism Dev Disord 2005;35(2):205–220. doi:10.1007/ s10803-004-1999-1.

[21] Diehl JJ, Paul, R. The assessment of prosodic disorders and neurological theories of prosody. Int J Speech-Lang Pathol 2009;11:287–292. doi:10.1080/17549500902971887.

[22] Green H, Tobin, Y. Prosodic analysis is difficult ... but worth it: A study in high functioning autism. Int J Speech-Lang Pathol 2009;11(4):308–315. doi:10.1080/17549500903003060.

[23] Peppé S. Why is prosody in speech-language pathology so difficult? Int J Speech-Lang Pathol 2009;11(4):258–271. doi:10.1080/17549500902906339.

[24] Edelson L, Diehl JJ. Prosody . In: Volkmar FR, Paul R, Pelphrey K, Powers MD, editors. Encyclopedia of autism spectrum disorders. New York: Springer, 2013:2413–2417.

[25] Chapman R. Children's language learning: An interactionist perspective. J Child Psychol Psychiatry 2000;41:33–54.

[26] Hirsh-Pasek K, Golinkoff RM. The origins of grammar. Cambridge, MA: MIT Press, 1996.

[27] Jusczyk PW. The role of speech perception capacities in early language acquisition. In: Mack MB, editor. Language: Multidisciplinary perspectives. Mahwah, NJ: Lawrence Erlbaum Associates, 2003:61–83.

[28] Moon C, Cooper RP, Fifer WP. Two-day olds prefer their native language. Infant Behav Dev 1993;16:495–500. doi:10.1016/0163-6383(93)80007-U

[29] Fernald A. The perceptual and affective salience of mothers' speech to infants. In: Feagans L, editor. The origins and growth of communication. New Brunswick, NJ: Ablex Publishing Corporation, 1983:5–29.

[30] Cooper RP, Aslin RN. Developmental differences in infant attention to the spectral properties of infant-directed speech. Child Dev 1994;65:1663–1677. doi:10.1111/j.1467-8624.1994.tb00841.x.

[31] Morgan JL. Prosody and the roots of parsing. In: Warren P, Editor. Prosody and parsing. United Kingdom: Psychology Press, 1996:69–106.

[32] Jusczyk, PW. Syntactic units, prosody, and psychological reality during infancy. In: Morgan JL, Demuth K, editors. Signal to syntax: bootstrapping from speech to grammar in early acquisition. Hillsdale, NJ: Erlbaum, 1993:389–408.

[33] Jusczyk PW, Houston DM, Newsome M. The beginnings of word segmentation in english-learning infants. Cogn Psychol 1999;39:159–207. doi:10.1006/cogp.1999.0716.

[34] Hobson R. Autism and emotion. In: Volkmar FR, Paul R, Klin A, Cohen D, editors. Handbook of autism and pervasive developmental disorders, vol 1: diagnosis, development, neuro-biology, and behavior, 3rd ed.Hoboken, NJ: John Wiley & Sons Inc., 2005:406–422.

[35] Lartseva A, Dijkstra T, Buitelaar JK. Emotional language processing in autism spectrum disorders: a systematic review. Front Hum Neurosci 2015;8:991.

[36] Erwin R, Van Lancker D, Guthrie D, Schwafel J, Tanguay P, Buchwald JS. P3 responses to prosodic stimuli in adult autistic subjects. Electroencephalogr Clin Neurophysiol 1991; 80(6):561–571.

[37] Globerson E, Amir N, Kishon-Rabin L, Golan O. Prosody recognition in adults with high-functioning autism spectrum disorders: from psychoacoustics to cognition. Autism Res 2015;8(2):153–163.

[38] Kleinman J, Marciano PL, Ault, RL. Advanced theory of mind in high-functioning adults with autism. J Autism Dev Disord 2001;31(1):29–36. doi:10.1023/A:1005657512379.

[39] Lindström R, Lepistö-Paisley T, Vanhala R, Alén R, Kujala T. Impaired neural discrimination of emotional speech prosody in children with autism spectrum disorder and language impairment. Neurosci Lett 2016;628:47–51.

[40] Peppé S, McCann J, Gibbon F, O'Hare A, Rutherford M. Assessing prosodic and pragmatic ability in children with high-functioning autism. J Pragmatics 2006;38(10):1776–1791. doi:10.1016/j.pragma.2005.07.004

[41] Rutherford MD, Baron-Cohen S, Wheelwright S. Reading the mind in the voice: A study with normal adults and adults with asperger syndrome and high functioning autism. J Autism Dev Disord 2002;32(3):189–194. doi:10.1023/A:1015497629971.

[42] Grossman RB, Bemis RH, Plesa Skwerer D, Tager-Flusberg H. Lexical and affective prosody in children with high-functioning autism. J Speech Lang Hear Res 2010b;53:778–793. doi:10.1044/1092-4388(2009/08-0127)

[43] Hobson RP, Ouston J, Lee A. Emotion recognition in autism – coordinating faces and voices. Psychol Med 1988;18:911–923.

[44] Prior M, Dahlstrom B, Squires TL. Autistic children's knowledge of thinking and feeling states in other people. J Child Psychol Psychiatry Allied Disciplines 1990;31:587–601. doi:10.1111/j.1469-7610.1990.tb00799.x

[45] Järvinen-Pasley A, Paisley J, Heaton P. Is the linguistic content of speech more salient than its perceptual features in autism? J Autism Dev Disord 2008;38:239–48. doi:10.1007/s10803-007-0386-0[46]Järvinen-Pasley A, Peppé S, King-Smith G, Heaton P. The relationship between form and function level receptive prosodic abilities in autism. J Autism Dev Disord 2008;38(7):1328–1340.

[47] Peppé S, McCann J, Gibbon F, O'Hare A, Rutherford M. Receptive and expressive prosodic ability in children with high-functioning autism. J Speech Lang Hear Res 2007;50 (4):101528. doi:10.1044/1092-4388(2007/071)

[48] Chevallier C, Noveck I, Happé F, Wilson D. From acoustics to grammar: Perceiving and interpreting grammatical prosody in adolescents with asperger syndrome. Res Autism Spectr Disord 2009;3:502–516. doi:10.1016/j.rasd.2008.10.004.

[49] Diehl JJ, Bennetto L, Watson D, Gunlogson C, McDonough J. Resolving ambiguity: A psycholinguistic approach to understanding prosody processing in high-functioning autism. Brain Lang 2008;106(2):144–152. doi:10.1016/j.bandl.2008.04.002.

[50] Grossman RB, Bemis RH, Plesa Skwerer D, Tager-Flusberg H. Lexical and affective prosody in children with high-functioning autism. J Speech Lang Hear Res 2010a; 53:778–93. doi:10.1044/1092-4388(2009/08-0127)

[51] Kargas N, López, B, Morris P, Reddy V. Relations among detection of syllable stress, speech abnormalities, and communicative ability in adults with autism spectrum disorders. J Speech Lang Hear Res 2016;59(2):206–215.

[52] Grossman RB, Tager-Flusberg H. Quality matters! differences between expressive and receptive non-verbal communication skills in adolescents with ASD. Res Autism Spectr Disord 2012;6(3):1150–1155. doi:10.1016/j.rasd.2012.03.006.

[53] Diehl JJ, Berkovits L. Is prosody a diagnostic and cognitive bellwether of autism spectrum disorders? In: Harrison A, editor. Speech disorders: causes, treatments, and social effects. New York: Nova Science Publishers, 2010:159–176.

[54] Diehl JJ Paul R. Acoustic and perceptual measurements of prosody production on the PEPS-C by children with autism spectrum disorders. Appl Psycholing 2013;34:135–61. doi:10.1017/S0142716411000646.

[55] Loca J, Wootton T. Interactional and phonetic aspects of immediate echolalia in autism – a case study. Clin Ling Phonetics 1995;9(2):155–184. doi:10.3109/02699209508985330.

[56] Paccia JM, Curcio F. Language processing and forms of immediate echolalia in autistic children. J Speech Hear Res 1982;25(1):42–47. Available at: http://jslhr.highwire.org/cgi/content/abstract/25/1/42. Accessed June 13, 2018.

[57] Diehl JJ, Paul R. differences in the imitation of prosidic patterns in children with autism spectrum disorders. Res Autism Spectr Disord 2012;6(1):123–134. doi:10.1016/j.rasd.2011.03.012.

[58] Paul R, Bianchi N, Augustyn A, Klin A, Volkmar FR. Production of syllable stress in speakers with autism spectrum disorders. Res Autism Spectr Disord 2008;2(1):110–124. doi:10.1016/j.rasd.2007.04.001.

[59] Diehl JJ, Watson DG, Bennetto L, McDonough J, Gunlogson C. An acoustic analysis of prosody in high-functioning autism. Appl Psycholing 2009;30(3):385–404. doi:10.1017/S0142716409090201

[60] Hubbard K, Trauner DA. Intonation and emotion in autistic spectrum disorders. J Psycholing Res 2007;36(2):159–173.

[61] Hubbard, DJ, Faso, DJ, Assmann PF, Sasson NJ. Production and perception of emotional prosody by adults with autism spectrum disorder. Autism Res 2017;10(12):1991–2001.

[62] Nadig A, Shaw H. Acoustic marking of prominence: how do preadolescent speakers with and without high-functioning autism mark contrast in an interactive task? Lang Cogn Neurosci 2015;30(1–2):32–47. doi:10.1080/01690965.2012.753150.

[63] Van Santen JP, Prud'hommeaux ET, Black LM, Mitchell M. Computational prosodic markers for autism. Autism 2010;14(3):215–236. doi:10.1177/1362361309363281.

[64] Nadig A, Shaw, H. Acoustic and perceptual measurement of expressive prosody in high-functioning autism: Increased pitch range and what it means to listeners. J Autism Dev Disord 2012;42(4):499–511. doi:10.1007/s10803-011-1264-3

[65] Dawson G, Jones EJ, Merkle K, Venema K, Lowy R, Faja S, ... Webb, SJ. (2012). Early behavioral intervention is associated with normalized brain activity in young children with autism. J Am Acad Child Adolesc Psychiatry 2012;51(11):1150–1159.

[66] Wetherby AM, Woods J, Allen L, Cleary J, Dickinson H, Lord, C. Early indicators of autism spectrum disorders in the second year of life. J Autism Dev Disord 2004;34(5):473–493. doi:10.1007/s10803-004-2544-y.

[67] Paul R, Fuerst Y, Ramsay G, Chawarska K, Klin, A. Out of the mouths of babes: Vocal production in infant siblings of children with ASD. J Child Psychol Psychiatry 2011;52(5):588–598. doi:10.1111/j.1469-7610.2010.02332.x.

[68] Patten E, Belardi K, Baranek GT, Watson LR, Labban JD, Oller, DK. Vocal patterns in infants with autism spectrum disorder: Canonical babbling status and vocalization frequency. J Autism Dev Disord, 2014;44(10):2413–2428.

[69] Schoen E, Paul R, Chawarska, K. Phonology and vocal behavior in toddlers with autism spectrum disorders. Autism Res 2011, online first, doi:10.1002/aur.183

[70] Sheinkopf SJ, Mundy P, Oller DK, Steffens M. Vocal atypicalities of preverbal autistic children. J Autism Dev Disord 2000;30(4):345. Available at: http://search.ebscohost.com/login.aspx?direct=true&db=aph&AN=11305520&site=ehost-live

[71] Esposito G, Hiroi N, Scattoni ML. Cry, baby, cry: expression of distress as a biomarker and modulator in autism spectrum disorder. Int J Neuropsychopharmacol 2017;20(6):498–503.

[72] Esposito G, Venuti, P. How is crying perceived in children with autism spectrum disorder? Res Autism Spectr Disord, 2008;2(2):371–384. doi:10.1016/j.rasd.2007.09.003.

[73] Esposito G, Venuti P. Comparative analysis of crying in children with autism, developmental delays, and typical development. Focus Autism Deve Disabilities 2009;24(4): 240–247. doi:10.1177/1088357609336449.

[74] Esposito G, Venuti P. Understanding early communication signals in autism: a study of the perception of infants' cry. J Intell Disability Res 2010b;54(3):216–223. doi:10.1111/j.1365-2788.2010.01252.x.

[75] Esposito, G., Venuti, P., & Bornstein, M. H. (2011). Assessment of distress in young children: A comparison of autistic disorder, developmental delay, and typical development. Research in autism spectrum disorders, 5(4):1510–1516.

[76] Esposito G, Nakazawa J, Venuti P, Bornstein MH. Perceptions of distress in young children with autism compared to typically developing children: a cultural comparison between Japan and Italy. Res Dev Disabilities 2012;33(4):1059–1067. doi:10.1016/j.rasd.2011.02.013.

[77] Sheinkopf, S. J., Iverson, J. M., Rinaldi, M. L., & Lester, B. M. (2012). Atypical Cry Acoustics in 6-Month-Old Infants at Risk for Autism Spectrum Disorder. Autism Research, 5(5): 331–339.

[78] Ghaziuddin M, Gerstein, L. Pedantic speaking style differentiates asperger syndrome from high-functioning autism. J Autism Dev Disord 1996;26(6):585–595. Available at: http://search.ebscohost.com/login.aspx?direct=true&db=aph&AN=9707073151&site=ehost-live

[79] Lord C, Rutter M, DiLavore, PC, Risi S, Gotham K, Bishop SL. Autism diagnostic observation schedule: ADOS-2. Torrance: Western Psychological Services, 2012.

[80] Rutter M, Le Couteur A, Lord C. Autism diagnostic interview-revised. Los Angeles: Western Psychological Services, 2003.

[81] Peppé S, McCann J. Assessing intonation and prosody in children with atypical language development: The PEPS-C test and the revised version. Clinical Linguistics and Phonetics, 2003;17(4–5):345–354. doi:10.1080/0269920031000079994.

[82] Shriberg LD, Kwiatkowski J, Rasmussen C. The prosody-voice screening profile (PVSP). Tucson, AZ: Communication Skill Builders, 1992.

[83] Esposito G, Venuti, P. Developmental changes in the fundamental frequency (f0) of infants' cries: a study of children with autism spectrum disorder. Early Child Dev Care 2010a;180(8):1093–1102. doi:10.1080/03004430902775633.

[84] Bolte E, Diehl, JJ. Measurement tools and target symptoms/skills used to assess treatment response in individuals with autism spectrum disorder. J Autism Dev Disord 2013;43 (11):2491–2501. doi:10.1007/s10803-013-1798-7.

[85] Dykstra J, Sabatos-DeVito MG, Irvin DW, Boyd, BA, Hume KA, Odom, SL. Using the language environment analysis (LENA) system in preschool classrooms with children with autism spectrum disorders. Autism 2013;17(5):582–594. doi:10.1177/1362361312446206.

[86] Oller DK, Niyogi P, Gray S, Richards JA, Gilkerson J, Xu D, ... Warren, SF. Automated vocal analysis of naturalistic recordings from children with autism, language delay, and typical

development. Proc Natl Acad Sci 2010;107(30):13354–13359. doi:10.1073/pnas.1003882107.

[87] Yoder PJ, Oller, DK, Richards, JA, Gray S, Gilkerson J. Stability and validity of an automated measure of vocal development from day-long samples in children with and without autism spectrum disorder. Autism Res 2013;6(2):103–107. doi:10.1002/aur.1271.

[88] Woynaroski T, Oller DK, Keceli-Kaysili B, Xu D, Richards JA, Gilkerson J, Gray S, Yoder P. The stability and validity of automated vocal analysis in preverbal preschoolers with autism spectrum disorder. Autism Res 2017;10(3):508–519.

[89] Warren, SF, Gilkerson J, Richards, JA, Oller, DK, Xu D, Yapanel U, Gray S. What automated vocal analysis reveals about the vocal production and language learning environment of young children with autism. J Autism Dev Disord 201140(5):555–569. doi:10.1007/s10803-009-0902-5.

[90] Van Santen, JPH, Sproat RW, Hill AP. Quantifying repetitive speech in autism spectrum disorders and language impairment. Autism Res 2013;6(5):372–383. doi:10.1002/aur.1301.

[91] MacFarlane H, Gorman K, Ingham R, Hill, AP, Papadakis K, Kiss G, van Santen J. Quantitative analysis of disfluency in children with autism spectrum disorder or language impairment. PloS one 2017;12(3):e0173936.

[92] McCoy K, Hermansen E. Video modeling for individuals with autism: a review of model types and effects. Educ Treat Children 2007;30(4):183–213. doi:10.1353/etc.2007.0029.

[93] Grynszpan O, Weiss, PL, Perez-Diaz F, Gal E. Innovative technology-based interventions for autism spectrum disorders: a meta-analysis. Autism 2014;18(4):346–361.

[94] Charlop-Christy, MH, Loc L, Freeman KA. A comparison of video modeling with in vivo modeling for teaching children with autism. J Autism Dev Disord 2000;30(6):537–552. doi:10.1023/A:1005635326276

[95] Macpherson K, Charlop MH, Miltenberger, CA. Using portable video modeling technology to increase the compliment behaviors of children with autism during athletic group play. J Autism Dev Disord 2015;45(12):3836–3845.

[96] Simmons, ES, Paul R, Shic F. Brief report: A mobile application to treat prosodic deficits in autism spectrum disorder and other communication impairments: a pilot study. J Autism Dev Disord 2016;46(1):320–327.

[97] Welkowitz L, Green, J. A study of the effects of speech feedback on conversational patterning and prosody in adults with autism spectrum disorders. Eastern Psychological Association, New York, NY, 2012.

Part III: **Assessing and Quantifying Speech Intelligibility in Patients with Congenital Anatomical Defects, Disabling Conditions, and Degenerative Diseases**

Xiyue Wang, Hua Huang, Jia Fu, Heng Yin and Ling He

8 Automatic assessment of consonant omission and speech intelligibility in cleft palate speech

Abstract: The effective assessment of cleft palate speech has a great significance in clinical practice. Two algorithms are proposed to automatically detect the consonant omission and assess the speech intelligibility in cleft palate speech. The cleft palate speech database contains 530 participants from the Hospital of Stomatology, Sichuan University. The vocabulary of speech database includes all initial consonants and the most widely used vowels in Mandarin. All the speech recordings are assessed and annotated by professional speech–language pathologists. Based on the differences between vowels and initial consonants in Mandarin, this work combines the short-time autocorrelation function and the hierarchical clustering model to realize the automatic detection of consonant omission. The average detection accuracy is 82.75%. Based on the automatic continuous speech-recognition algorithm, the evaluation of speech intelligibility is completed. The recognition accuracy of automatic speech-recognition system is proportional to the speech intelligibility. And the hypernasality grades and speech intelligibility are in inverse proportion. For the normal speech, the recognition accuracy of automatic speech recognition system is 96.41%. With the increase of hypernasality grades, the accuracy of automatic speech-recognition system reduces.

Keywords: Cleft palate speech, consonant omission, speech intelligibility, automatic continuous speech recognition

8.1 Introduction

The cleft palate is a common congenital craniofacial deformity. The existence of velopharyngeal insufficiency (VPI) is the main factor that affects the pronunciation of cleft palate patients. The VPI indicates that the soft palate posterior wall and the pharynx wall are not completely joined in the speech-pronouncing process. More intuitively, there is an open connection between the nasal cavity and the oral cavity. The airflow overflows from the oral cavity to the nose cavity, which destroys the resonance balance and results in the hypernasality. The surgery can repair the velopharyngeal function. However, the cleft palate patients might still suffer the speech disorders, such as hypernasality,

https://doi.org/10.1515/9781501502415-009

consonant omission, and consonant substitution, etc. In clinic, the invasive and non-invasive techniques are utilized to assess hypernasality. The invasive method evaluates hypernasality with some invasive instruments, such as nasendoscopy, videofluoroscopy, etc. And the non-invasive technique is performed by the professional speech–language pathologists. The computer-based automatic evaluation algorithm in cleft palate speech can provide objective and convenient assessment.

In recent years, speech signal-processing technology, as a non-invasive technique, has been used in the study of the cleft palate speech. Many works have studied the automatic hypernasality detection methods in cleft palate speech. These methods are mainly based on: Teager Energy Operator (TEO) [1, 2], all-pole vocal tract model [3], pole-zero vocal tract model [4], the formant characters of hypernasality sound [5–7], and the combination of acoustic features and classifiers [8–11].

The consonant omission is a common dysarthria disorder in cleft palate speech, which is caused by the lack of air pressure during the pronunciation of consonant in the cleft palate patients. When the consonant omission occurs, the meaning of speech conveyed by cleft palate patients will be greatly changed. This may seriously affect their daily communication. In anatomical structure, the pronunciation of different consonants is corresponding to different articulation places, which can reflect the velopharyngeal function.

Most of current researches investigate clinical profile of consonant omission in cleft palate speech by clinicians. Luyten et al. [12] analyze five cleft palate patients and conclude that consonant omission and consonant substitution in English are more frequently occurred in /s/ and /z/. In Zhu's work, 40 unrepaired cleft children, 28 repaired cleft children and 32 normal children are participated in the experiment. The experimental results indicate that the highest occurrence frequency of consonant omission is/j/and/d/in Mandarin [13]. Jiang et al. [14] and Li et al. [15] have the similar conclusion, that is, the consonant omission mainly occurs in /z/, /zh/, /j/, and /g/. After studying 100 patients with cleft palate, Yin et al. [16] discover the consonant /d/, /g/,/ j/, and /z/ are omitted more frequently. Hu's work indicates that the omissions of consonant /p/ and /b/for VPI patients have the occurrence frequency of 12% and 14%, respectively [17]. Zhou et al. [18] and Wang et al. [19] show that younger patients with cleft palate are more likely to have consonant omission than the older ones. Bruneel et al. [20] analyze the speech utterances spoken by 15 cleft palate patients and 15 control samples. The experimental results indicate that the frequency of consonant omission is higher in cleft palate patients than the control group.

The automatic evaluation of the consonant omission can provide assistant diagnose for doctors. A rare work has been done to investigate the automatic consonant omission algorithm in cleft palate speech. In [8], an automatic consonant omission detection algorithm is proposed based on the difference between the initial consonants and finals in Mandarin. And a satisfactory accuracy is obtained. However, the number of the speech utterances tested in that work is limited. It only considers 11 initial consonants according to the acoustic characteristic of cleft palate speech. Consonant omission is one type of the misarticulation disorders in cleft palate speech. A few articles have studied other types of misarticulation disorders in cleft palate speech, such as consonant substitution and consonant distortion. Vijayalakshmi et al. [21] assess the dysarthric speech based on the isolated speech-recognition system. From the experiment results of speech recognition, they conclude that the consonants /p/ and /d/ can sometimes be identified as the nasalized consonant/m/. Laitinen et al. [22] indicate that the consonant misarticulation and distortion have the largest probability to occur, and the consonant substitution has small probability among the dental consonants (/r/, /s/ and /l/).

The resonance disorders and articulation disorders greatly affect the speech intelligibility of cleft palate patients. If the speech intelligibility is too low, it is difficult for audiences to understand. The articles [23, 24] indicate that there are modest correlations between speech intelligibility and size of velopharyngeal gap. Therefore, the effective evaluation of cleft palate speech intelligibility has great significance in clinical practice. At present, the most frequently used methods to measure cleft palate speech intelligibility are rating scale [25–28], transcription task [23, 24, 29], articulation test score [30] and subjective judgment by the parents of the patients [31], inexperienced listeners [32], or experienced speech pathologists [33]. However, these methods are not precise and depended on the abilities of speech–language pathologists. Since the subjective judgment does not have a fixed standard, the results of the evaluation cannot be utilized by doctors. In addition, subjective judgment depends upon cognitive factors, such as affection, emotion, context, etc.

In recent years, a computer-based method using the automatic speech recognition (ASR) technique has been studied to achieve the automatic speech intelligibility assessment. The ASR system builds an acoustic model, which is the Hidden Markov Models (HMM), and it is independent from auditory perception of audience [34–36]. However, the experiment of [34] is just based on the word recognition. Schuster et al. [35] have carried out experiment to show that there are correlations between the recognition accuracy of ASR and the speech intelligibility. That is, low speech-recognition accuracy of ASR is corresponding to the low speech intelligibility. Our previous work has also applied the ASR system to evaluate the grades of the speech intelligibility [9]. In addition to the ASR-based approach, Bocklet et al. [37] also propose a speech intelligibility assessment method based on Gaussian Mixture Model (GMM) and Support Vector Regression (SVR) in 2009. First, the Mel-Frequency Cepstral Coefficients (MFCCs) are extracted as the feature. Then, GMMs are used to model the feature. Finally, the components of GMM are used as the input of SVR and the speech intelligibility score could be obtained. The correlation between the raters and this speech intelligibility assessment system is around 0.8.

In this chapter, two algorithms are proposed to automatically detect the consonant omission and assess the speech intelligibility in cleft palate speech. 1) The algorithm for automatic detection of consonant omission is proposed based on the differences between vowels and initial consonants in Mandarin. The vowels have obvious periodicity, while the initial consonants are non-periodic, except /m/, /n/, /l/, and /r/. Based on the hierarchical clustering algorithm, this chapter calculates the threshold value to detect the consonant omission. 2) The algorithm for automatic assessment of cleft palate speech intelligibility is proposed. It utilizes the automatic continuous speech-recognition algorithm to realize the speech intelligibility evaluation. The experimental results show that the recognition accuracy of ASR is proportional to the speech intelligibility. However, the hypernasality grades and the speech intelligibility are in inverse proportion.

The rest of the chapter is organized as follows. In the next section, the cleft palate speech database is described in detail. Section 8.3 describes the algorithm of automatic consonant omission detection. And Section 8.4 describes the algorithm of automatic speech intelligibility assessment. The experiments and results are presented in Section 8.5. The conclusions and discussions are presented in Section 8.6.

8.2 Cleft palate speech (CPS) database

The collection of cleft palate speech recordings is limited by various factors, such as the rare number of patients, the various accent of speakers, and the design of vocabulary list, which highly reflects the characteristics of cleft palate speech [8]. Moreover, most of the cleft palate patients are children, who are not easy to cooperate with doctors for data acquisition. In this work, an abundant cleft palate speech database is applied, which is collected by the Hospital of Stomatology, Sichuan University, which has the largest number of cleft lip and palate patients in China. A total of 530 patients are included in this database.

Only the speech utterances recorded from 120 out of 530 speakers are annotated at phoneme-level with both hypernasality grades and articulation error. Thus, the speech recordings of these 120 speakers are tested in this chapter. The block diagram of speech collection is shown in Figure 8.1.

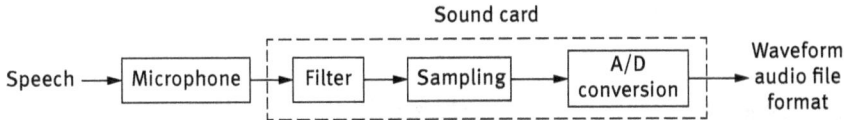

Figure 8.1: The block diagram of speech collection.

The detailed process of cleft palate speech collection is illustrated as follows. 1) Doctors inform the patients and their parents the main purpose and the general process of speech recordings' acquisition; 2) The patients or their parents sign the consent form, which includes the agreement of recording process and speech data sharing; 3) The speech–language pathologists guide the patients to read the "vocabulary list" [8], which includes all 84 commonly used words in Mandarin; 4) After the patients are familiar with the "vocabulary list," they read it aloud themselves' 5) The whole recording process is completed in a professional speech-recording chamber, with the Sennheiser professional wired microphone in the sampling rate of 44,100 Hz and resolution of 16 bits. The microphone is located directly ahead of the lips and away from the lip at 15 cm; 6) The speed of reading is controlled as one single word per second, which is operated by the gesture signal of speech–language pathologists. The details of the 120 cleft palate patients are described in Table 8.1.

Table 8.1: Details of the 120 cleft palate patients.

	Male	Female
children (5–12 years old)	39	38
teenagers (13–17 years old)	11	8
adults (beyond 18 years old)	12	12

There are two types of disorders in cleft palate speech, namely, resonance disorders and articulation disorders. The typical resonance disorders include hypernasality, nasal air emission, etc. The symptom of hypernasality is an excessive nasal sound. The nasal air emission denotes that the air leaks through the nose during the speech production procedure. And the articulation disorders include consonant omission, consonant substitution, consonant distortion, etc. The consonant omission, substitution, and distortion mean the consonants are omitted, substituted, and distorted, respectively. All speech recordings in this database are labeled by three professional speech–language pathologists. Only the recordings that all the three speech–language pathologists are consistent with the assessment results could be incorporated into this database.

8.2.1 Dataset-I: Dataset for automatic consonant omission detection

A Mandarin syllable consists of two parts, namely, initial and final. The structure of Mandarin is shown as follows (*from en.wikipedia.org/wiki/Syllable*).

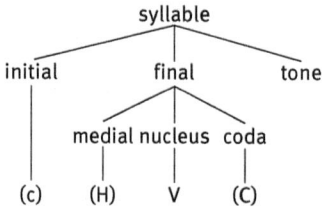

Figure 8.2: Traditional Mandarin syllable structure.

Almost all the studies about speech signal processing do not take into account coda in the Mandarin syllable. Therefore, the coda is not considered in the consonant omission and ASR-based speech intelligibility assessment algorithms.

The initials are all consonants, and there are 21 initials. The finals are composed of vowels or compound vowels. Consonant omission is a typical articulation disorder, which can greatly change the meaning of the speech. It is caused by the lack of air pressure during the pronunciation of initials. In Dataset-I, 420 syllables with consonant omission selected from 120 patients and 420 syllables without consonant omission are included. These syllables cover all the 21 initial consonants and the most widely used vowels (*a, i, u, o*) in Mandarin [8]. The consonant omission occurs when a cleft palate patient omits the initial consonant phoneme in a Mandarin syllable. As a result of individual differences, different cleft palate patients might omit different initial consonants. And some cleft palate patients might not have the speech disorder of consonant omission at all. Therefore, in this CPS database, only a part of speech recording is with consonant omission. All the speech recordings with consonant omission in the CPS database are included in Dataset-I, and the equal number of controlled recordings are included in Dataset-I as well.

8.2.2 Dataset-II: Dataset for automatic speech intelligibility assessment

Due to the articulation disorders, the cleft palate patients have difficulty in pronouncing certain syllables, causing some speech syllables to sound distorted or mushy. The resonance disorders make the cleft palate speech hoarse or breathy. These cleft palate speech disorders seriously affect the speech intelligibility. In Dataset-II, 1,440 sentences collected from 120 patients are included. The time duration of one sentence is around 5 s.

8.3 Automatic detection of consonant omission

This chapter proposes an algorithm to recognize consonant omission in cleft palate speech automatically, combining short-time autocorrelation function and the hierarchical clustering model.

A Mandarin syllable consists of the initial and the final. In Mandarin phonetics [38], the structure of the Mandarin syllable is C+V (consonant + vowel). There are 21 initial consonants in Mandarin. When the cleft palate patient is lack of oral pressure during the pronunciation process, the initial consonant omission occurs. In Mandarin, most initial consonants are voiceless, except /m/, /n/, /l/, and /r/ [38]. In the pronunciation of voiceless consonant, the speech sequence is non-periodic. Thus, its short-time autocorrelation function waveform shows the similar characteristics to noise signal. Vice-versa, the vowel is voiced. Its speech sequence is periodic and its short-time autocorrelation function is also periodic. To demonstrate this, Figure 8.3 shows the waveforms of the short-time autocorrelation function for different type of speech signal units.

Observed from Figure 8.3, the short-time autocorrelation function of unvoiced speech shows the non-periodic characteristics, to the contrary, the short-time autocorrelation function of voiced speech is periodic. Based on these differences between vowels and initial consonants in Mandarin, an automatic consonant omission detection method in cleft palate speech is proposed. The flowchart is shown as follows.

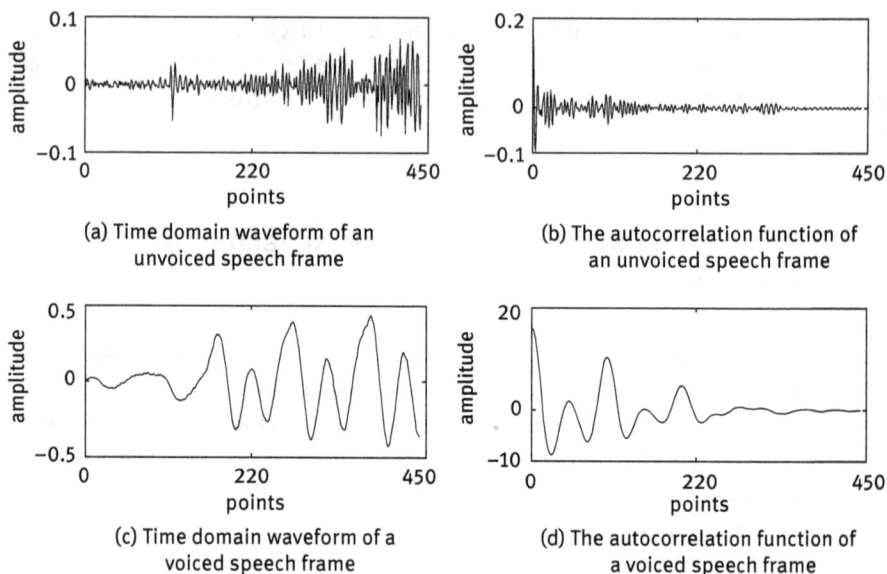

Figure 8.3: The contrast of autocorrelation function for unvoiced and voiced speech signals.

where $R_i(k)$ represents the short-time autocorrelation function of the ith frame speech signal. P denotes the maximum value of peaks' number. T is a threshold which can be calculated by the hierarchical clustering model. In Figure 8.4, the speech signal is normalized and segmented into frames first. Then, for each speech frame signal, the short-time autocorrelation function can be calculated. And then, the number of peaks and the max local peaks of the short-time autocorrelation function for each speech frame can be obtained. Finally, the threshold T is set to detect the consonant omission. The detail pseudocode is shown in Figure 8.5.

8.3.1 Preprocessing

The cleft palate speech signal is normalized first. Then, the Hamming window is applied to obtain the speech frame with the length of 20 ms and the duration of frame shift is 10 ms.

8.3.2 Short-time autocorrelation function

For each speech frame, the short-time autocorrelation function is calculated:

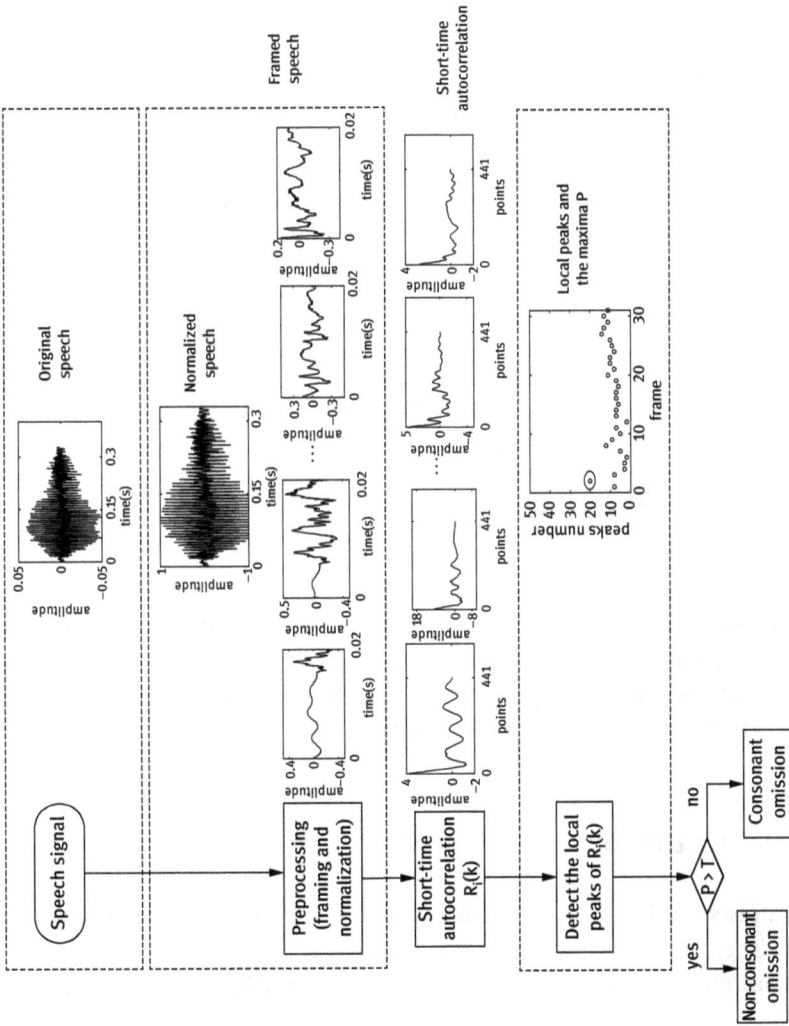

Figure 8.4: Flowchart of consonant omission detection method.

Algorithm for consonant omission detection	
1: Begin	Input speech signal x(n) with length L
2: Framing	Frame length 20 ms; frame shift 10 ms
	$x_i \leftarrow x(n)$
3: Short-time autocorrelation	For (i = 1 to f)
	$\{ R_i(k) \leftarrow \sum\limits_{m=0}^{N-K-1} x_i(m) \, x_i(m+k), \quad 0 \leq m \leq N-1, \quad i = 1,2,3,...f \; /\}$
4: Detecting peaks	For (i = 3 to f −3)
	$\{ P_i \leftarrow$ Detect the local peaks of $R_i(k) /\}$
5: Max local peaks	$P \leftarrow \max(P_i)$
6: Detecting consonant omission	If $P > T$ Then
	$\{$ Non-consonant omission $/\}$
	else
	$\{$ Consonant omission $/\}$
7: End	

Figure 8.5: Pseudocode of consonant omission detection algorithm.

$$R_i(k) = \sum_{m=0}^{N-k-1} x_i(m)x_i(m+k), 0 \leq m \leq N-1, \quad i = 1, 2, 3, \ldots f \qquad (8.1)$$

where i represents the ith frame, $x_i(m)$ represents the ith speech signal, $R_i(k)$ denotes the short-time autocorrelation function of the ith frame speech signal, N is the length of one frame speech signal, k represents the delay points, and f denotes the frame number of speech signal.

8.3.3 Detect the local peaks of $R_i(k)$

The local peaks of $R_i(k)$ are the local maxima of the short-time autocorrelation function. The calculation algorithm is as follows:

It is assumed that a point call k_0 is included in the interval (k_1,k_2). Make k_0 satisfy:

$$\begin{cases} R_i(k_0) > R_i(k_0 - 1) \\ R_i(k_0) > R_i(k_0 + 1) \end{cases} k_1 < k_0 < k_2 \qquad (8.2)$$

where $R_i(k_0)$ is called a local maxima of short-time autocorrelation function, and it is called peak of the short-time autocorrelation function in this chapter. Then, the number of peaks can be summed, which is represented by P_i.

8.3.4 Calculation of threshold based on hierarchical clustering

Hierarchical clustering is a bottom-up classification method. Before clustering, each original clustering object is regarded as an independent subclass. We calculate the degree of similarity between two objects and cluster two objects with the maximum similarity into the same class until the termination condition is satisfied [39]. Three implementation steps of the hierarchical clustering are as follows:

Step I: Calculate the distance between two objects. The Euclidean distance is used.

Step II: Divide the objects into r clusters. Calculate the sum of squares in intra-cluster [39]:

$$sum_t = \sum_{i=1}^{n_t} (g_l(t) - \overline{g(t)})^T (g_l(t) - \overline{g(t)}), \qquad (8.3)$$

where sum_t represents the sum of squares in intra-cluster, G_t represents the tth clusters, $g_l(t)$ represents the lth object in G_t, n_t denotes the objects number in G_t, and $\overline{g(t)}$ represents the center of G_t, that is the mean of the total objects in G_t.

Based on equation (8.3), the sum of squares of total r clusters can be calculated:

$$sum = \sum_{t=1}^{r} sum_t = \sum_{t=1}^{r} \sum_{i=1}^{n_t} (g_l(t) - \overline{g(t)})^T (g_l(t) - \overline{g(t)}), \qquad (8.4)$$

Step III: The classification criterion is to realize the minimum sum of squares in intra-cluster.

In this work, P_i is the peaks' number of the short-time autocorrelation function, which is calculated frame-by-frame. Then, for a Mandarin syllable, the maximum value of the peaks' number represented by P is calculated. The consonant omission can be detected by

$$P = \begin{cases} P > T, \text{non} - \text{consonant omission}, \\ P \leq T, \text{consonant omission}, \end{cases} \tag{8.5}$$

where P represents the maximum value of the peaks' number for a Mandarin syllable. T is a threshold for detecting the consonant omission, which can be obtained by the hierarchical clustering model. Figure 8.6 shows the results of hierarchical clustering. The empty circles represent the speech with consonant omission, and the solid circles denote the speech without consonant omission. The experimental samples come from the Hospital of Stomatology, Sichuan University, which include all the initials and widely used finals. The total number of samples is 387 Mandarin syllables: there are 166 syllables with initial consonant omission and 221 syllables with non-consonant omission.

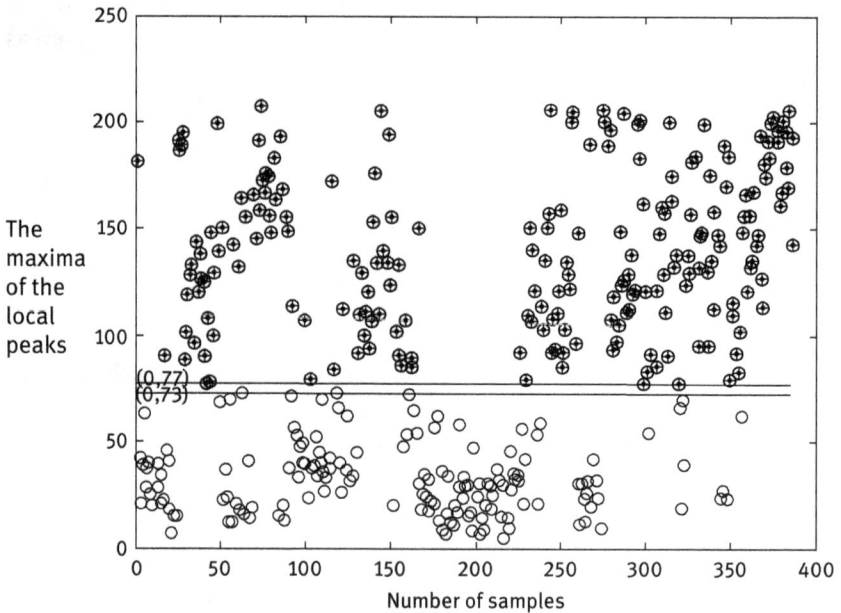

Figure 8.6: Hierarchical clustering results.

The values of P for the syllables with consonant omission are smaller than that of syllables with non-consonant omission. Thus, syllables with consonant omission are shown in the lower part of Figure 8.6. From Figure 8.6, it can be seen that when the value of T is between 73 and 77, a good classification performance can be obtained.

8.4 Automatic assessment of speech intelligibility

Low speech intelligibility for cleft palate speech is a typical characteristic. This chapter adopts the automatic continuous speech-recognition algorithm to realize the speech intelligibility evaluation, utilizing the HMM. In this work, the experiment platform is based on the HTK toolbox, which is widely used in ASR. The accuracy of cleft palate speech recognition has a positive relation with the speech intelligibility. However, the hypernasality grades and speech intelligibility are in inverse proportion. The process of the continuous speech recognition is illustrated as follows.

8.4.1 Hidden Markov models (HMM)

As shown in Figure 8.7, a Markov model can be regarded as a finite state machine [40].

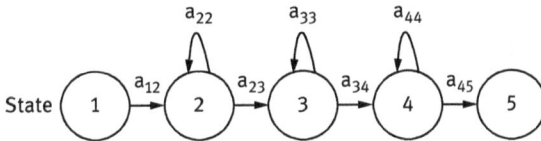

Figure 8.7: A simplified HMM model.

where a_{ij} denotes the state transition probability. It should be noticed that the states in the head and tail are non-emitting. They are used only for connections between two HMM models.

On the one hand, the implicit state corresponds to the stable pronunciation unit in the acoustic layer. And the change of pronunciation is described by state transition. The state transition of HMM is controlled by the state transition probability matrix A, which is illustrated in equation (8.6).

$$A = \begin{bmatrix} a_{11} & \cdots & a_{1N} \\ \cdots & \cdots & \cdots \\ a_{N1} & \cdots & a_{NN} \end{bmatrix}, \tag{8.6}$$

where N represents the state number, a_{ij} denotes the transition probability from the ith state to the jth state.

On the other hand, the probability and statistics model are introduced. The probability density function is used to find the recognition result. In HMM, it is assumed that the sequence of observed speech vectors corresponding to each speech signal unit is generated by this Markov model [40]. The sequence of observed speech vectors is the extracted feature. The MFCC parameter is the most widely used acoustic feature. The output observation probabilities are denoted as the set $\{b_{ij}(k)\}$. With the state transferring from the ith state to the jth state, $b_j(o_t)$ indicates the probability distribution. The form of $b_j(o_t)$ is shown in equation (8.7).

$$b_j(o_t) = \sum_{k=1}^{N} c_{jk} f(o_t, u_{jk}, U_{jk}), \ 1 \le j \le N \tag{8.7}$$

where $f(O_t, u_{jk}, U_{jk})$ represents the Gauss function, o_t denotes the observed sequence vector, k represents the number of Gauss functions, c_{jk} represents the proportion of the kth Gauss function in all the Gauss functions, u_{jk} denotes the mean value of the kth Gauss function, and U_{jk} is the variance of the kth Gauss function.

8.4.2 The process of continuous speech recognition

The continuous speech recognition based on HTK is usually composed of four steps, namely, preliminary data processing, model revaluation, recognition test, and result evaluation.

Step 1: Preliminary data processing
In the early stage of data processing, there are five items to complete, namely, the original data acquisition, data transcription files creation, task grammar definition, dictionary establishment, and feature extraction.
1) *Original data acquisition:* the original speech is collected by the Hospital of Stomatology, Sichuan University, which is made up of short sentences. The time durations of these sentences are around 5s.
2) *Data transcription files creation:* there are two kinds of transcription files. The first file is written by hand, which describes the sentence information. That is, the syllable transcription of each sentence. However, the boundary of these syllables is not included. The second transcription file is used to annotate the syllable-level and phoneme-level (initials/finals) information based on the first transcription file. It can be realized by the script file

named *prompts2mlf* and the tool *HLEd*, which are both included in the HTK toolbox.

3) *Task grammar definition:* the main purpose of the task grammar is to constrain the pronunciation of vocabulary by a specific grammar structure. In this chapter, the transcription files, such as *HParse, HBuild*, are used to complete the definition of Bigram language model.

4) *Dictionary establishment:* The dictionary can be defined according to the practical needs. In this chapter, the structure of initial+final is adopted. That is, the training unit is the initial/final unit. Note that all the syllables in the original speech must be included in the dictionary to train a robust acoustic model.

5) *Feature extraction:* the feature extraction is also called data coding in the ASR. A configure file is needed, which includes the sampling frequency, window size, acoustic feature, frame periodicity, number of MFCC coefficients, function for windowing frames, pre-emphasis coefficient, and the number of filter bank channels. In this chapter, the 13 MFCC coefficients and its 13 delta and 13 acceleration coefficients are chosen [40].

Step 2: model revaluation

The main purpose of the model revaluation is to train a stable and efficient HMM. The HTK provides two sets of revaluation tools, namely, *HInit/HRest+HERest* and *HCompV+HERest*, which are, respectively, corresponding to the bootstrap and flat-start training method. Due to the boundary information of syllables in sentences is unknown, the flat-start training method is chosen. The main purpose of the *HCompV* and *HERest* is to complete the generation and training of the monophones model. The creation of the thiphones model is a key step to make the model more stable.

Step 3: recognition test

The recognition process is based on the tool *HVite*. The input of the HMM includes the testing speech recording, grammar file, and dictionary. According to the identification probability, the output of the model is the corresponding text files with sentence boundary information.

Step 4: result evaluation

In this stage, it compares the sentence text file produced in step 3 with the previous transcription file produced in step 1, and finally outputs the corresponding recognition correct rate. The used HTK tool is *HResult*.

8.5 Experimental results

8.5.1 Results for automatic consonant omission detection

Based on the differences between vowels and consonants in Mandarin, we propose the automatic consonant omission detection algorithm in cleft palate speech. The results of consonant omission detection are listed in Table 8.2.

Table 8.2: Results for automatic consonant omission detection.

Actual speech category	Automatic detected speech category (%)		
	Non-consonant omission		Consonant omission
Non-consonant omission	76.92		23.08
Consonant omission	11.43		88.58
Average accuracy		82.75	

The average accuracy is 82.75%. The detection accuracy for consonant omission is 88.58% and the detection accuracy for non-consonant omission is 76.92%. Totally, 23.08% of speech recordings with non-consonant omission are detected as the consonant omission. The reason is that the speech utterances all the 21 consonant initials, where the /m/, /n/, /l/, and /r/ belong to the voiced sounds. And the short-time autocorrelation function of voiced consonants and vowels has similar periodicity.

In our previous study [8], the accuracy of consonant omission detection is over 94%. However, only 11 initial consonants are considered. This chapter includes all 21 initial consonants, and the detection accuracy is 82.75%. The majority of current studies investigate the dysarthria features of consonant omission. This chapter proposes an automatic consonant omission detection algorithm. It aims to provide a more objective and efficient assistant aid.

8.5.2 Results for automatic speech intelligibility assessment

This chapter adopts the automatic continuous speech-recognition algorithm to realize the automatic speech intelligibility evaluation. The 10-fold cross-validation

Table 8.3: Results for automatic speech intelligibility assessment.

Actual hypernasality grade (%)	ASR accuracy (%)
Normal	96.41
Mild	74.59
Moderate	73.77
Severe	65.82

is applied 10 times to the experiment. The results of the automatic speech recognition are shown in Table 8.3.

From Table 8.3, it is seen that when the actual hypernasality grade is normal, the accuracy of ASR reaches up to 96.41%. With the increase of hypernasality grades, the accuracy of automatic speech recognition reduces. When the hypernasality grade is severe, the accuracy is the lowest, which is 65.82%. The higher hypernasality grades bring lower speech intelligibility.

There are three studies on cleft palate speech intelligibility based on ASR [34–36]. The ASR system converts the speech signal into the acoustic features, such as MFCC and its delta coefficients. Then, combined with the Unigram language model, they adopt the word-based semi-continuous HMM to train the speech recordings. Literature [35] includes 111 cleft palate patients, and the highest word accuracy is 76.8%. Literature [34] and literature [36] include only 31 cleft palate patients, and the highest word accuracies are around 75.8% and 72.9%, respectively.

Compared with the state-of-the-art studies, this chapter: (1) instead of using word-based semi-continuous HMM adopts sentence-based continuous HMM, considering that the sentences contain more acoustic information; (2) adopts the Bigram language model instead of Unigram language model, since the Bigram language model needs to estimate more parameters; (3) uses the more abundant cleft speech recordings. The number of cleft palate patients in literatures [34–36] is 111, 31, and 31, respectively. In the experiment of this chapter, the speech utterances recorded from 120 patients are included.

8.6 Conclusions and discussions

There are many factors that can affect perceptual evaluation of speech–language pathologists, such as the level of experience, affection, emotion, thought, context, and so on. The proposed system can assist objectively speech–language pathologists in evaluation of cleft palate speech. In some countries, cleft palate care is well developed. The speech–language pathologists are distributed in public or private hospitals, educational institutions, community, home health-care, and hospice [41]. The speech assessment by speech–language pathologists is a relatively new field in many other countries, where the speech–language pathologists are not sufficient. The automatic cleft palate speech assessment system proposed in this chapter can provide a convenient and economical assistant diagnose for these patients.

This chapter proposes two algorithms to study the two speech disorders in cleft palate speech, which are the automatic detection of consonant omission and assessment of cleft palate speech intelligibility, respectively. Currently, most of the experimental samples are small for the study of cleft palate speech [1–7]. In this chapter, the speech utterances are collected by the Hospital of Stomatology, Sichuan University. The datasets in this chapter are based on a database with a total of 530 patients.

The consonant omission detection algorithm is based on the differences between vowels and initial consonants in Mandarin. The vowels have obvious periodicity, while the initial consonants are non-periodic, except /m/ ,/n/, /l/, and /r/. The algorithm detects the local peaks of the short-time autocorrelation function and calculates the maxima of the peaks' number for a Mandarin syllable. This chapter utilizes the hierarchical clustering algorithm to determine the threshold value for the consonant omission detection. Table 8.2 lists the results for automatic consonant omission detection. The average detection accuracy is 82.75%. In the previous study [8], the correct identification of consonant omission is over 94%. However, it only considers 11 initial consonants according to the acoustic char-acteristic of cleft palate speech. This chapter includes all 21 initial consonants. When the actual speech is non-consonant omission, the accuracy is slightly low. The reason is that the speech utterances with non-consonants contain the voiced sounds:/m/, /n/, /l/, and /r/. The short-time autocorrelation functions of these voiced consonants have the similar periodic characteristics to the Mandarin vowels. Thus, the voiced consonants cannot be detected precisely.

The automatic cleft palate speech intelligibility evaluation is performed using the automatic continuous speech recognition method. The core of the algorithm is to build an acoustic model, which is the HMM. The experiment platform is based on a widely used HTK toolbox. The accuracy of cleft palate speech recognition has a positive relation with the speech intelligibility. However, the hypernasality grades and the speech intelligibility are in inverse proportion. As known that the higher hypernasality grades of cleft palate patients have, the more difficult for audiences to understand in auditory percep-tion. In clinical practice, the hypernasality grades are obtained by the auditory assessment of the speech–language pathologists. The hypernasality sounds like that the speech is leaked through the nasal cavity, which may make some speech sounds distorted and mushy [42]. Therefore, the speech intelligibility can be affected by the different degree of hypernasality, and this affection can be represented by the auditory perception. This is coincident with the experiment results listed in Table 8.3. For normal speech, the recognition accuracy of ASR is the highest, which is 96.41%. With the increase of hypernasality grades, the recognition accuracy of ASR reduces. For the speech utterances with severe hypernasality, the recognition accuracy is the lowest, which is 65.82%. The results are consistent with the human auditory perception. If the hypernasality grade is higher, the speech intelligibility is lower. For the evaluation of the cleft palate speech intelligibility, some previous works are judged by the parents of patients [31], some inexperienced listeners [32], or experienced speech pathologists [33]. Manual evaluation is subjective and time consuming. Although the evaluation of speech–language pathologists can be regarded as a gold standard, however, it is not convenient. The ASR system of literature [34] is just based on the words recognition. Sentences contain more speech information, thus sentence-based ASR can better reflect the speech intelligibility. In this chapter, the automatic continuous speech recognition is based on a large number of sentences. Compared with our previous studies [9], this chapter has greatly improved the accuracy of the ASR system.

Due to the limited cleft palate speech utterances, this chapter chooses the HMM-based ASR instead of deep neural network (DNN)-based system. The DNN model requires a large amount of training samples. Generally, DNN model requires 24–400 h training samples [43–45]. The Dataset II in this chapter is about 2 h. The data acquisition process of cleft palate speech is difficult. The acquisition process of cleft palate speech is affected by a variety of factors, such as the different examination settings, perceptual rating methods, accent of speakers, the articulation skills, and vocabulary list. Moreover, the majority of cleft palate patients are children. It is difficult for children to quietly follow the instructions of doctors. Therefore, for a child, it usually takes half a day or more time to collect satisfactory speech data.

Acknowledgement: This work is supported by the National Natural Science Foundation of China 61503264.

References

[1]   Cairns DA, Hansen JH, Riski JE. A noninvasive technique for detecting hypernasal speech using a nonlinear operator. IEEE Trans Biomed Eng 1996;43(1):35.

[2] Nieto RG, Marín-Hurtado JI, Capacho-Valbuena LM, et al. Pattern recognition of hyper-
     nasality in voice of patients with Cleft and Lip Palate. 2014 XIX Symposium on Image,
     Signal Processing and Artificial Vision (STSIVA), Armenia, Colombia, 2014:1–5.
[3] Rah DK, Ko YI, Lee C, et al. A Noninvasive estimation of hypernasality using a linear
     predictive model. Ann Biomed Eng 2001;29(7):587–594.
[4] Akafi E, Vali M, Moradi N. Detection of hypernasal speech in children with cleft palate. in 2012
     19th Iranian Conference of Biomedical Engineering (ICBME), Tehran, Iran, 2012:237–41.
[5] Vijayalakshmi P, Reddy MR, O'Shaughnessy D. Acoustic analysis and detection of hyper-
     nasality using a group delay function. IEEE Trans Biomed Eng 2007;54(4):621–629.
[6] Haque, S., Ali MH, Haque AF. Cross-gender acoustic differences in hypernasal speech and
     detection of hypernasality. International Workshop on Computational Intelligence (IWCI),
     Dhaka, Bangladesh, 2016:187–191.
[7] Vijayalakshmi P, Nagarajan T, Rav J. Selective pole modification-based technique for the
     analysis and detection of hypernasality. TENCON 2009–2009 IEEE Region 10 Conference.
     Singapore, Singapore, 2009:1–5.
[8] He L, Zhang J, Liu Q, et al. Automatic evaluation of hypernasality and consonant misarti-
     culation in cleft palate speech. IEEE Signal Processing Letters, 2014, 21(10):1298–1301.
[9] He L, Zhang J, Liu Q, et al. Automatic evaluation of hypernasality and speech intelligibility
     for children with cleft palate. 8th IEEE Conference Industrial Electronics and Applications
     (ICIEA), Melbourne, Australia, 2013:220–223.
[10] He L, Tan J, Hao H, et al. Automatic evaluation of resonance and articulation disorders in
     cleft palate speech. IEEE China Summit and International Conference on Signal and
     Information Processing (ChinaSIP), Chengdu, China, 2015:358–362.
[11] Liu Y, Wang X, Hang Y, et al. Hypemasality detection in cleft palate speech based on
     natural computation. 12th International Conference on Natural Computation, Fuzzy
     Systems and Knowledge Discovery (ICNC-FSKD), Changsha, China, 2016:523–528.
[12] Luyten A, Bettens K, D'Haeseleer E, et al. Short-term effect of short, intensive speech
     therapy on articulation and resonance in Ugandan patients with cleft (lip and) palate. J
     Commun Disord 2016;61:71–82.
[13] Zhu HP, Sun YG. Acoustic features of consonants articulated by children with cleft palate. J
     Mod Stomatol 1998;12(3):181–183.
[14] Jiang LP, Wang GM, Yang YS, et al. The study on articulation characteristics of the patients
     after pharyngoplasty. China J Oral Maxillofacial Surgery 2005;3(1):48–50.
[15] Li F, Li XM, Zhao JF, et al. The observation on articulation characteristics of 48 patients
     after pharyngoplasty. J Zhengzhou University (Medical Sciences), 2008;43(1):173–175.
[16] Yin H, C.L. G, B. S, et al. A preliminary study on the consonant articulation of older patients
     with cleft palate. West China J Stomatol 2013;31(2):182–185.
[17] Hu MF., F. L, L.N. X, et al. Phonological characteristics and rehabilitation training of
     bilabial consonant articulation disorders in patients repaired cleft plate. Chin J Rehabil
     Theory Pract 2017;23(2):211–216.
[18] Zhou QJ, H. Y and B. S. Error analysis of functional articulation disorders in children. West
     China J Stomatol 2008;26(4):391–395.
[19] Wang XM, K.H, H.Y. L, et al. A comparative study on the consonant articulation place of
     preschool and older patients with cleft palate. Int J Stomatol 2017;44(1):37–40.
[20] Bruneel L, Luyten A, Bettens K, et al. Delayed primary palatal closure in resource-poor
     countries: Speech results in Ugandan older children and young adults with cleft (lip and)
     palate. J Commun Disord 2017;69:1–14.

[21] Vijayalakshmi P, Reddy MR. Assessment of dysarthric speech and an analysis on velo-pharyngeal incompetence. International Conference of the IEEE Engineering in Medicine & Biology Society, New York, 2006:3759.

[22] Laitinen J, Haapanen ML, Paaso M, et al. Occurrence of dental consonant misarticulations in different cleft types. Folia Phoniatrica et Logopaedica 1998;50(2):92–100.

[23] Subtelny JD. Intelligibility and associated physiological factors of cleft palate speakers. J Speech Lang Hear Res 1959;2(4):353.

[24] Subtelny JD, Koepp-Baker H, Subtelny JD. Palatal function and cleft palate speech. J Speech Hear Disord 1961;26(3):213.

[25] Forner LL. Speech segment durations produced by five and six year old speakers with and without cleft palates. Cleft Palate J 1983;20(3):185–198.

[26] Jr MW, Sommers RK. Phonetic contexts: their effects on perceived nasality in cleft palate speakers. Cleft Palate J 1975;27(6):410.

[27] Maegawa J, Sells RK, David DJ. Speech changes after maxillary advancement in 40 cleft lip and palate patients. J Craniofacial Surg 1998;9(2):177.

[28] Subtelny JD, Van Hattum RJ, Myers BB. Ratings and measures of cleft palate speech. Cleft Palate J 1972;9(1):18.

[29] Mcwilliams BJ. Some factors in the intelligibility of cleft-palate speech. J Speech Hear Disord 1954;19(4):524.

[30] Kent RD, Weismer G, Kent JF, et al. Toward phonetic intelligibility testing in dysarthria. J Speech Hear Disord, 1989;54(4):482.

[31] Van Lierde K, Luyten A, Van Borsel J, et al. Speech intelligibility of children with unilateral cleft lip and palate (Dutch cleft) following a one-stage Wardill–Kilner palatoplasty, as judged by their parents. Int J Oral Maxillofacial Surg 2010;39(7):641–646.

[32] Konst EM, Weersink-Braks H, Rietveld T, et al. An intelligibility assessment of toddlers with cleft lip and palate who received and did not receive presurgical infant orthopedic treatment. J Commun Disord 2000;33(6):483–501.

[33] Witt PD, Berry LA, Marsh JL, et al. Speech outcome following palatoplasty in primary school children: do lay peer observers agree with speech pathologists? Plastic Reconstr Surg 1996;98(6):958–965.

[34] Maier, A., Hacker C, Noth E, et al., Intelligibility of children with cleft lip and palate: Evaluation by speech recognition techniques. 18th International Conference on Pattern Recognition (ICPR), Hong Kong, China, 2006:274–277.

[35] Schuster M, Maier A, Bocklet T, et al. Automatically evaluated degree of intelligibility of children with different cleft type from preschool and elementary school measured by automatic speech recognition. Int J Pediatr Otorhinolaryngol 2012;76(3): 362–369.

[36] Schuster M, Maier A, Haderlein T, et al., Evaluation of speech intelligibility for children with cleft lip and palate by means of automatic speech recognition. Int J Pediatr Otorhinolaryngol 2006;70(10):1741–1747.

[37] Bocklet T, Maier A, Riedhammer K, et al. Towards a language-independent intelligibility assessment of children with cleft lip and palate. In The Workshop on Child (ACM), Cambridge, USA, 2009:1–4.

[38] Bao HQ, Lin MC. Shiyan yuyinxue gaiyao (Enlarged Edition). Beijing: Higher Education Press, 2016:457–483.

[39] Sharma A., Boroevich K, Shigemizu D, et al. Hierarchical Maximum Likelihood Clustering Approach. IEEE Transactions on Bio-medical Engineering, 2016;64(1):112–122.

[40] Young S, Evermann G, Gales M, et al. The HTK book (for HTK version 3.4). Cambridge University Engineering Department, 2006;2(2):2–3.

[41] Pollens R. Role of the speech-language pathologist in palliative hospice care. J Palliative Med 2004;7(5):694–702.

[42] Wyatt R, Sell D, Russell J, et al. Cleft palate speech dissected: a review of current knowledge and analysis. Br J Plast Surg 1996;49(3):143–149.

[43] Zhou P, Jiang H, Dai LR, et al. State-clustering based multiple deep neural networks modeling approach for speech recognition. IEEE/ACM Transactions on Audio Speech & Language Processing, 2015, 23(4):631–642.

[44] Xue S, Abdel-Hamid O, Jiang H, et al. Fast adaptation of deep neural network based on discriminant codes for speech recognition. IEEE/ACM Trans Audio Speech Lang Process 2014;22(12):1713–1725.

[45] Dahl GE, Acero A. Context-dependent pre-trained deep neural networks for large-vocabulary speech recognition. IEEE Trans Audio Speech Lang Process 2012;20(1):30–42.

Kamil L. Kadi and Sid Ahmed Selouani

9 Distinctive auditory-based cues and rhythm metrics to assess the severity level of dysarthria

Abstract: Millions of children and adults suffer from acquired or congenital neuromotor communication disorders that affect their speech intelligibility. Automatic characterization of the speech impairment can improve the patient's quality of life and assist experts in the assessment and treatment of the impairment. In this chapter, we present different techniques for improving the analysis and classification of disordered speech to automatically assess the severity of dysarthria. A model simulating the external, middle and inner parts of the ear is presented. The model provides relevant auditory-based cues that are combined with conventional Mel-Frequency Cepstral Coefficients (MFCCs) and rhythm metrics to represent atypical speech utterances. The experiments are carried out using data from the Nemours and Torgo databases of dysarthric speech. Gaussian mixture models (GMMs), support vector machines (SVMs), and multinomial logistic regression (MLR) are tested and compared in the context of dysarthric speech assessment. The experimental results show that the MLR-based approach using multiple and diverse input features offers a powerful alternative to the conventional assessment methods. Indeed, the MLR-based approach achieved the best correct classification rate of 97.7%, while the GMM- and SVM-based systems achieved 93.5% and 76.8% correct classification rate, respectively.

Keywords: rhythm metrics, Dysarthria, acoustic analysis, Cepstral acoustic features, logistic regression, prosodic features, auditory distinctive features

9.1 Introduction

Communication is a multidimensional dynamic process for expressing thoughts, emotions, and needs, thus allowing interactions between people and their environment. Cognition, hearing, speech production, and motor coordination are involved in the communication process. Impairment of one or more of these aspects causes disordered communication. This can have a great impact on quality of life, preventing individuals from expressing their needs, wants, and opinions. It also reduces the capacity to express personality and exercise autonomy, and often has an impact on relationships and self-esteem [1]. Therefore, it is necessary to

https://doi.org/10.1515/9781501502415-010

improve the communication of individuals suffering from a verbal communication disability by offering them more opportunities to interact with their environment.

Over the years, there has been an increasing interest in offering automated frameworks to measure the quality and to process the pathological speech. The goal is to provide accurate and reliable systems that can help clinicians to diagnose and monitor the evolution of speech impairments. Researchers have extensively investigated different issues related to the pathological speech evaluation. These studies reveal that the evaluation of the pathological speech intelligibility and quality is a difficult task.

In the context of these research efforts, Kim et al. in [2] performed feature-level fusions and subsystem decision to capture abnormal variation in the prosodic, voice quality, and pronunciation aspects in pathological speech. They obtained the best automatic intelligibility classification performance of 73.5% on the The Netherlands Cancer Institute (NKI)-Concomitant Chemoradiotherapy (CCRT) corpus, which contains recordings and perceptual evaluations of speech intelligibility before treatment and after treatment of speakers by means of chemoradiotherapy [3]. The features were designed in sentence-independent fashion to correspond to the sentence-level running speech and, therefore, the vowel segments of each utterance were concatenated. On the same corpus, Fang et al. tested a multi-granularity combined feature scheme composed of conventional acoustic features, Mel S-transform cepstrum coefficients, and chaotic features and obtained a correct intelligibility classification rate of 84.4% using a support vector machine-based system [4]. In [5], a system was designed to capture the pronunciation, rhythm, and intonation of speech utterances to assess the aphasic speech intelligibility. The results demonstrated the potential for the computerized treatment using support vector machine and logistic regression and thus contributed for bridging the gap between human and automatic intelligibility assessment.

Our research focuses on dysarthria, one of the most common speech communication disorders associated with a neurological impairment. Millions of adults and children throughout the world are affected by dysarthria, which reduces the intelligibility of their speech. Dysarthria is a motor speech disorder resulting from disturbed muscular control of the speech mechanism, caused by damage to the central or peripheral nervous system. Dysarthria has various causes including Parkinson's disease, head injury, stroke, tumor, muscular dystrophy, and cerebral palsy [6].

Numerous tools and methods have been developed to help dysarthric speakers. Indeed, prominent achievements have been made in the fields of speech recognition, speech intelligibility enhancement, and automatic evaluation. For instance, in [7], an adaptive system is proposed to match dysarthric speech to the normal speech to provide intelligible verbal communication. The proposed mechanism adapts the tempo of sonorant part of dysarthric speech with respect to the level of severity. A good performance in the recognition of tempo-adapted dysarthric speech, using a GMM as well as a Deep neural network was obtained using the Universal Access Speech Corpus. To identify the acoustic features underlying each listener's impressions of speaker's similarity, a perceptual similarity-based approach to dysarthria characterization by utilizing multinomial logistic regression with sparsity constraints was proposed in [8]. This approach permitted an examination of the effect of clinical experience on listeners' impressions of similarity. To perform an intelligibility assessment of dysarthria, a technique based on iVectors was proposed in [9]. This study showed that the major advantage of iVectors is that they compress all acoustic information contained in an utterance into a reduced number of measures, and then they are suitable to be used in conjunction with simple classifiers. In this application, the correlation between intelligible perceptual ratings and the automatic intelligibility assessments reached 0.9. In the field of dysarthric speech recognition, Rudzicz improved the intelligibility of dysarthric speech before performing the speech recognition using the Torgo database [10]. The Torgo database of dysarthric articulation is distributed by the Linguistic Data Consortium and can be accessed through a licensing agreement (https://catalog. ldc.upenn.edu/LDC2012S02).

Several approaches have been developed to automatically assess the severity of dysarthria. In [11], feedforward artificial neural networks (ANNs) and support vector machines (SVMs) with phonological features were used to design discriminative models for dysarthric speech. Statistical GMMs were combined with the ANN soft-computing technique along with Mel-Frequency Cepstral Coefficients (MFCCs) and speech rhythm metrics in [12], and 86% accuracy was achieved over four levels of severity. In [13], a classifier based on Mahalanobis distance and discriminant analysis was developed for the classification of dysarthria severity using acoustic features, and 95% accuracy was achieved over two levels of severity. Linear discriminant analysis was combined with an SVM automatic classifier using prosodic features. This method achieved a classification rate of 93% over four severity levels of dysarthria [14]. In [15], an automatic intelligibility assessment system performed an effective binary classification after capturing the atypical variations in dysarthric speech and using linear discriminant analysis and SVM-based classifiers. Most recently, a global average classification accuracy of 97.5% (over 2 databases) was obtained by an ANN that was trained to classify speech into various severity levels within the Dysarthric Speech Database for Universal Access and the Torgo database [16].

Recent clinical studies concluded that in the case of dysarthria assessment, we still need more tools and frameworks that can capture the most prominent audible symptoms and that are capable to perform an efficient assessment of intelligibility and impairment severity level [17, 18].

In this study, different acoustical analyzers were used to assess the level of severity of dysarthria performed by different classifiers. The severity levels were classified using both the Nemours dysarthric speech corpus [19] and the Torgo database of acoustic and articulatory speech [20].

The remainder of this chapter is structured as follows. Section 9.2 describes the auditory-based cues, the MFCCs, and the rhythm metrics that were used as acoustical analyzers. Section 9.3 presents the principle of the Frenchay dysarthria assessment used as a reference in our experiments. Section 9.4 presents the background on the GMM, SVM, and multinomial logistic regression (MLR), which are the three techniques used to assess dysarthric speech. In Section 9.5, the experiments and their outcomes are presented and discussed. Finally, Section 9.6 concludes the chapter.

9.2 Acoustic analysis

The extraction of reliable parameters to represent the speech utterance waveform is an important issue in pattern recognition. This extraction process aims to extract the relevant information contained in the speech signal while excluding the irrelevant part. Several features can be used as input parameters in speech recognition and disorder characterization systems, including Linear Predictive Coding (LPC) coefficients, MFCCs, short-time spectral envelope, short-time energy, and zero-crossing rate. Numerous studies have shown that the use of human hearing properties can provide a potentially useful front-end speech representation [21]. These studies also showed that these features involve different levels of perception, ranging from low-level features, such as the acoustic and phonetic components of speech to high-level features, such as pronunciation, prosody, and semantic information.

This chapter presents an approach that combines different sources of information related to the speech signal to improve its representation by selecting relevant and complementary cues. These sources consist of the conventional MFCCs, rhythm measures, and auditory-based indicative features.

9.2.1 Cepstral acoustic features

A mapping of the acoustic frequency to a perceptual frequency scale can be defined in the *bark* scale or *mel* scale. Mel-scale filter banks are used to compute the MFCCs that have been shown to be robust in automatic speech recognition.

The short-term MFCC approach is also found appropriate for the parameterization of dysarthric speech. MFCCs have been often used in the front-end signal processing of applications, such as the recognition of dysarthric speech and classification of speech disorders in general [22]. The Mel scale introduced by Davis and Mermelstein maps from a linear to a non-linear frequency scale based on human auditory perception [23]. The Mel scale approximation is

$$Mel(f) = 2595.\log_{10}\left(1 + \frac{f}{700}\right), \qquad (9.1)$$

where f represents the linear frequency scale (in Hz).

To compute the MFCCs, a discrete cosine transform (DCT) is applied to the outputs of M critical band-pass filters. These filters are triangular and ranged on the Mel frequency scale, which is linear below 1 kHz and logarithmic above. Between 15 and 24 filters can be used; in this work, approximately two filters per octave were used. The MFCCs are defined as:

$$MFCC_n = \sum_{m=1}^{M} X_m \, \cos\left(\frac{\pi \, n}{M}(m - 0.5)\right), \; n = 1, 2, \ldots, N, \qquad (9.2)$$

where M is the analysis order, N represents the number of cepstral coefficients, and X_m ($m = 1, 2, \ldots, M$) is the log-energy output of the mth filter applied to the log-magnitude spectrum of the signal. An illustration of the filters used throughout our experiments is shown in Figure 9.1. Several cross-validation experiments were carried out to determine the optimal frame duration. In the proposed framework, the MFCCs were calculated using a 16 ms Hamming window that contained 256 samples with an overlap of 50%. This frame size value was found to be effective as it satisfies the stationary criterion, which is required when processing random signals to achieve a good trade-off between complexity and quality. The same frame length was used to calculate the auditory-based cues presented below, which simplified the combination of the two feature sets obtained independently.

9.2.2 Speech rhythm metrics

Speech rhythm is defined as the pattern of variation in the duration of intervals. An important advantage of defining rhythm as patterns of durational variability is that it identifies specific units that can be measured objectively and compared. Researchers have developed a number of metrics that quantify speech rhythms in different languages. There are two main families of rhythm metrics, both of

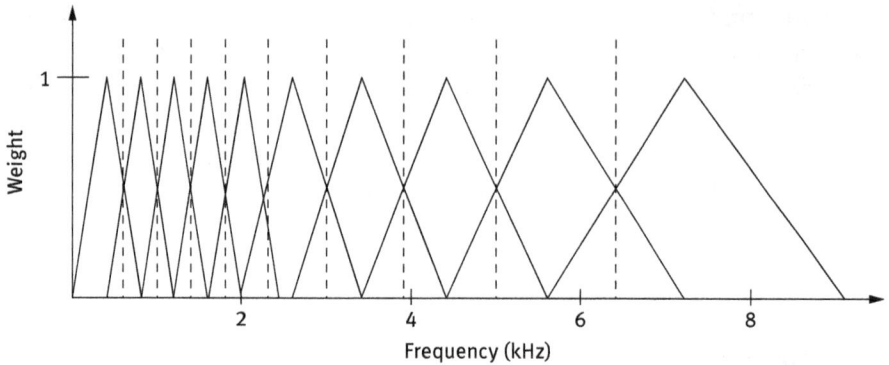

Figure 9.1: An illustration of the Mel-filter bank generating the short-term MFCCs.

which use measures of speech timing that are based on the segmentation of the speech signal into vocalic and consonantal intervals. Pairwise variability indices (PVI) measure the difference in duration between immediately consecutive intervals and average these differences over an utterance [24]. Interval-based metrics quantify variation in individual vocalic or consonantal interval durations [25] using their standard deviations (deltaV and deltaC) over an utterance. A related measure considers the proportion of vowel durations (% V) over the utterance. Both types of indices have normalized measures that reduce the potential effects of speech tempo on raw measures. For the PVI-based measures, normalization is based on the mean duration of the two intervals being compared. Researchers tend to use raw durations when measuring consonantal effects (rPVI-C) but normalized measures for vowels (nPVI-V). To examine whether rhythm metrics are sensitive to the observed durational differences among dysarthric speakers, we measured the durations of the vocalic, consonantal, voiced, and unvoiced segments for each sentence of each speaker. The following seven metrics were used throughout the experiments: %V, deltaC, deltaV, rPVI-V, nPVI-V, rPVI-C, and nPVI-C.

9.2.3 Auditory-based modeling

The ability of the auditory system to efficiently process and interpret speech, even unintelligible dysarthric speech, makes auditory modeling a promising approach in the field of pathological speech analysis. Usually, the aim of acoustical analysis based on auditory modeling is to examine the response of the basilar membrane and the auditory nerve to various sounds. An advanced level of processing that simulates the auditory cortex can also be performed. Flanagan in [26], proposed a computational model to estimate the basilar membrane movement. This model has been found to be useful for reporting the subjective auditory behavior and acousto-mechanical process of the ear. Other well-known models, such as the cochlea model proposed by Lyon [27], the mean synchrony auditory representation proposed by Seneff [28], and ensemble interval histogram processing presented by Ghitza in [29], have been applied in many contemporary approaches. All of these models use a band pass filter bank to simulate cochlear filtering.

In recent years, there has been renewed interest in improving front-end processing to compute robust features, inspired by auditory modeling [30]. In the area of speech recognition, psychoacoustics and auditory physiology-based processing have become the main components of robust feature extraction methods, such as Gammatone features proposed by Schluter *et al.* [31] and Power Normalized Cepstral Coefficients (PNCC) presented by Kim and Stern in [32].

The auditory model used throughout the experiments simulates the external, middle, and inner parts of the ear. A band pass filter is used to model the various adaptive ossicle motions in the external and middle ear. A non-linear filter bank stimulates the basilar membrane (BM) that acts within the inner ear. The BM model also considers the electro-mechanical transduction of hair cells and afferent fibers from which the encoding signal is generated at the synaptic endings. Different regions of the various organs involved in perception and hearing are responsive to the sounds with different spectral properties. Thus, every part along the BM has given a resonance frequency for a certain input sound [33]. The BM is simulated using 24 overlapping filters that represent the cochlear filter bank. For the output of each channel, the absolute energy is denoted by W_i ($i = 1$, $2, 3, \ldots, 24$). Details of this auditory model can be found in [34]. The following eight auditory-based features were extracted from the speech signal to perform the dysarthria-level assessment: grave/acute (G/A), open/closed (O/C), diffuse/compact (D/C), flat/sharp (F/S), mellow/strident (M/S), continuous/discontinuous (C/D), tense/lax (TL), and mid-external energy (W_{md}). Table 9.1 defines the eight auditory cues and the formula used for their calculation, and Figure 9.2 represents the ear model used in this work.

9.3 Dysarthric speech assessment

The intelligibility of dysarthric speech can range from near normal to unintelligible, depending on the severity of the impairment. Usually, a large set of tests is used to measure the level of intelligibility and, thus, assess the severity of the

Table 9.1: Description of the auditory-based cues.

Auditory-based Cue	Description
(G/A)	measures the difference of energy between low frequencies(50–400 Hz) and high frequencies (3,800–6,000 Hz): $(W_1 + \ldots + W_5) - (W_{20} + \ldots + W_{24})$
(O/C)	a phoneme is considered closed if the energy of low frequencies(230–350 Hz) is greater than that of the middle frequencies(600–800 Hz). Hence, the O/C cue is calculated by: $W_8 + W_9 - W_3 - W_4$
(D/C)	compactness reflects the prominence of the central formantregion (800–1,050 Hz) compared with the surroundingregions (300–700 Hz) and (1,450–2,550 Hz): $W_{10} + W_{11} - (W_4 + \ldots + W_8 + W_{13} + \ldots + W_{17})/5$
(F/S)	a phoneme is considered sharp if the energy in (2,200–3,300 Hz)is more important than the energy in (1,900–2,900 Hz): $W_{17} + W_{18} + W_{19} - W_{11} - W_{12} - W_{13}$
(M/S)	strident phonemes are characterized by a presence of noisebecause of a turbulence at their articulation point which leadsto more energy in (3,800–5,300 Hz) than in (1,900–2,900 Hz): $W_{21} + W_{22} + W_{23} - W_{16} - W_{17} - W_{18}$
(C/D)	quantifies the variation of the spectrum magnitude by comparingthe energy of current and preceding frames. $\sum_{i=1}^{N_c} \lvert W_i(T) - W_a(T) - W_i(T-1) + W_a(T-1) \rvert$ $W_i(T)$ is the energy of channel i of current frame T. $W_a(T)$ is the energy average over all channels of current frame T.
(T/L)	measures the difference of energy between middle frequencies(900–2,000 Hz) and relatively high frequencies (2,650–5,000 Hz): $(W_{11} + \ldots + W_{16}) - (W_{18} + \ldots + W_{23})$
(W_{md})	measures the log-energy of the signal received from the external and middle ear: $W_{md} = 20 \ log \sum_{k=1}^{K} \lvert S'(k) \rvert$

disorder or progress of rehabilitation. Automatic methods of assessment can help clinicians to monitor dysarthria.

The *Frenchay Dysarthria Assessment* (FDA) is used to assess the severity of dysarthria [35]. For both the Nemours and Torgo databases, an assessment of the motor functions for each dysarthric speaker was carried out according to the standardized FDA (Enderby 1983). This section gives details about the Nemours and Torgo databases and FDA.

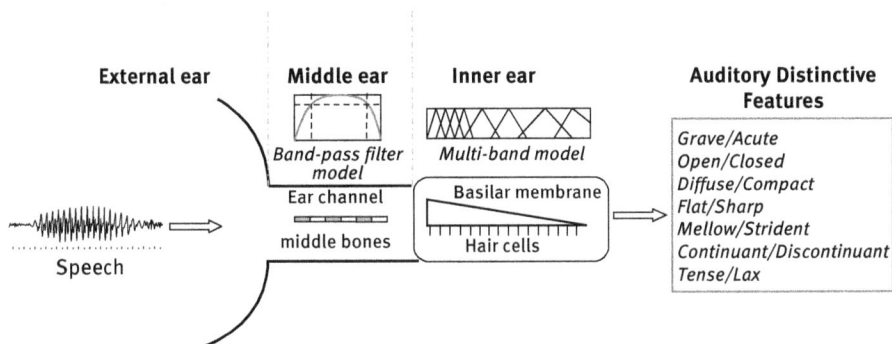

Figure 9.2: Block diagram of the ear model that generates the auditory distinctive features.

9.3.1 Nemours database

The Nemours is one of the few available databases of dysarthric speech than can be obtained through a licensing agreement. It includes recordings of 11 American patients who suffer from dysarthria with different degrees of severity. The dysarthric speakers produced 814 short and non-sensical sentences. The database contains two commonly used passages, the connected-speech paragraphs, "Grandfather" and "Rainbow," pronounced by each dysarthric patient. Every sentence in the database has the following form: "*The S is Ying the Z*," generated by randomly selecting S and Z, without substitution, from an ensemble of 74 monosyllabic nouns and selecting Y from an ensemble of 37 disyllabic verbs without substitution. This process produced 37 sentences, from which 37 additional sentences were generated by swapping the nouns S and Z. Thus, through the entire set of 74 sentences, each patient pronounced each noun and verb twice. The complete database was transcribed at the word-level and at the phoneme-level for 10 patients' sentences. Finally, the speech pathologist who conducted the recording sessions produced the whole speech corpus to serve as the healthy control.

9.3.2 Torgo corpus

The Torgo corpus was developed by the department of Computer Science and Speech Language Pathology at the University of Toronto, Canada, in collaboration with the Holland–Bloorview Kids Rehabilitation Hospital in Toronto. It includes about 23 hours of English speech data collected between 2008 and 2010 from eight dysarthric speakers (three females and five males) with different levels of intelligibility and seven non-dysarthric speakers (three females and four males) as a control group. The acoustic data were recorded through two different microphones:

the first was an array microphone with eight recording elements placed 61 cm in front of the speaker, and the second microphone was a head-mounted electret. The sampling rate was 44.1 kHz for the first microphone and 22.1 kHz for the second. A down-sampling at 16 kHz was performed on the acoustic signals by the database designers. The Torgo database is structured by speaker and by session. In our experiments, we reorganized the database by creating a new directory for each speaker. We sorted all of the audio recordings of the dysarthric speakers according to the type of speech text consistency as follows: non-words, short words, and restricted sentences. Thus, the dysarthric speaker's directory contained one folder for each of the script types plus another folder for the unrestricted spoken sentences, after renaming all of the speech wave files.

9.3.3 Frenchay Dysarthria Assessment

The FDA was first published in 1983, following a study that identified the patterns and characteristics of speech production and oromotor movements associated with proven neurological diseases. The test protocol can be used to assist with diagnosis and to guide treatment, and has good validity and reliability. The FDA second edition (FDA-2) has been amended to integrate more recent knowledge about motor speech disorders and their contribution to the neurological diagnoses. Some of the original items were dropped from the second edition (2008) as they were considered inadequate or redundant for management and diagnosis [36]. Files containing the detailed FDA results of dysarthric speakers are available from the Nemours and Torgo databases. To determine the global score of each dysarthric speaker, we relied on the research in [19].

The FDA test is divided into eight sections namely, reflex, respiration, lips, jaw, palate, laryngeal, tongue, and intelligibility. It also contains a section on influencing factors, such as sensation and rate. The eight sections assess a global set of 28 perceptual dimensions using a nine-point rating scale. To build our automatic system for assessing dysarthria severity, we required a single numerical value to represent the global FDA-score of each patient. The FDA score expresses the intelligibility level, which corresponds inversely to the dysarthria severity level. The highest percentages correspond to the most severe cases of dysarthria. Based on [19], the severity level percentages of the dysarthric speakers in the Nemours database are shown in Table 9.2.

These scores are not available from the Torgo database, which only provides a file containing the nine-point scale ratings of the 28 perceptual dimensions. Therefore, in our previous work in [37], a new global FDA-score was proposed for the eight dysarthric participants in the Torgo database, based on the perceptual

Table 9.2: Severity levels of dysarthric speakers from the Nemours database reflecting the FDA [19].

Patients	KS	SC	BV	BK	RK	RL	JF	LL	BB	MH	FB
Severity (%)	–	49.5	42.5	41.8	32.4	26.7	21.5,	15.6	10.3	7.9	7.1

Table 9.3: The new proposed Frenchay Dysarthria Assessment (FDA) scores of dysarthric speakers from the Torgo database [37].

Patients	M04	M01	M02	F01	M05	M03	F03	F04
Severity (%)	44.35	49.79	49.79	55.87	57.96	94.29	96.67	96.67

dimension scores on the basis of the recent FDA-2 protocol [36]. Table 9.3 shows the final results of this new score estimation method for the Torgo database patients.

The FDA score expresses the level of intelligibility, which is inversely correspondent to the severity of dysarthria. All of the dysarthric speakers were divided into three subgroups based on their assessment: "mild L1" includes patients F04, F03, M03, FB, MH, BB, and LL; "severe L2" includes M05, F01, JF, RL, RK, BK, and BV; and "severe L3" includes M02, M01, M04, SC, and KS. The details of the patients' naming are given in Section 9.5.

9.4 Feature selection and classification

In this section, we present the techniques designed to automatically assess the severity of dysarthric speech. Relevant features based on distinctive auditory-based cues, MFCCs, and rhythm metrics were used as inputs for the classification systems. The classification performance of the GMMs, SVMs, and MLR were compared in various experimental conditions.

9.4.1 GMM-based classifier

The efficiency of GMMs for modeling speech characteristics results from their ability to model arbitrary densities by capturing spectral forms [38]. For each class, c_i, which represents one of the severity levels, the training is initiated to obtain a model composed of the parameters of every Gaussian distribution, denoted by m, of a given class. This model includes the mean vector $\mu_{i,m}$, the covariance matrix $\sum_{i,m}$, and the weight for each Gaussian $w_{i,m}$. These characteristics are computed after performing a sufficient number of iterations to ensure the convergence of the expectation-maximization (EM) algorithm [39]. As illustrated in Figure 9.3, one model is generated to represent each dysarthric speech severity level.

During the test step, each processed signal is represented by an input acoustical vector $\boldsymbol{x}$. The size d of the $\boldsymbol{x}$ vector is the number of acoustical parameters extracted from the signal. The probability density function of each feature vector for a given class c_i is estimated as follows:

$$p(\boldsymbol{x}/C_i) = \sum_{m=1}^{M} w_{i,m} \cdot \frac{1}{\sqrt{(2\pi)^d |\sum_{i,m}|}} \cdot e^{A_{i,m}}, \tag{9.3}$$

$$\text{where } A_{i,m} = \left(-\frac{1}{2}(\boldsymbol{x} - \boldsymbol{\mu}_{i,m})^T \cdot \frac{1}{\sum_{i,m}} \cdot (\boldsymbol{x} - \boldsymbol{\mu}_{i,m}) \right)$$

and M is the dimension of the Gaussian distribution.

The algorithm computes the likelihood that the acoustical vector $\boldsymbol{x}$ corresponds to the class c_i. The prior probability of each class is assumed to be the same. Therefore, the maximum probability density function indicates the class to which $\boldsymbol{x}$ belongs.

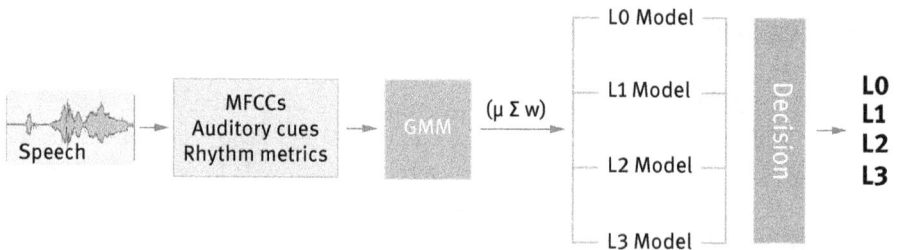

Figure 9.3: Block diagram of the dysarthric speech assessment process using GMMs.

9.4.2 SVM-based classifier

The SVM was proposed as a machine-learning approach by Vapnik [40]. Using a kernel function, the SVM projects the data onto a new high-dimensional space allowing linear separation. The classifier establishes a linear hyperplane separator that maximizes the margin between two data groups.

The kernel function is the key constituent of the SVM classifier. The learning and the generalization capabilities depend on the type of kernel function. In our experiments, a radial basis function (RBF) is applied as the kernel function, formulated by the following equation:

$$k(x, y) = exp\left(-\frac{||x - y^2||}{2 \times \sigma^2}\right),$$

(9.4)

where the σ parameter represents the Gaussian width that is optimized in the experiments. A multiclass-SVM using the "one-against-one" method is performed to discriminate the severity levels of dysarthria. As illustrated by Figure 9.4, binary classifiers are set to distinguish classes c_i and c_j, knowing that $0 < i \le L$, and $0 < j < i$, where L is the number of groups. $(L (L-1))/2$ binary SVMs are needed to classify L groups [31].

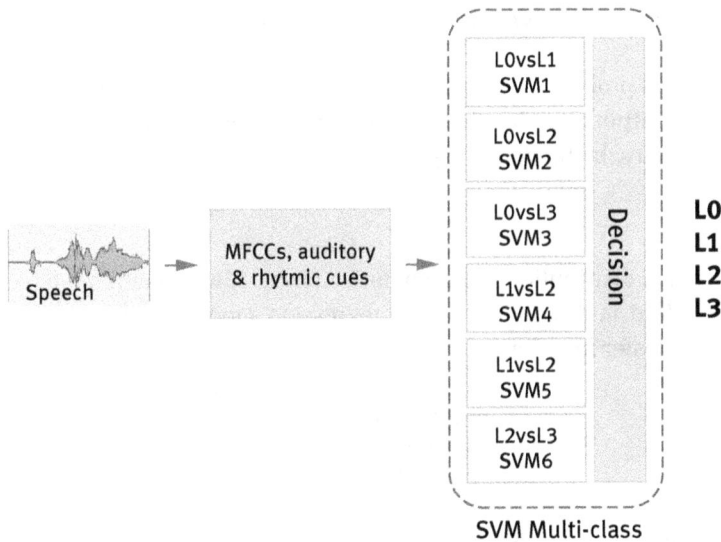

Figure 9.4: Block diagram of the dysarthric speech assessment process using SVMs.

9.4.3 Multinomial logistic regression

A combination of different input parameters is frequently used to improve the performance of classifiers. In the field of speech recognition, Zolnay et al.

showed in [41] that the log-linear combination of different feature streams leads to good performance. The concomitant use of various types of features is expected to extract complementary knowledge from each individual type of feature set.

In the framework presented in this study, both the MFCCs and the auditory-based cues are calculated on the basis of a typical temporal resolution of a 16 ms using a Hamming window that contains 256 samples with an overlapping of 50%. However, each of the rhythm metrics is calculated over sequences composed of several vocalic and consonantal intervals that span a whole sentence (several tens of milliseconds). To deal with the different resolutions of the acoustical analyzers, we propose to combine the sets of features obtained independently for the three acoustic streams, namely, the MFCCs, the auditory indicative features, and the rhythm metrics.

The MLR method is used to optimize the feature combination. Logistic regression is considered to be a useful alternative to GMMs and SVMs in the context of speaker identification [42]. We have also successfully used this technique in the context of native versus non-native accent discrimination [34].

For our multi-class problem, which consists of classifying dysarthria severity levels, we draw the output class label $\hat{y}$ as a multinomial distribution, which is the posterior probability, by the following formulation:

$$\hat{y} \sim mult(\hat{\varphi}), \tag{9.5}$$

where the multinomial distribution is parameterized by φ. If we assume we have L classes, the standard multinomial logistic regression model can be applied using the *softmax* transfer function as follows:

$$\hat{\varphi}_{c_i} = \frac{\exp\left(\boldsymbol{\beta}_{c_i}^T \boldsymbol{x}\right)}{\sum_{i=1}^{L} \exp\left(\boldsymbol{\beta}_{c_i}^T \boldsymbol{x}\right)}, \tag{9.6}$$

where $\boldsymbol{\beta}$ is the weight vector, $\boldsymbol{x}$ is the acoustic vector, and c_i is the class index. The goal is to estimate the optimal weights. If we have a total of K instances for the training, the log-likelihood is expressed by:

$$\ell(\hat{\varphi}) = \sum_{k=1}^{K} \sum_{i=1}^{L} \hat{y}_{kc_i} \log \hat{\varphi}_{kc_i}. \tag{9.7}$$

The optimization aims to find the best set of weights, $\boldsymbol{\beta}$, by minimizing $\ell(\hat{\varphi})$, which is done by setting its derivative to zero. The Iteratively Reweighted Least

Squares (IRLS) algorithm, described in detail in [43], can be used to find the optimal weights. The following algorithm summarizes the finding of optimal weights β:

IRLS Algorithm

Input $k = 1$, $A_{\beta_{ci}} = diag\ (p(x)(1 - p(x)))$, x, β_{ci}^1
While not meet the stop criterion do

$\quad$ Update β : $\beta_{ci}^{k+1} = \beta_{ci}^k + \left(x' A_{\beta_{ci}}\ x \right)^{-1} x' \left(\hat{y} - P_{\hat{\varphi}_{c_i}} \right)$

$\qquad\qquad = \left(x' A_{\beta_{ci}}\ x \right)^{-1} x' A_{\beta_{ci}} \left(x\beta_{ci}^k + A_{\beta_{ci}}^{-1} \left(\hat{y} - P_{\hat{\varphi}_{c_i}} \right) \right)$

$\qquad\qquad = \left(x' A_{\beta_{ci}}\ x \right)^{-1} x' A_{\beta_{ci}} Z^k$

$\quad k = k + 1$
end while

The IRLS algorithm is used by assuming the distribution of the acoustic vector $p(x)$ as Gaussian and $P_{\hat{\varphi}_{c_i}}$ is a Bernoulli distribution. The last equation form of the algorithm is a weighted regression of the vector Z^k which is expressed by:

$$Z^k = x\beta_{ci}^k + A_{\beta_{ci}}^{-1} \left(\hat{y} - P_{\hat{\varphi}_{c_i}} \right). \tag{9.8}$$

It is worth mentioning that MLR has the advantage of being able to perform the feature selection in addition to the classification task.

9.5 Experiments

9.5.1 Speech material

To train and test the classification systems, we combined the recordings of the Nemours database of dysarthric speech and the Torgo database of acoustic and articulatory speech from speakers with dysarthria. It is important to control the differences across databases to minimize the data combination effects on the experiments. For the Nemours database, the recording sessions were con-ducted in a small sound-dampened room, while for the Torgo database an acoustic noise reduction was performed. For both databases, the Pulse Code Modulation (PCM) was used for speech coding, and the speech signal was sampled at a rate of 16 kHz with a 16 bit sample resolution. The Resource

Interchange File Format (RIFF) was used for audio files. Furthermore, normalization and silence removal were carried out at the pre-processing stage on all the recording materials.

9.5.2 Subjects

The speakers from the Nemours database were 11 young adult males[1] affected by different categories of dysarthria as a consequence of either cerebral palsy (CP) or head trauma (HT), and one male adult as a control speaker. Of the seven patients who had CP, two had athetoid CP (one quadriplegic), three had spastic CP with quadriplegia, and two had a combination of athetoid and spastic with quadriplegia. Each dysarthric speaker is referred to by a two-letter code: BB, BK, BV, FB, JF, KS, LL, MH, RK, RL, and SC.

The Torgo database of dysarthric articulation consists of aligned acoustics from speakers with either CP or amyotrophic lateral sclerosis (ALS), which are the two recurrent causes of speech disability [44]. Torgo speakers were between the ages of 16 and 50 years old. Each of these eight dysarthric speakers recorded approximately 500 utterances, while every speaker in the control group recorded about 1,200 utterances [20]. All participants were assigned a code beginning with "F" or "M" for female and male speakers. The last two digits designate the order in which the participant was enrolled. Thus, the eight dysarthric speakers considered over our experiments are referred to as F01, F03, F04, M01, M02, M03, M04, and M05.

9.5.3 Results and discussion

The experimental dataset contained 1,330 sentences, comprising 70 sentences recorded by each dysarthric speaker, in particular, 11 from the Nemours database and eight from the Torgo database. Silence removal and segmentation of the audio streams containing speech were applied to all the recordings. The process was based on the signal energy (i.e., L^2 norm) and spectral centroid characteristics, using a threshold method to detect the speech segments [45].

To train the different classifiers to discriminate the L0, L1, L2, and L3 severity levels, we used 539 and 392 sentences from Nemours and Torgo, respectively. These sentences were obtained by regrouping the first 49 sentences pronounced by each speaker. To perform the test experiment, we used 231 sentences from

---

1 The age of the Nemours database speakers is not provided

Nemours and 168 sentences from Torgo. The test sentences were unseen during the training. The data used in the test represent 30% of the total amount of available data. In the following metric, the correct classification rate, was used to evaluate the performance of the assessment systems:

$$\text{Correct classification rate} = \left(\frac{\text{number of correct severity classifications}}{\text{total number of severity classification trials}} \right) \times 100.$$

$$(9.9)$$

Table 9.4 presents the results of an extensive set of experiments. The optimal number of Gaussians used by the GMM-based system was obtained after multiple validation experiments using different numbers of Gaussians. The same approach was used to find the best C and σ parameters of the SVM-based system. To obtain the results presented in Table 9.4, the GMM system used 128 Gaussians. This number was found to be adequate for all GMM-based classification experiments using different features.

Table 9.4: Correct classification rate (in %) of different input features used by the GMM- multi class SVM- and MLR- based classification systems (classifiers) to perform the dysarthria severity level assessment. The "+" symbol indicates the concatenation of the features involved in the acoustical analysis.

Feature Set Classifiers	MFCCs	MFCCs + Auditory cues	MFCC + Rhythm metrics	MFCCs + Auditory cues + Rhythm metrics
GMMs	92.3%	93.2%	90.1%	93.5%
multiclass-SVMs	76.6%	75.3%	77.7%	76.8%
MLR	–	95.1% (19)	91.8% (16)	**97.7%** (22)

The GMM method using MFCCs, auditory distinctive features, and rhythm cues correctly classified 93.5% of the dysarthria severity levels: L0, L1, L2, and L3.

The multiclass-SVM includes binary SVMs. A "majority voting" method (best candidate) was used as the decision strategy of the system. The best performance of the SVM assessment system (76.8%) was achieved using the combination of the three types of input features.

The GMM achieved a higher correct classification rate than the SVM. This difference can probably be explained by the ability of the GMM, and statistical-based methods in general, to deal with variable time lengths in the input data. This suggests that the SVM cannot efficiently process utterances that have different and variable durations, especially when these utterances are provided by two different corpora (Nemours and Torgo). This effect was somewhat attenuated by the use of rhythm metrics, as these features are segmental and are calculated at the sentence-level. The speech rhythm relates to tempo and timing of segmental units. Therefore, the quantitative rhythm measure is performed on a variable length utterance which is usually a sentence composed of several syllables. The mean length of the utterances used in our experiments is ranging from 2 s to 7 s. Each rhythm measure is then considered as segmental as it is calculated for the whole utterance length.

The results showed that the MLR-based approach performed better than the GMMs and SVMs with respect to each type of feature and combination. When the MFCCs, auditory, and rhythm cues were combined, the MLR method significantly improved the classification rate and achieved the best score of 97.7%. As shown in Table 9.4, the MLR was carried out when at least two different types of acoustic vectors were used. Therefore, the MLR method was not applied, when only the MFCCs were used.

The performance reached by the MLR method demonstrates the ability of this method to optimize the combination of features at different resolution levels. Indeed, both MFCCS and auditory features are calculated at a frame basis while the rhythm metrics are segmental and are calculated at the sentence level. We kept the feature fusion as simple as possible by performing a concatenation of the feature vectors having different resolutions. The MLR is expected to optimize this concatenation and this is the reason why we opted for this method in the context of variable resolution of the acoustical parameters.

The detailed analysis of the MLR results revealed that based on the Hosmer–Lemeshow criterion [46], some parameters affected the classification performance more than the others. In the case where the MLR used all of the features (best score), two auditory cues (C/D and W_{md}) and three rhythm metrics (DeltaV, rPVI-V, and rPVI-C) were discarded from the set of selected features to perform the classification task. This suggests that to a certain extent, the information related to the mid-external energy and discontinuities provided by the auditory model, as well as the raw versions of the PVI metric, were less relevant for the classification task, when the 22 other input parameters were used.

It is important to emphasize that the discarded parameters differed, when two streams of features were considered. Indeed, it appears that both the raw and normalized rhythm variations in the PVI were significant for the classification, when the rhythm metrics were used together with the MFCCs. Therefore, for this latter configuration, 16 input parameters were used for the classification. In the case where auditory cues were combined with the MFCCs, 19 parameters were used as input parameters. Only the W_{md} was found to be non-significant. These results confirm that the use of a combination of

MFCCS, auditory-based features, and rhythm metrics provides a very effective solution for the classification of dysarthria severity. These results also suggest that the MLR-based technique could constitute a powerful approach to concomitantly select relevant features and perform the classification of dysarthric speech.

9.6 Conclusion

This chapter presented original approaches for improving the analysis and classification of dysarthric speech. The front-end signal processing used a model to simulate the external, middle, and inner parts of the ear to provide relevant auditory-based cues, which were combined with conventional MFCCs and rhythm metrics to provide a multidimensional feature representation. These features were used by the GMM-, SVM-, and MLR-based systems to perform automatic assessment of dysarthria severity. The experiments were conducted using data from both the Nemours and Torgo corpora of dysarthric speech. The results showed that the integration of rhythmic and auditory-based features together with conventional MFCCs as inputs to a multinomial logistic regression significantly improved the performance of the dysarthric assessment system. This suggests, first, that the MLR-based approach offers a powerful alternative to well-established methods. Our current research effort is focused toward the improvement of this method by investigating its combination with deep neural networks to expand the classification task (more levels) and to efficiently perform accurate speech recognition of the dysarthric speech. Second, the MLR-based method offers a new perspective that integrates additional features, such as those based on the speech rhythm and auditory model, into a unified framework to improve the classification performance.

Although the use of human judgments is a fairly common approach to evaluate such assessment tool, this study does not provide such evaluation. It is important to mention that a human evaluation is systematically subjective, which may account for some of the discrepancies among exams. This justifies our approach to restrain our study to the automatic classification rate, which is considered as an objective measure. However, in a clinical context, the objective measures are often considered less useful for analyzing and portraying the dynamics of the patients with respect to their environments and past interactions (before the impairment).

In a future work, we plan to investigate the inclusion of prosodic features and acoustic parameters based on the empirical mode decomposition into a complete speech impairment evaluation and recognition system. This approach opens the doors toward the design of personalized assistive speech systems and devices based on robust and effective speech recognition that are still not available for people who live with speech impairments. The automatic assessment systems presented in this chapter may be useful for clinicians who can easily and efficiently perform the monitoring of rehabilitation programs for dysarthric patients. A fast, simple, and cost-effective alternative to the manual FDA test is available through this tool. It can also be used to prevent incorrect subjective diagnoses and reduce the time required to assess the severity dysarthric speech disorder.

References

[1]   Roth C. Dysarthria. In: Caplan B, Deluca J, Kreutzer JS, editors. Encyclopedia of Clinical Neuropsychology. Springer, 2011:905–8.

[2]   Kim J, Kumar N, Tsiartas A, Li M, Narayanan SS. Automatic intelligibility classification of sentence-level pathological speech. Comput Speech Lang 2015;29:132–44.

[3]   Clapham R, Molen LV, Son RV, Brekel MV, Hilgers F. NKI-CCRT Corpus – speech intelligibility before and after advanced head and neck cancer treated with concomant chemoradiotherapy, Proceedings of the Eight International Conference on Language Resources and Evaluation, European Language Resources Association, 2012:3350–5.

[4]   Fang C, Haifeng L, Ma L, Zhang M. Intelligibility evaluation of pathological speech through multigranularity feature extraction and optimization, computational and mathematical methods in medicine, Published online January 17. 2017:1–8.

[5]   Le D, Licata K, Persad C, Mower E. Automatic assessment of speech intelligibility for individuals with aphasia. IEEE Trans Audio, Speech, Lang 2016;24:2187–99.

[6]   Enderby P. Disorders of communication: dysarthria. In: Tselis AC, Booss J, editors. Handbook of clinical neurology. Elsevier, New York, United States, 2013:110–273.

[7]   Vachhani B, Bhat C, Das B, Kopparapu SK. Deep autoencoder based speech features for improved dysarthric speech recognition. Interspeech, Stockholm, Sweden, 2017:1854–8.

[8]   Lansford KL, Berisha V, Utianski RL. Modeling listener perception of speaker similarity in dysarthria. J Acoust Soc Am 2016;139:EL209–EL215.

[9]   Martinez D, Lleida E, Green P, Christensen H, Ortega A, Miguel A. Intelligibility assessment and speech recognizer word accuracy rate prediction for dysarthric speakers in a factor analysis subspace. ACM Trans Accessible Comput 2015;6:1–21.

[10] Rudzicz F. Adjusting dysarthric speech signals to be more intelligible. Comput Speech Lang, Elsevier, 2013;27:1163–77.

[11] Rudzicz F. Phonological features in discriminative classification of dysarthric speech. IEEE International Conference on Acoustics, Speech and Signal Processing, Taipei, Taiwan, 2009:4605–8.

[12] Selouani SA, Dahmani H, Amami R, Hamam H. Using speech rhythm knowledge to improve dysarthric speech recognition. Int J Speech Technol 2012;15:57–64.

[13] Paja MS, Falk TH. Automated dysarthria severity classification for improved objective intelligibility assessment of spastic dysarthric speech. Interspeech, Portland, OR, 2012:62–5.

[14] Kadi KL, Selouani SA, Boudraa B, Boudraa M. Automated diagnosis and assessment of dysarthric speech using relevant prosodic features. In: Yang G, Ao S, Gelman L, editors. Trans Eng Technol, Springer, 2013:529–42.

[15] Kim J, Kumar N, Tsiartas A, Li M, Narayanan S. Automatic intelligibility classification of sentence-level pathological speech. Comput Speech Lang, Elsevier, 2014; 29:132–44.

[16] Bhat C, Vachhani B, Kopparapu SK, Automatic assessment of dysarthria severity level using audio descriptors. IEEE International Conference on Acoustics, Speech and Signal Processing (ICASSP), New Orleans, LA, 2017:5070–4.

[17] Barkmeier-Kraemer JM, Clark HM. Speech–language pathology evaluation and management of hyperkinetic disorders affecting speech and swallowing function. Tremor and other hyperkinetic movements, Published online Sep. 2017:7–489.

[18] Wannberg P, Schalling E, Hartelius L. Perceptual assessment of dysarthria: comparison of a general and a detailed assessment protocol. Logopedics Phoniatrics Vocol 2015;41:159–67.

[19] Menendez-Pidal X, Polikoff JB, Peters SM, Leonzio JE, Bunnell HT. The Nemours database of dysarthric speech. Fourth International Conference on Spoken Language, Philadelphia, PA, 1996, 3:1962–5.

[20] Rudzicz F, Namasivayam AK, Wolff T. The TORGO database of acoustic and articulatory speech from speakers with dysarthria. Lang Resour Eval J Springer, 2012;46:523–41.

[21] O'Shaughnessy D. Speech communications: human and machine. 2nd ed. Wiley-IEEE Press, Hoboken, New Jersey, United States, 1999.

[22] Shahamiri SR, Salim SS. Artificial neural networks as speech recognizers for dysarthric speech: identifying the best-performing set of MFCC parameters and studying a speaker-independent approach. Adv Eng Inf J Elsevier 2014;28:102–10.

[23] Davis S, and Mermelstein P, Comparison of parametric representation for monosyllabic word recognition in continuously spoken sentences. IEEE Trans Acoust Speech Signal Process 1980;28:357–66.

[24] Grabe E, Low EL. Durational variability in speech and the rhythm class hypothesis. Lab Phonol 2002;7:515–46.

[25] Ramus F, Nespor M, Mehler J. Correlates of linguistic rhythm in the speech signal. Cogn Elsevier 2000;75:AD3–AD30.

[26] Flanagan JL. Models for approximating basilar membrane displacement. Bell Syst Technol J 1960;39:1163–91.

[27] Lyon RF. A computational model of filtering, detection, and compression in the cochlea. IEEE International Conference on Acoustics, Speech and Signal Processing (ICASSP), Paris, France, 1982:1282–5.

[28] Seneff S. A joint synchrony/mean-rate model of auditory speech processing. J Phonetics 1988;16:55–76.

[29] Ghitza O. Auditory models and human performance in tasks related to speech coding and speech recognition. IEEE Trans Speech Signal Process 1994;2:115–32.

[30] Stern R, Morgan N. Hearing is believing: biologically inspired methods for robust automatic speech recognition. IEEE Signal Process Mag 2012;29:34–43.

[31] Schluter R, Bezrukov L, Wagner H, Ney H. Gammatone features and feature combination for large vocabulary speech recognition. Acoustics, Speech and Signal Processing, (ICASSP), Honolulu, Hawaii, USA, 2007;4:649–52.

[32] Kim C, Stern RM. Power-normalized cepstral coefficients (pncc) for robust speech recognition. IEEE/ACM Trans Audio, Speech Lang Process 2016;24:1315–29.

[33] Caelen J. Space/time data-information in the ARIAL project ear model. Speech Commun 19854:467.

[34] Selouani SA, Alotaibi Y, Cichocki W, Gharssallaoui S, Kadi KL. Native and non-native class discrimination using speech rhythm and auditory-based cues. Comput Speech Lang 2015;31:28–48.

[35] Enderby PM, Frenchay dysarthria assessment. PRO-ED, Austin, Texas, United States, 1983.

[36] Enderby PM, Palmer R. Frenchay dysarthria assessment. 2nd ed. (FDA-2), PRO-ED, Austin, Texas, United States, 2008.

[37] Kadi KL, Selouani SA, Boudraa B, Boudraa M. Fully automated speaker identification and intelligibility assessment in dysarthria disease using auditory knowledge. Biocybern Biomed Eng J Elsevier 2016;36:233–47.

[38] Reynolds DA, Rose RC. Robust text-independent speaker identification using Gaussian mixture speaker models. IEEE Trans Speech Audio Process 1995;3:72–83.

[39] Dempster AP, Laird NM, Rubin DB, Maximum-likelihood from incomplete data via the EM algorithm. J Acoust Soc Am 1977;39:1–38.

[40] Vapnik VN. An overview of statistical learning theory. IEEE Trans Neural Netw 1999;10:988–99.

[41] Zolnay A, Schlüter R, Ney H. Acoustic feature combination for robust speech recognition. IEEE International Conference on Acoustics, Speech, and Signal Processing (ICASSP), Philadelphia, PA, 2005:457–60.

[42] Katz M, Schaffoner M, Andelic E, Kruger S, Wendemuth A. Sparse kernel logistic regression using incremental feature selection for text-independent speaker identification, Proceedings of Speaker and Language Recognition Workshop, IEEE Odyssey, San Juan, Puerto Rico, 2006.

[43] Wolke R, Schwetlick H. Iteratively reweighted least squares: algorithms, convergence, and numerical comparisons. SIAM J Sci Stat Comput 1988;9:907–21.

[44] Kent RD, Rosen K. Motor control perspectives on motor speech disorders. In Maassen B, Kent RD, Peters H, Van LP, Hulstijn W, editors. Speech motor control in normal and disordered speech. Oxford University Press, Oxford, United Kingdom, 2004:285–311.

[45] Giannakopoulos T, Pikrakis A. Introduction to audio analysis, 1st ed. Elsevier Academic Press, Cambridge, Massachusetts, United States, 2014.

[46] Hosmer DW, Lemeshow S. A goodness-of-fit test for the multiple logistic regression model. Commun Stat J 1980;9:1043–69.

Abdelilah Jilbab, Achraf Benba and Ahmed Hammouch

10 Quantification system of Parkinson's disease

Abstract: Technological advances in signal processing, electronics, embedded systems, and neuroscience have allowed the design of devices that help physicians to better assess the evolution of neurological diseases. In this context, we are interested in the development of an intelligent system for the quantification of Parkinson's disease (PD). To achieve this, the system contains two parts: a wireless sensor network and an embedded system. The wireless sensor network is used to measure motor defects of the patient; it is constituted of several nodes which communicate among themselves. These nodes are intelligent sensors; they contain accelerometers, EMG, and blood pressure sensors to detect any malfunction of the patient's motor activities. As regards to the embedded system, it allows analyzing the patient's voice signal to extract a descriptor that characterizes PD. The network detects the patient's posture and measures his or her tremors. The voice analysis system measures the degradation of the patient's condition. The embedded system combines the three decisions using the Chair–Varshney rule. The data fusion between the sensor network and the embedded system will quantify the disease to facilitate the diagnostic for the physician, while providing the ability to effectively assess the evolution of the patient's health.

Keywords: Embedded System, Parkinson's Disease, Sensors network, Signal processing

10.1 Introduction

Due to the increasing life expectancy and aging population, Parkinson's disease (PD) is becoming more common worldwide. The disease usually affects people over 55 years of age; it is estimated that one in 100 people would be reached at age 65, and two out of every 100 at age over 70 [1].

PD is characterized by muscle contraction, limb tremor, and slow motion; these symptoms are due to the degeneration of certain nerve cells in the brain. This disease, also known as agitating paralysis, is a neurological pathology that has an impact on motor control systems, such as walking, talking, writing, or completing other simple tasks.

https://doi.org/10.1515/9781501502415-011

Research in this field gives hope to compensate the motor losses of the patients. Indeed, it has been proved that an acoustic stimulus makes it possible to recover the balance of the inner ear, which reinforces the regulation of motor actions of patients.

The use of a smart electronic device for generating these stimuli will thus accurately regulate the orientations of PD patients. In addition, real-time archiving and analysis of the patient's condition will help the physician to prescribe an accurate and effective diagnosis to improve his or her condition.

Cognitive impairment in patients is useful to deliver pertinent information to quantify the levels of the progression of PD. To achieve this goal, we have implemented a method that classifies this disease in four classes, according to its degree of evolution. This method is based on the analysis of the patient's speech signal; by quantifying the particular characteristics of the voice, which form a voice characteristic of PD. Thus, by analyzing the voice of the patients, it will be possible to make the following interventions:

- Early detection of the PD disease;
- Prevention and treatment of its long-term complications;
- Effective management and monitoring the patient's state.

The physician can, therefore, adapt the frequency and the dose of the drugs or the stimulus, according to her state of health of patients which is determined in real-time. Next, an embedded system will compute a quantum that reflects the evolution of the disease and merge the analysis of the patient's voice with the results of the wireless sensor network. Finally, the diagnosis can be sent immediately to the physician for assessment and prescription of the treatment to follow.

10.2 Related works

To identify people with Parkinson's disease, a voice analysis, based on the detection of dysphonia, was presented by Max Little et al. [2]. In their work, they used the pitch period entropy, which allows a robust measure against the noisy environment. The problem of speech analysis will become complex when we consider other factors, such as gender and the variable acoustic environment. Max Little et al., used a database of 23 patients with Parkinson's disease and eight healthy individuals, all aged between 46 and 85 years (an average age of 65.8 years with a standard deviation of 9.8). The database has 195 continuous vowel type phonations, where each participant has given an average of six length records ranging from 0 to 36 seconds [3]. On this basis, the authors applied a Support Vector Machines (SVM) kernel method.

In addition to the SVM, other authors have used statistical learning methods, such as the Linear Discriminative Analysis (LDA) [4]. These methods make it possible to discriminate patients from healthy people, by selecting the best analytical characteristics. Theoretical studies have shown that the accuracy of the classification degrades, when a large number of characteristics are used [4]. The choice of attributes does not always guarantee optimal functionality [5].

A non-linear model was introduced by Shahbaba et al. [6] for the detection of Parkinson's disease. This classification model uses the Dirichlet process mixtures. The authors compared three methods, namely, the Multinomial Logit Models (MLM), the decision trees, and the SVM. They obtained a classification accuracy of 87.7%. Resul Das [7] studied four classification methods, namely, neural networks, DMneural, the regression tree, and the decision tree [7]. The authors used the SAS software [8], which makes the data retrieval process simpler and supports all the essential tasks within an integrated solution. In his experiments, Resul Das was able to reach a precision of 92.9% in the case of neural networks. These are interesting results compared to the previous studies [9].

Based on the common characteristics of the voice, Guo et al. [10] proposed learning functions genetic programming and the expectation maximization algorithm (GP-EM) that combine GP gene programming with the EM algorithm. They were able to achieve a classification accuracy of 93.1%.

Sakar et al. [11] focused on reducing the set of characteristics; they looked for those that maximize the discrimination of Parkinsonian patients compared with the healthy people. For this purpose, they applied a joint information measure with a permutation test to evaluate the statistical importance between dysphonia characteristics and discriminant results. The authors were able to classify the characteristics according to the criterion of Minimum Redundancy Maximum Relevance (mRMR), with an algorithm SVM for the classification.

Ozcivit et al. [12] constructed a set of classifiers of automatic learning algorithms. These algorithms were assembled using rotation forest. A classification accuracy of 87.13% was achieved using mRMR-4 applied to Parkinson's.

Astrӧm et al [13] have created a parallel neural network (parallel feed forward neural network). A classification accuracy of 91.20% was obtained with nine networks. To optimize the set of features, Spadoto et al [14] applied a scalable classifier based on the OFP algorithm. They obtained an accuracy of 84.01% by combining the OFP with a gravity search algorithm (GSA-OPF) for only eight attributes.

The problem of the optimization of the set of characteristics was also studied by Li et al [15]. The authors proposed a non-linear SVM-based fuzzy logic transformation method for classification. They were able to reach an accuracy of 93.47%.

Mandal et al [16] proposed different methods, such as the Bayesian network [17, 18], Sparse Multinomial Logistic Regression [19], SVM, boosting methods, neural networks, [20, 21] and other machine learning models. In addition, they used RF [22, 23], which is a regression logistic [24], to achieve a classification accuracy of 96.93%. Other authors have used Haar wavelets as a projection filter [25, 26]. For example, Oscift [27] has been able to achieve the maximum classification accuracy of 100%.

Wan-li Zuo et al. [28] proposed a method based on the optimization of Particle Swarm Optimization (PSO) particles, reinforced by a fuzzy logic KNN. The PSO technique was developed by Eberhart and Kennedy [29] to treat each individual as a particle in a d-dimensional space in which the position and velocity of the particle are represented. Wan-li Zuo et al, therefore, adopted the PSO-FINN method [30, 31] and adapted it to maximize the classification performance of Parkinsonians compared with the healthy people [28]. They reached a maximum accuracy of 97.47%, using the 10-fold-CV method.

Hui-Ling Chen et al [32] used a FKNN (fussy KNN) method 33], using a cross-SVM-based method. They achieved a classification accuracy of 96.07 percent. Hariharan et al [34] have improved the classification with an intelligent hybrid system, reaching the maximum accuracy of 100%.

Betul et al [35] performed voice tests on several topics. They took samples for continuous vowel phonations and speech samples [35]. After applying different tools to learning machine based on the data, they found that the most discriminative features are extracted from continuous vowel phonations. They also compared cross-validation methods, such as Leave One Subject Out (LOSO). Their best accuracy of classification is 85%, using a database of 40 individuals, namely:
−   20 patients with Parkinson's disease, including six women and 14 men. Patients' ages ranged from 43 to 77 years, with an average of 64.86 and a standard deviation of 8.97;
−   20 healthy people, including 10 women and 10 men. The ages of healthy subjects varied from 45 to 83 years, with an average of 62.55 and a standard deviation of 10.79.

Jaafari [36] presented a combinatorial method for extracting the characteristics of the samples. It has combined seven non-linear features with 13 MFCC. The seven non-linear features are as follows:
−   the pitch period to entropy;
−   the recurrence period density of the entropy;
−   the noise to harmonic ratio;
−   detrended fluctuation analysis;
−   fractal dimension;
−   the energy distribution coefficient of the pointed indices series;
−   the energy distribution coefficient of the series of amplitude peaks .

The last two characteristics are robust with several uncontrollable effects, such as noisy environment [36]. MFCCs have been widely used in speech processing, such as speech recognition and speaker identification. The extracted features were combined in a multi-layer perception (MLP), which uses a hidden layer neural network classifier. The classification accuracy obtained is 97.5%. The database used is 200 voice samples, taken from a group of:

- 25 Parkinsonian patients, including five women and 20 men, having different levels of severity. Their ages range from 49 to 70 years with an average of 58.64;
- 10 healthy people, including two women and eight men. Their ages range from 39 to 63 years with an average of 50.7.

10.3 Diagnosis of Parkinson's disease using voice analysis

10.3.1 The characteristics of the voice signal

The characteristics of the speech signal are strongly affected by the temporal properties of the signal. It can be seen that the speech signal is stationary for durations from 20 ms to 30 ms. The characteristics of the speech signal can thus be determined in time windows varying between 20 and 30 ms. Models using fenestration and cepstral characteristics have been applied in several domains, going from classification [37] to speech recognition [38–41].

In addition to the cepstral characteristics, there are other characteristics that can be extracted from a speech signal. Many of them are used to identify particular classes. In our case, we are interested in the general characteristics, which are not related to particular classes.

10.3.1.1 Cepstral analysis

The analysis, using the basic Fourier transform, leads to the decomposition of the speech signal into a spectral sequence [42]. Thus, the Discrete Fourier Transform of a speech signal (k) gives a series of complex values (n). In general, the coefficients $|(n)|$ are correlated; which gives redundancy of information.

In contrast, analysis using cepstrum is an improved way to obtain an uncorrelated version of the spectral vector. Moreover, the calculation of the cepstrum gives an interpretation of the speech production model. The idea is to consider that the v_k constituting a speech signal is the result of the convolution of the signal of the source by the filter modeling the vocal tracts:

$$v(k) = u(k) * b(k), \tag{10.1}$$

where $v(k)$ is the time signal, $u(k)$ the exciter signal, and $b(k)$ the contribution of the vocal tracts. The problem consist of separating the signals (k) and (k) by applying a deconvolution.

The Z-transform of the equation gives:

$$V(z) = U(z) \times B(z), \tag{10.2}$$

$$\Rightarrow log \ |V((z)| = log \ |U(z)| + log \ |B(z)|, \tag{10.3}$$

The cepstrum is obtained by inverse transformation [43]. The actual expression of the cepstrum [44] is obtained by replacing the Z transformation with a discrete Fourier transform:

$$C(k) = TFD^{-1}(log(TFD(v(k)))), \tag{10.4}$$

With the cepstral coefficients, (k) we can, therefore, dissociate the effects of the vocal tract from the source excitation. Theoretically, the channel of the voice affects the envelope of the frequency spectrum: the first coefficients (k) tell us about this effect. The excitation source generally has a finer character: the coefficients (k) of higher orders describe this phenomenon.

The MFCC technique

To normalize the coefficients (k) to the human perception, filtering is carried out using a filter bank in accordance with the MEL scale (Figure 10.1) [45].

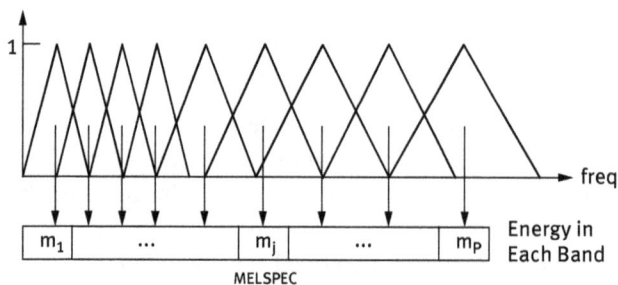

Figure 10.1: Filterbank for the Mel scale.

We then obtain the MFCC coefficients to describe a scale that reflects human perception with different frequency precisions. In this scale, the high frequencies are seen with less accuracy than the low frequencies, in accordance with the human eye.

Fraile et al [46] propose Mel scale cepstral frequency coefficients for the measurement of Parkinsonian vocal disorders. The use of MFCCs has been shown to reduce the effect of noise, reducing measurement size, and simplifying classification [47, 48]. Other related works, such as Kapoor et al. [49] and Bemba et al. [50], used vector quantized MFCCs.

Initially, the MFCC technique was used in speech recognition systems. It uses attributes of high dimensions, extracted from the frequency domain. The effectiveness of this technique for voice analysis has been proven experimentally [36]. The use of MFCCs can be justified by two empirical reasons. The first is that the calculation of the MFCC does not require the determination of the "pitch" [36, 51–95]. The second is that the analysis in the cepstral-domain for this application is justified by the presence of noise information in this domain [36, 96], and that the MFCC technique compresses this information on the first cepstral coefficient, which reduces the analysis dimension and simplifies the classification [47, 48, 97].

The PLP technique
Another technique, called perceptual linear prediction (PLP) and proposed by Hermansky in 1990 [98], was used in speech recognition. This technique is similar to classical linear prediction (LP), to which is added the psychophysical properties of human hearing to estimate the auditory spectrum [98]. This was done using three main concepts, namely,
- The critical band resolution curves;
- The curve with equal loudness;
- The law of power of the intensity (loudness).

The advantage of the PLP on the conventional LP is that it retains only the relevant information of the voice signal.

Loudness is a characteristic related to the intensity of the speech signal, it also depends on the frequency. To have isosonic curves (Figure 10.2), the curves of Fletsher and Munson are often used [99, 100].

These curves make it possible to take into account the human perception of loudness, they are standardized by ISO [101].

The loudness is calculated in the frequency domain via the expression of the energy of the speech signal, which is weighted by coefficients ω_n in each frequency band, that is,

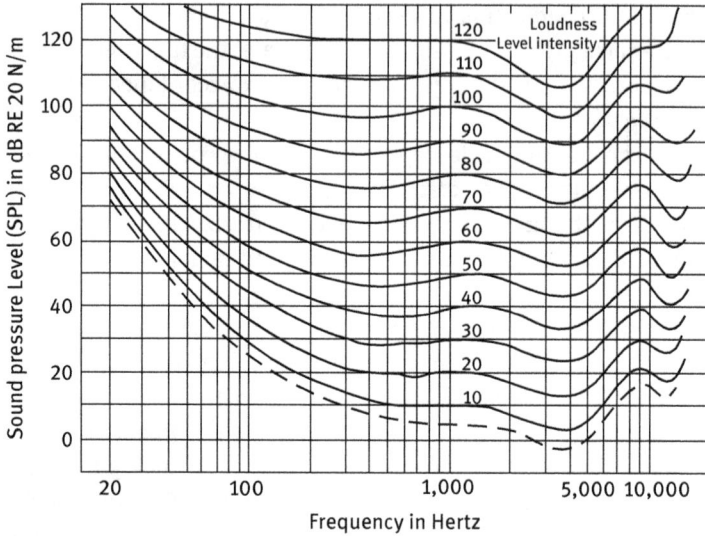

Figure 10.2: Isosonic curves [99].

$$E_T = \frac{1}{N} \sum_{n=1}^{N} \omega_n V^2(n),\qquad(10.5)$$

The weights, ω_n, are estimated from the isosonic curves, allowing the consideration of human perception.

10.3.1.2 The pitch attribute

The characteristics of the speech signal are affected by the source parameters, which are related to the vibrations of the vocal folds, such as voicing and fundamental frequency F0. The pitch is one of the fundamental parameters in the production, analysis, and perception of speech. This parameter is a main revealer of phonetic, lexical, syntactic, and emotional information. Various advanced techniques, analysis, and interpretation of the speech signal are based on this attribute; The pitch goes into their development and becomes, in this sense, an essential element in the implementation of applications dedicated to automatic speech processing.

The pitch is a psychoacoustic characteristic allowing to dissociate the women's voice from the men's voice. This characteristic is determined according to two models [102]:

- The first is a location model, for which a spectral analysis is performed in which the value of the pitch is estimated according to the relationship between the frequency peaks [103].
- The second is a time model, for which the pitch is calculated by temporal analysis of the periodicity in each frequency band [104, 105].

10.3.1.3 Other attributes for Parkinson's patients

The fundamental frequency F0
The fundamental frequency of the speech signal can be calculated via the auto-correlation function. This function () of the time signal (n) is calculated by:

$$\psi_T = \sum_{t=t_0}^{t_0+N} v(t) \times v(t+T), \tag{6}$$

The algorithm, computing the fundamental frequency fo, is based on the following formula:

$$f_0 = \frac{1}{\arg\ \max\ (\psi_T)}, \tag{7}$$

The Jitter
Short-term fluctuations characterize, in particular, morphological damage of the vocal cords. These fluctuations are the jitter of the fundamental frequency fo. There are different representations of Jitter, which is calculated as the average absolute difference between two consecutive periods [90, 91].

Relative Jitter is defined as the mean difference between two consecutive periods, divided by the average duration of the signal [90, 91]. The HBP represents the relative average of the disturbances. It is calculated as the difference between the mean of a period and the mean of the period and its two neighbors, divided by the average duration of the signal [90, 91].

Finally, the Jitter PPQ5 represents the five points "Period Perturbation Quotient" is defined as the average absolute difference between a period and the mean of the latter and its four nearest neighbors, divided by the average duration of the signal [90, 91]. There are many problems with Jitter measurement because there is no formal definition [51]. Its value depends on the technique of measurement of the fundamental frequency [72].

The Shimmer

The Shimmer (shimmer or shimmer) also has several definitions. It represents the variation of the peak-to-peak amplitude in decibels, calculated by the mean of the differences between the amplitudes of the consecutive periods multiplied by 20 [90, 91]. As for the relative Shimmer, it is expressed as the average difference between the amplitudes of the consecutive periods, divided by the average amplitude of the signal. The ratio is expressed in percent [90, 91]. The Shimmer APQ11 represents the quotient of the perturbations of 11 amplitude points, defined as the difference between the mean of the amplitude of a period and the mean of the amplitudes and its 10 nearest neighbors, divided by the average amplitude of the signal [90].

The Harmonicity

The instability of the signal appears as a noise added to it. It can, therefore, be calculated by considering the ratio between the energy of the harmonics present in the signal spectrum and the energy of the noise. There are several methods for measuring the aperiodic part of the speech signal. In our context, two methods are used:

- The HNR ratio expresses the relative energy of the harmonics on the noise energy (expressed in dB). This method has been proposed by Yumoto et al. [92].
- The NNE coefficient proposed by Katsuya et al [93].

In the case where the vibration frequency is not stable, the HNR and NNE coefficients do not give an accurate measurement. To resolve this problem, Qi et al [94] proposed a method for measuring HNR that minimizes the effects of vibrational instability (Jitter) [72].

The Phonetogram

The main idea of the Phonetogram is to represent, in a Cartesian plane, the voice dynamic range, that is, the intensity as a function of the frequency [72]. This representation is used to identify the limits of the voice function. The length of the graph informs us about the dynamics of the frequencies. The thickness of the graph informs us about the dynamics of the intensity [72].

Figure 10.3 shows the Phonetogram of a 58-year-old normal person. As can be seen, the tone dynamics of the person is 576 Hz (almost three octaves), and the dynamic range of the intensity is 40 dB. This person has a good tonal dynamics but his dynamics of intensity is insufficient. The center of gravity is at the point (220 Hz, 56 dB) [72].

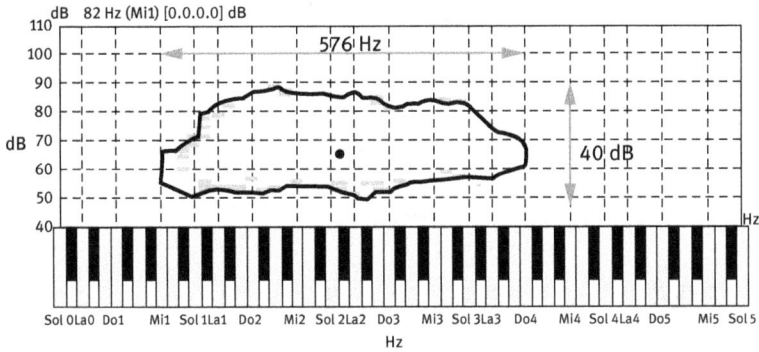

Figure 10.3: Phonetogram of a normal person.

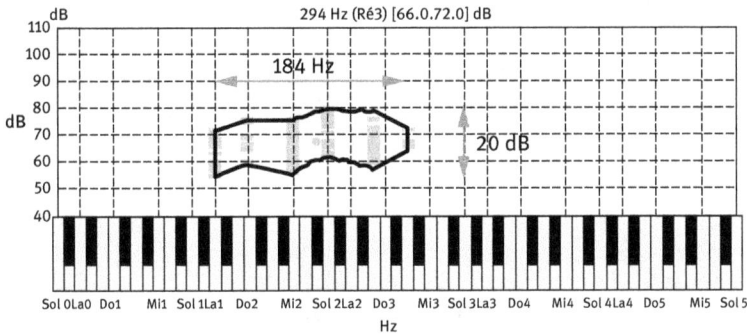

Figure 10.4: Phonetogram of a Parkinsonian patient.

Figure 10.4 shows the Phonetogram of a patient with Parkinson's disease. Its tone dynamics range between 110 and 294 Hz, which is less than two octaves and its intensity range is 20 dB [72]. The center of gravity is on the point (196 Hz, 57 dB) [72].

The MPT

The measurement of MPT provides information on the capacity of the voice organs and on the performance of the voice source [72]. It consists of measuring the phonation time of the continuous vowel, /a/ [72].

The Intensity

The symptom associated with voice disorders and the reduction of subglottic pressure is one of the important factors that reduce the intensity. The variation of the value of the intensity as a function of time is calculated by the mean square root of the acoustic speech signal for each window of 10 milliseconds and it is presented in the form of a curve [52]. The mean value of the intensity is about 70 dB at 30 cm from the mouth of a normal person. It is 85 dB if it raises its voice and 105 dB if it cries [52].

10.3.2 Classification of Parkinson's disease

10.3.2.1 Subjective measures of voice characteristics

The perceptual measures of the voice disorders are realized by listening to the patient when he speaks. The physician focuses on simple aspects of the patient's voice production, such as pitch, intensity, rhythm, and intelligibility of speech [80]. Numerous methods of perceptual analysis have been proposed, to evaluate the quality of the voice [81–83]. Among these, the GRBAS [82] scale is the most widely used method [52, 72]. Dysarthria, in Parkinson's disease, can be measured with a reference grid of voice; it is a multidimensional grid called UPDRS [84–86]. The UPDRS grid is interesting for the surveillance of Parkinson's disease. It describes the severity in five stages according to the voice [52]:
- 0 = normal voice;
- 1 = slight decrease in intonation and volume;
- 2 = monotonous speech, blurry but comprehensible, clearly disturbed;
- 3 = disruption of the path difficult to understand;
- 4 = unintelligible speech.

In addition to the UPDRS, neurologists have been involved in other multidisciplinary approaches, which aim to group the anomalies of different interferences in the functioning of the voice production system (respiration, phonation, resonance, articulation), without ignoring the cognitive and psychological dimensions of voice communication [80]. For this reason, they prefer methods that are more objective.

10.3.2.2 Objective measures of voice characteristics

Aerodynamic methods
Aerodynamics are fundamental in the production of voice. It is at the origin of all the sound events. Indeed, the pulmonary air column is the source of the speech signal, which is modulated by the different constituents of the vocal tract [80].

Aerodynamic parameters are formed by the air currents at the mouth and nostrils, in addition to intra-buccal and subglottic pressures [80]. ROUSSELOT (1895) [87] is the first to propose objective aerodynamic measurements. The determination of the variations of aerodynamic parameters, as a function of pronunciations, provides information on the movements of the organs of the patient's vocal apparatus [80, 88, 89].

The time-frequency measurements of the acoustic signal
In this section, we present the most commonly used acoustic measurements to detect speech disorders in the context of Parkinson's disease. Acoustic measurements depend on many dysfunctions of a patient's voice, for example, the breath is correlated with the ratio of harmonics on noise, asthenia with the vocal intensity, and a forcing voice with a higher fundamental frequency F0. The instability of glottis vibration is the main cause of dysphonia. Therefore, the measurement of these fluctuations is used to quantify dysphonia.

10.4 The diagnosis of Parkinson's disease

Parkinson's patients suffer from hypokinetic dysarthria, which manifests in all aspects of speech production: breathing, phonation, articulation, nasalization, and prosody. Clinicians rely on the quality of speech and try to find the causes of its degradation using phonological and acoustic indices. Voice signal analysis will develop techniques for classifying and quantifying neurological diseases. Thus, specialists will have more reliable techniques of diagnosis allowing the evaluation of the effects of the disease and the monitoring of its evolution. We have found that the origins of voice are from aerodynamic and acoustic phenomena, which are produced on a flow of air from the lungs. We consider that this phenomenon is the excitatory signal (k). It is directed toward the exterior of the human body through various organs, which are responsible for the production of speech; the effect of these organs is modeled by the signal (k), which is the contribution of the vocal tract. Thus, Parkinson's disease is only a degenerative condition represented by a particular model of dysfunction of the system.

Parkinson's disease is one of the many neurological disorders such as Alzheimer's disease and epilepsy. These diseases cause uncontrollable physical and psychological effects in patients. Parkinson's disease generally affects people over the age of 60 [106]. Globally, nearly 10 million people suffer from this disease [35, 107].

Patient care is very costly, and costs may increase in the future [2, 108]. To date, there is no effective cure for this disease; therefore, patients require periodic monitoring and treatment. For a Parkinsonian patient, moving to doctors is very difficult. To this end, the development of a monitoring and telemonitoring solution is necessary. The significant evolution in information and telecommunication technologies facilitates the implementation of telemonitoring and telemedicine systems [109, 110] to simplify the diagnosis of patients. In addition, these new technologies can improve the effectiveness of intervention in medical centers [16, 111, 141].

Currently, the main challenge for medicine is to correctly and prematurely detect Parkinson's disease [112–114], to avoid patient suffering, caused by late diagnoses and interventions [115]. Some studies have shown that this disease causes speech impairment in approximately 90% of patients [2, 116–118], and this may reveal the early stages of the disease [109]. Due to the present signal-processing possibilities, these speech impairments can be used to detect Parkinson's patients [61, 119, 120]. Indeed, Parkinson's disease represents a particular mode of dysfunction of the central nervous system (CNS) [35, 121, 122]. It is characterized by a progressive degradation of nigrostriatal dopaminergic, leading to chronic dysfunction of the basal ganglia system [122, 123]. This system is essential to control the performance of motor reflexes [122]. Consequently, loss of CNS efficiency causes partial or complete loss in motor reflexes, speech, and other vital functions [35, 121]. Research in the field of Parkinson's disease is oriented toward diagnosis, such as DNA [124], deep brain stimulation [125], transcription phase [126], and gene therapy [127].

James Parkinson [128] has described the symptoms of Parkinson's disease; this includes vibrations in the hands, arms, legs, face, and jaw [32]. Voice production, in particular, is an effective means of demonstrating a model of the sequential or simultaneous organization of motor plans [122]. The model must be dynamic with an instantaneous behavior that depends on its previous states [122]. The complex organization of articulatory gestures of speech is under the control of the CNS and basal ganglia in particular [122]. The dysfunctions of the production of vocal sounds, called dysphonia [36], lead to a reduction in loudness, breathiness, and roughness. In addition, they reduce energy in the upper parts of the harmonic spectrum, causing an exaggerated vocal tremor [2, 35, 51].

There are other vocal dysfunctions caused by this disease, for example, hypophonia (low volume), dysarthria (problems in the voice articulations), and monotony (reduced pitch range) [35]. Dysarthria is considered to be the most important characteristic of voice disorders observed in Parkinson's disease. In fact, this characteristic causes the reduction of the articulatory movements and the decrease of the prosodic modulation of the speech [52]. One of the treatment methods used is the injection of a small amount of botulinum toxin [53] into the larynx area. This treatment provides temporary rehabilitation for 3 to 4 months then the dysphonic symptoms will return [16].

Recently used methods aim to adjust the vocal intensity of Parkinson's patients, such as:
–   "Lee Silverman Voice Treatment" (LSVT) [54, 55]: this method increases the vocal intensity by phonatory and respiratory efforts,
–   "Pitch Limiting Voice Treatment" (PLVT) [56]: This method improves speech intensity and keeps the pitch level lower.

Speech symptoms can tell us about the severity of the disease [2, 36]. To quantify these symptoms, numerous tests have been introduced [2, 36]. The most used approaches are as follows:
–   Patients are asked to pronounce continuous vowels at a comfortable level with continuous phonation [6, 36, 57, 58].
–   Patients are asked to say standard sentences that are constructed from representative linguistic units and to be held as long as possible in the course of execution [2, 36, 58, 41].

Real-time voice tests are considered the more realistic for diagnosis. But the problem is that they may contain many linguistic components in addition to the effects of joint confusion [2, 36]. Long and durable vowels represent the more stable speech performances, and thus, they allow a relatively simple acoustic analysis. Therefore, several researchers prefer to use the first approach to detect symptoms of dysphonia [2, 59, 120, 59, 63].

In general, speech samples are recorded using a microphone and then analytical algorithms are applied. There are several software packages implementing these algorithms, such as PRAAT [44] and MDVP [45].

The main characteristics used to detect speech disorders in Parkinson's are [2, 35, 16, 28, 32, 36, 66]:
–   the fundamental frequency F0;
–   the loudness, which indicates the relative intensity of the voice;
–   the jitter measurement, which represents the cycle-to-cycle variation of the F0;
–   the shimmer, which represents the cycle-to-cycle variation of the amplitude in speech;
–   the harmonic to noise ratio, which represents the degree of periodicity of the vocal acoustic signal.

Many differences have been reported by comparing the measures of these characteristics for a Parkinsonian patient with those of a holy person [24, 68].

10.4.1 Proposed methods

10.4.1.1 Methods for classification

In our studies, we used different methods to detect Parkinson's disease. Thus, in a first stage [50], we extracted 20 dimensional MFCC from a database of 34 subjects (Figure 10.6) (17 Parkinsonian patients and 17 healthy people). The process for extracting MFCC coefficients is shown in Figure 10.5

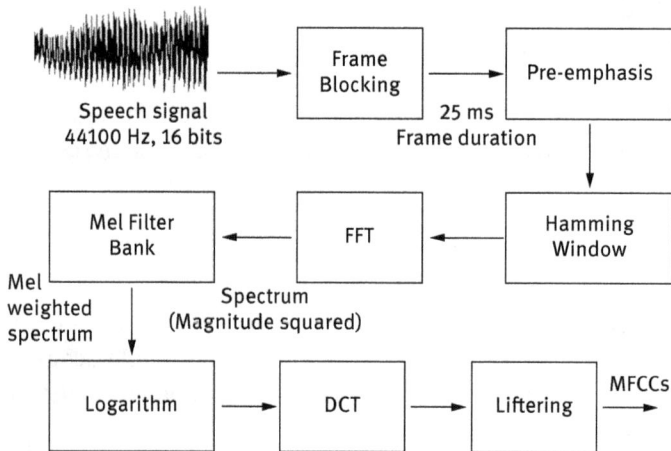

Figure 10.5: Extraction diagram of the MFCC coefficients.

We then compressed the MFCC frames using a vector quantization (VQ), with six sizes for codebooks (1, 2, 4, 8, 16 and 32) (Figure 10.7).

The maximum classification accuracy achieved is 100% and the accuracy of the average classification is 82% (Table 10.1 and 10.2).

For the classification of people with Parkinson's disease, compared with the healthy one, we used the LOSO system with an SVM classifier.

In the same context, in a second study [75], we replaced the MFCC with the PLP technique. The accuracy of the maximum classification achieved in this case is 91.17% and the average precision is 75.79% (Table 10.3).

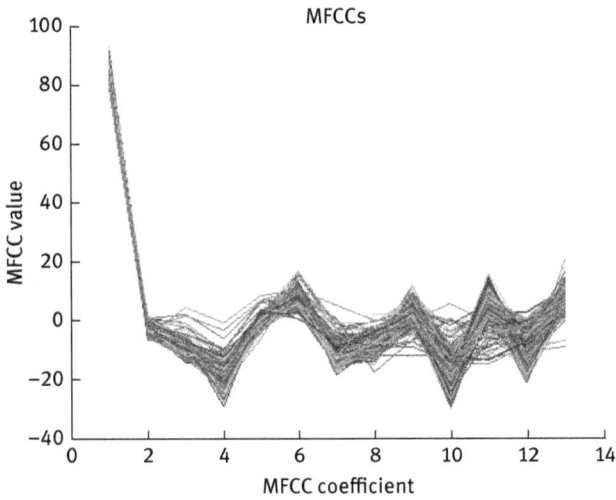

Figure 10.6: The MFCCs of a parkinsonion patient.

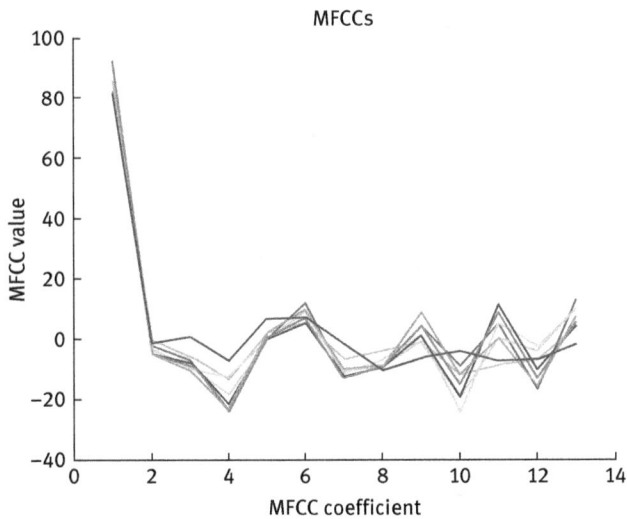

Figure 10.7: The MFCCs of a parkinsonion patient with a codebook size of 8.

In a third study [76], we compressed the PLP (Figure 10.8) frames by calculating their average value to extract the relative speech imprint for each subject.

With this method, we were able to achieve an average classification accuracy of 82.35% (Figure 10.9).

Table 10.1: Classification results for different codebook sizes using MFCC.

Codebook	Max accuracy (%)	Min accuracy (%)	Mean accuracy (%)
1	100	73.52	81.85
2	70.58	70.58	70.58
4	71.32	71.32	71.32
8	69.85	69.85	69.85
16	70.22	70.22	70.22
32	67.64	67.64	67.64

Table 10.2: Calculated coefficients for the SVM classifier.

Codebook	Maximum accuracy coefficients	Minimum accuracy coefficients	Kernels
1	13	3 2 4 5 7 10	Linear
2	8 9 10	8 9 10	Linear
4	5	5	Linear
8	8	8	Linear
16	8	8	Linear
32	15	15	Linear

Table 10.3: Classification results for different codebook sizes using PLP.

Codebook	Max accuracy (%)	Min accuracy (%)	Mean accuracy (%)
1	91.17	67.64	75.79
2	75	75	75
4	68.38	68.38	68.38
8	63.60	63.60	63.60
16	62.31	62.31	62.31
32	61.85	61.85	61.85

For the RBF SVM classification, we have found, based on the obtained results, that when we consider a large number of coefficients, the classification accuracy decreases. This is also true for sensitivity and for specificity. The maximum precision obtained with the RBF classification is 70.59%, using the first coefficient.

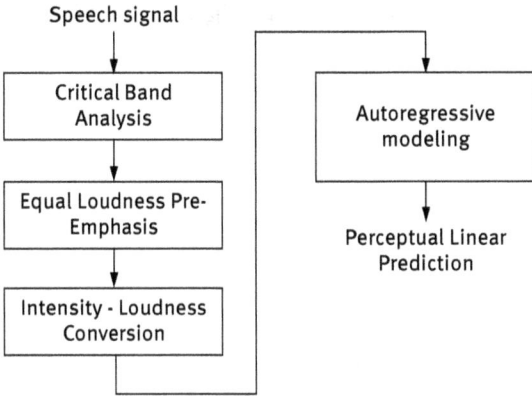

Figure 10.8: The process of calculating PLP coefficients.

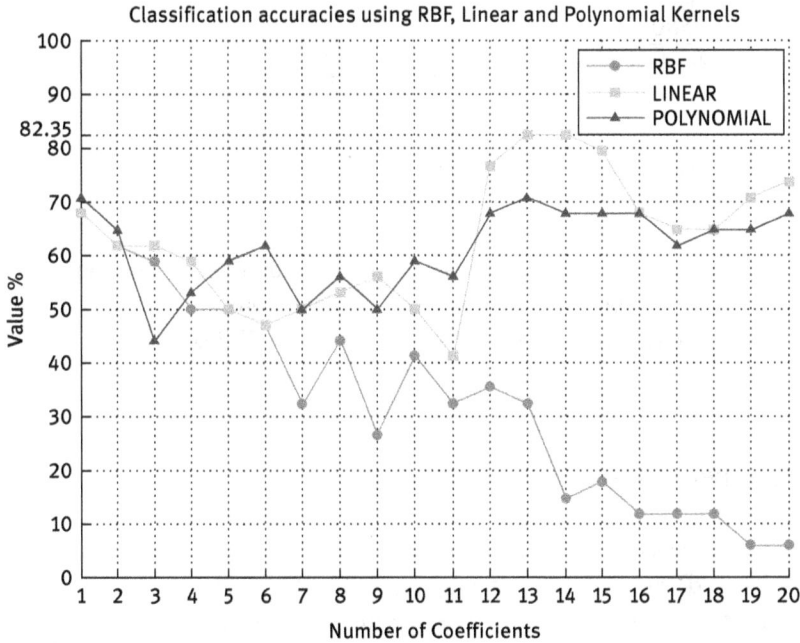

Figure 10.9: Classification accuracy using RBF, linear and polynomial kernels.

The results of the polynomial SVM classification are shown in Figure 10.10. A maximum classification accuracy of 70.59% was obtained using only the 1st and 13th PLP coefficients.

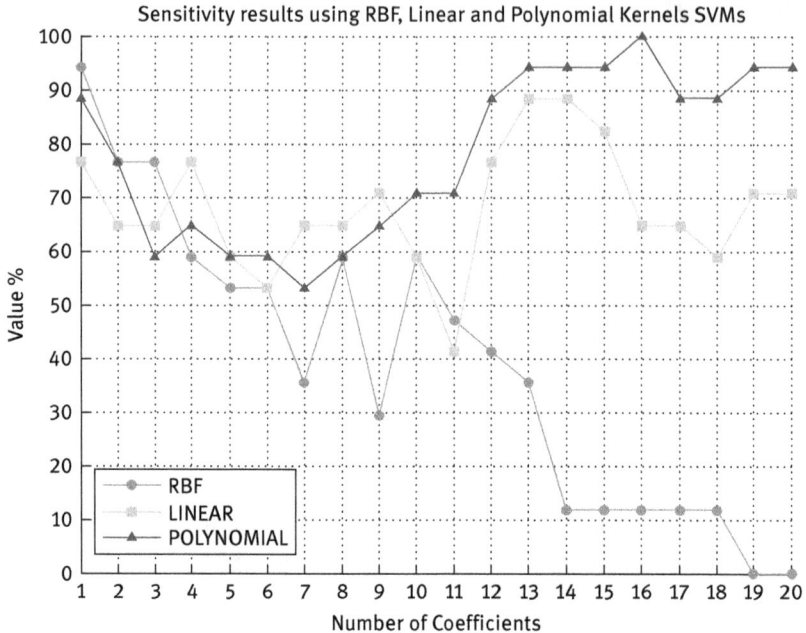

Figure 10.10: Classification sensitivity using linear and polynomial RBF kernels.

With the PLP, we obtained the same maximum precision of classification using the RBF kernel. It can be seen in Figure 10.11 that a maximum classification accuracy of 82.35% is reached using the first 13 and 14 PLP coefficients with a linear kernel.

10.4.1.2 Quantification of Parkinson's disease

Parkinson's disease symptoms do not appear suddenly, they are the result of a slow process and the early stages may go unnoticed [77]. To this end, the development of an earlier diagnosis is a crucial issue for patients and for researchers; it will make it possible to act faster and to better understand the disease to be able to cure it or even prevent it.

Studies have shown a strong relationship between voice degradation and progression of Parkinson's disease [78]. The severity of the disease can be measured using different empirical tests and physical examinations. The measurements are standardized using one of the famous clinical parameters, known as the Unified Parkinson's Disease Rating Scale (UPDRS) [66]. Recently, there have been

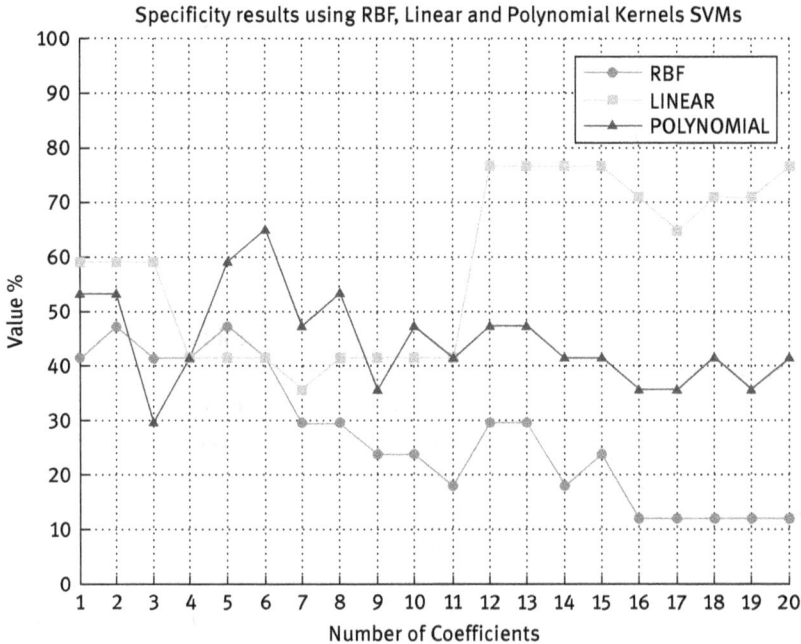

Figure 10.11: Classification specificity using the RBF, linear and polynomial kernels.

numerous research studies to quantify Parkinson's disease and represent it according to the UPDRS [36, 66, 78, 79]. Voice analysis is a useful way to detect the severity of Parkinson's disease if the patient is already affected.

To achieve this goal, Tsanas et al. [66] used the Praat software [64] to calculate classical characteristics, such as Jitter, Shimmer, and harmonic-to-noise ratio HNR. They also used MDPV prefixes to associate their measurements with Kaypentax results [65]. In addition, they found that the log-transformed classical measurements carrying clinical information and that are selected by an automatic algorithm are more appropriate for UPDRS prediction. The database used by the authors is composed of 42 patients including 14 women and 28 men with Parkinson's disease. They have an average age of 64.4 years with a standard deviation of 9.24. The average UPDRS engine is 20.84 ± 8.82 points with a total UPDRS of 28.44 ± 11.52 points.

The authors of [51] studied the possibility of using vowel phonation/a/to automatically quantify Parkinson's disease. These authors were able to extract the relevant characteristics, thus, reducing their number from 309 to 10 characteristics. The maximum performance achieved is 90%, using an SVM classifier. The database used in this study was 14 patients with Parkinson's disease, including six women and eight men. The age of the patients varies between 51 and 69 years, with an average of 61.9 and a standard deviation of 6.5. Each patient recorded nine phonations, 25% of which were repeated to qualify them intra-rat-ratability, giving a total of 156 speech samples.

10.4.1.3 Critics and limitations

Voice disorders are caused by physical problems, such as nodules or vocal polyps that affect the vocal folds, paralysis of the vocal folds due to blows or surgery, or ulcers of the vocal folds. These disorders can also be caused by improper use of vocal organs, such as using the voice at too high or too low "pitch." In some cases, dysphagia manifests as a cross between poor use of the vocal organs and some physiological problems [7].

According to Teston [72], dysphonia in the context of neurological disorders can be caused by multiple factors, such as

- hypotonia, which is manifested by low muscle tone that can lead to a reduction in muscular strength and, therefore, a reduced level of voice and fundamental frequency F0 [143];
- hypertonia, which causes an abnormal increase in muscle tone, leading to breaks and difficulties in the vocal signal [144];
- trembling, which causes a trembling voice [145] and the instability of the fundamental frequency F0 during continuous phonation [146];
- spasmodic dysphonia, which causes sudden changes in the pitch, pauses, non-intelligibility, and a trembling voice;
- laryngeal palsy, where the vocal cord remains more or less in an open position after poor neuromotor control [72].

Dysphonia may also be due to anatomical changes in the glottis, changes due to the appearance of nodules, polyps or cysts that are benign lesions of the vocal folds [72].

Anatomical changes may also be caused by inflammations, such as laryngitis of the vocal cords. As a result, the voice becomes deeper, with difficulties in the higher "Pitch"; it becomes slightly deaf and may even disappear completely [72].

In addition, there may be anatomical changes in the glottis, caused by surgical trauma, following elimination of a tumor, for example. As a result, the voice becomes seriously degraded, deeper, of lower intensity, however, intelligible in a noiseless place [72].

So far, there are few effective methods capable of distinctly distinguishing between Parkinson's disease and other neurological diseases. Being able to distinguish between Parkinson's disease among patients with other neurological disorders is a challenge.

10.5 Sensor networks in the service of Parkinson's patients

10.5.1 The constraints associated with wireless sensor networks

10.5.1.1 Standard of biomedical

Sensor networks, used in biomedical, are called the BAN (Body Area Network); they are networks carried on the human body (Figure 10.12). These networks have been designated by the IEEE802.15.6 standard, created to set up the necessary guidelines for the realization of biomedical applications.

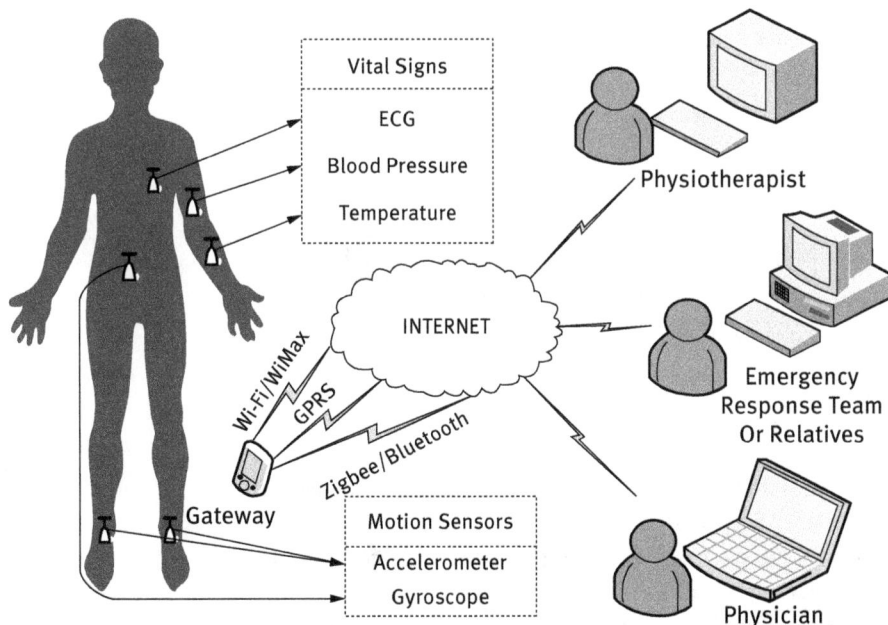

Figure 10.12: Example of a BAN application [129].

The IEEE802.15.6 standard specifies the technical requirements for each application, from the study and modeling of the BAN propagation channel, to the study of the physical and MAC layers. Several constraints have been taken into account by this standard; in particular, the following orientations:

- *Energy consumption:* the life-time of the batteries is several months or even years. The network must be defined so that energy consumption is minimal. This results in a low consumption of the transmission and reception elements of the physical layer and by mechanisms established at the level of the MAC layer.
- *Antennae:* the nature of the antenna and its location on the body affects the propagation losses of the signal. The antenna of a knot can be integrated there and can be located on the skin or inside the clothing.
- *Mobility:* the human body regularly undergoes great motilities of the members; this introduces variations of the propagation channel. These changes are causing a degradation in communications' performance.
- *Coexistence:* the standard recommends the coexistence of 10 BAN networks in a space of 6 m³. These networks must also be able to operate in a polluted environment with electromagnetic waves of various kinds.

10.5.1.2 Energy Consumption in Sensor Networks

In a network sensor, the sequencing of a sensor node is illustrated in the Figure 10.13:

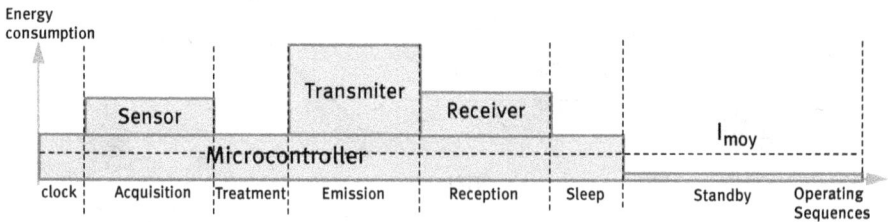

Figure 10.13: Energy consumption sequence of a sensor node.

The acquisition energy is dissipated during the measurements made by the sensors. The acquisition can be clocked by a sampling frequency or activated per event. In general, this energy is negligible compared with the overall energy consumed by the node.

The processing energy is an energy consumed by the microcontroller during the execution of the data processing algorithms. Although this energy depends on the complexity of the used algorithms, it is generally low compared with that required for transmission.

The transmission energy consists of two possible types of consumption, namely, the energy consumed during a transmission and/or the energy consumed during a reception. In both the cases, this energy depends on the amount of data to be communicated, the transmission range, and the physical properties of the radio module. The emission is characterized by its power. Thus, when the power of a transmitted signal is high, the range will be large, and the energy consumed will obviously be higher. We notice in Figure 10.13 that the transmission energy represents the largest portion of the energy consumed by a node in the network. For this, we are particularly interested in optimizing this energy. The diagram in Figure 10.14 represents the consuming elements of the transmission energy.

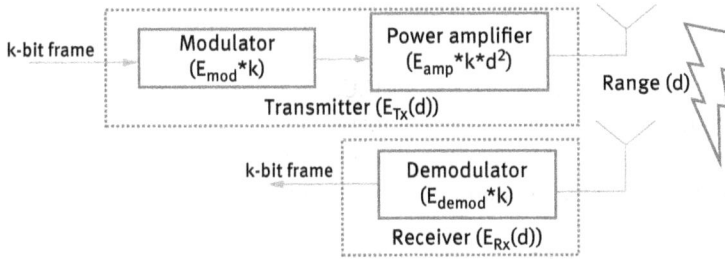

Figure 10.14: Representative diagram of the energy consuming blocks.

The energy consumption model can be described by the following equations:

$$\begin{cases} E_{Tx}(k,d) = k \times E_{mod} + k \times E_{amp} \times d^2 \ \textit{for the distances } d < d_0 \\ E_{Tx}(k,d) = k \times E_{mod} + k \times E_{amp} \times d^4 \ \textit{for the distances } d \geq d_0 \\ E_{Rx}(k) = k \times E_{mod}, \qquad\qquad\qquad (E_{mod} = E_{demod}). \end{cases} \quad (10.6)$$

The coefficient k represents the number of bits in the frame. The distance, d, between two communicating nodes is less than the threshold d_0, then the power amplifier will provide less effort, and the energy consumed will be proportional to d^2. In contrast, if the range exceeds the threshold d_0, the consumed energy will become proportional to d^4. We note in this model that the equation of the reception energy does not depend on the range d. The use of network sensors in a medical context requires low-energy operation, caused mainly by power limitation. Indeed, uncontrolled power to a certain limit can be negative for human health. In addition, the sensor nodes must operate at reasonable temperatures. Therefore, limited energy consumption is required. Consequently, energy is one of the most crucial constraints in designing nodes.

10.5.1.3 Reliability of measurements

In addition to energy consumption, there is a second constraint that is related to the reliability of information measured by the network. In fact, the state of health of a patient is paramount and any error of treatment, coming from a node, can distort the diagnosis. An error correcting encoder is, therefore, necessary for our application. Moreover, the coding must be chosen so as to optimize the energy consumption.

The distribution of processing on several nodes, followed by a merge of information, is a higher level to enhance the reliability of the network. The fusion of data is the subject of several scientific researches. Thus, the authors of [147] propose a data fusion system for fire prevention. The system is based on the aggregation of sensors using cumulative sums (CUSUM). The author in [148] used the retro-propagation theorem for the classification and fusion of multi-sensor data, its algorithm is based on learning error correction. The author in [149] quantified the nodes by local decision bits and studied three quantization algorithms based on weight, statistics, and redundancy. It is then observed that the last two algorithms are adapted to networks, which have a limited number of nodes and which corresponds perfectly to our case. The algorithms, based on statistical calculations, have a better stability, whereas the algorithms based on the redundancy have better performances if the degree of quantification is high.

10.5.2 A network of sensors for Parkinson's detection

10.5.2.1 The sensor nodes

A node is organized around a microcontroller. It can ensure the acquisition of one or more sensors and even communicate with neighboring nodes in single, half, or full-duplex. We propose three types of nodes:
- Type 1: nodes based essentially on accelerometers, and gyroscopes (Figure 10.15);
- Type 2: nodes containing accelerometers, and blood pressure sensors (Figure 10.16);
- Type 3: nodes for sensing electromyogram signals (Figure 10.17).

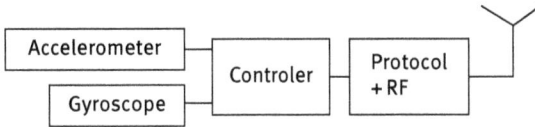

Figure 10.15: Node Type1.

The nodes of the first type are mounted on the patient's limbs. These nodes can provide the information of his or her posture when sitting, standing, or moving.

The nodes of the second type are mounted on the patient's legs. They measure nervous disorders that lead to an abnormal reaction in the muscles.

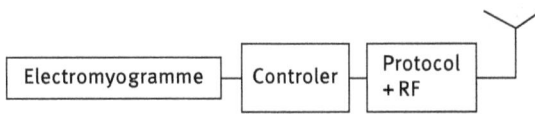

Figure 10.16: Node Type2.

The nodes of the third type are mounted on the patient's arm. They measure the applied force and tremor while at the rest.

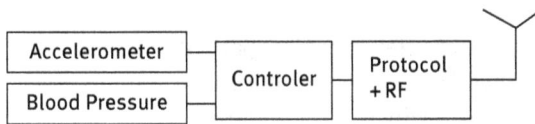

Figure 10.17: Node Type3.

10.5.2.2 BAN network architecture

The BAN network is structured around the collaboration of a dozen nodes operating autonomously. Each node performs its own measurements and communicates, wirelessly with the other nodes, for a more reliable decision. Our application consists of a network of cooperative wireless sensors, to measure the gestures, and the efforts provided by the Parkinsonian patient. In addition to the sensor nodes, the network has a sink node that collects various information to send to the embedded diagnostic system. The sink node can also be used to send the patient's physiological information remotely, so that they can be archived or diagnosed in real-time. This will give rise to simpler and more reliable diagnoses to better understand disease states in the patients.

The proposed BAN network (Figure 10.18) is characterized by a cooperative aspect of its various nodes. Each node is a small embedded system that integrates a processor to perform simple processing operations. Instead of

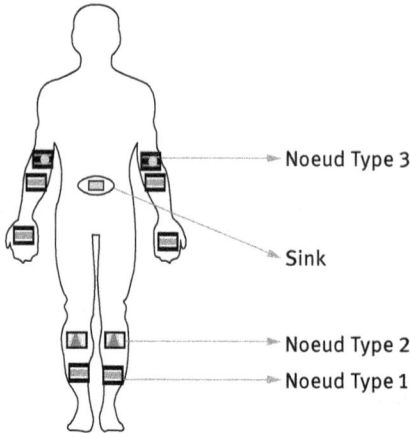

Figure 10.18: BAN network for PD patients.

transmitting all the sensed measures, a node transmits only the necessary data, and partially processed it.

10.5.2.3 Correction of errors

The use of sensor networks, in a medical context, requires particular vigilance for errors due to the transmission channel. The choice of error control systems is very critical in the case of a BAN network, for which good reliability is required. For our medical application, the network requires a better measurement reliability, with minimal energy consumption. The appropriate error-correction code must be selected based on the Bit Error Rate (BER) and the power consumption.

In several published works, the authors use error-correcting codes, such as Automatic Repeat reQuest (ARQ) and Forward Error Correction (FEC) techniques. The ARQ technique does not require additional data processing at the intermediate nodes of the network. It consists of detecting the errors by a standard error detector code and then sends an automatic request of repeating ARQ, requesting the retransmission of missing packets. The FEC technique is used to protect against loss of packets on sensor networks. Its basic principle is to intelligently add redundancy and take advantage of this super information to determine the reliability of the message. In some cases, this technique also makes it possible to reconstruct the original message, even if the reception has been erroneous. This possibility of error correction is due to redundancy, in particular, the more the redundancy, the easier it is to detect and correct any errors.

The authors [130] and [131] have shown that the use of the ARQ is limited for the sensor networks, this is because of the additional retransmission. However, it can be seen in the reference [132] that the energy efficiency of the ARQ, compared to that of BCH, is better for short distances.

Another category of error-correcting coders, called Fountain codes, is well suited to our context. Indeed, these coders potentially have an infinite yield, which means that the number of encoded packets can be theoretically unlimited. Thus, the transmission of the encoded packets continues until the complete reception of the information, and this is independent of the number of lost packets [155]. For this technique, the transmission of a combination of information is completed only by the acknowledgment, which is sent by the receiver. This principle is appropriate in our case, because it makes it possible to improve the reliability of the communications, without needing a priori knowledge of the channel that often changes.

Studies have shown that the convolution, Hamming and Reed Solomon codes are better, in terms of BER, than all the other existing codes. However, the complex decoder associated with these codes consumes considerable energy. These encoders are, therefore, not advantageous in the case of wireless sensor networks. In addition, "Fountain" codes (Figure 10.19) have been shown to significantly improve the efficiency and reliability of the network. In reference [133], for example, there is a study on the impact of "Fountain" codes on energy consumption in a wireless sensor network.

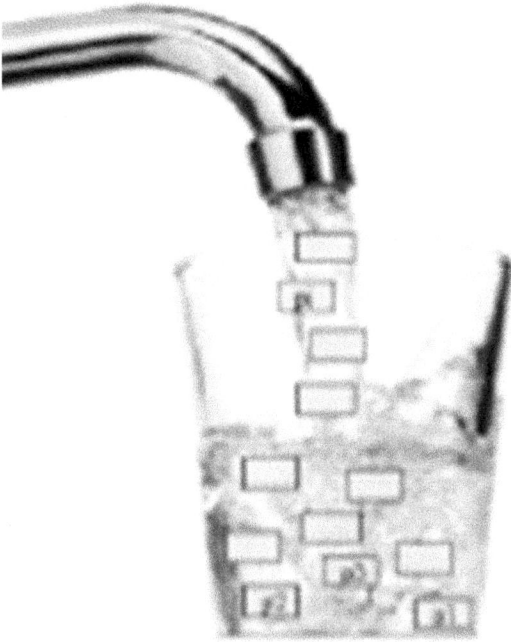

Figure 10.19: Analogy of the code 'Fountain' [134].

The class of "Fountain" codes can be implemented with simple coding and decoding algorithms. These encoders, therefore, consume little energy. In addition, they are adaptive to the instantaneous states of the channels, which avoid the need for feedback. Indeed, these codes make it possible to send as many packets as necessary so that the decoder can recover the source data. Among the known, "Fountain" codes are of three categories: RLF (Random Linear Fountain), LT (Luby Transform), and RC (Raptor Code). For the experimental implementation, we implemented the LT code (Figure 10.20) considering a BAN network, whose constraints respect the standard IEEE802.15.6.

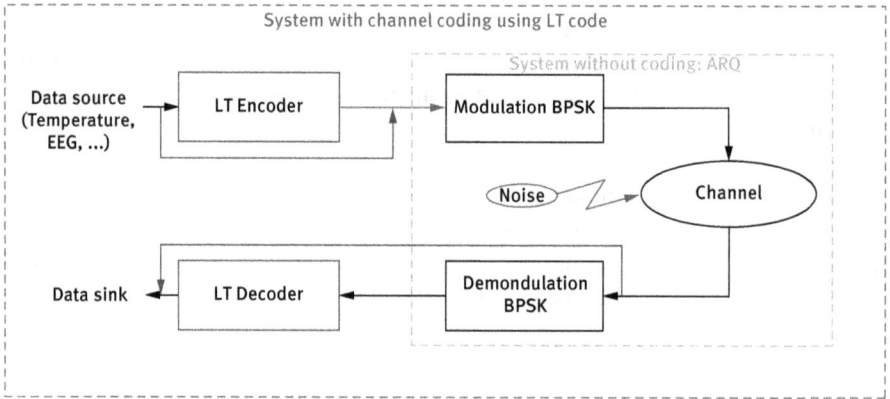

Figure 10.20: Mounting for LT coding simulation.

The simulation parameters according to IEEE802.15.6 are summarized in Table 10.4:

Table 10.4: Simulation parameters [135].

Parameter	Type or value
R (Transmission rate)	20 Kbit/s
F (Frequency carrier)	868 MHz
N_b (Number of bits per packet)	100 octets (uncoded channel) 105 octets (with LT coding)
E_{Ele}	50 nJ/bit
E_{amp}	10 pJ/bit/m^2 0.0013 pJ/bit/m4

In the first step, we analyzed the performance of the LT code in terms of BER and the results of the simulation are shown in Figure 10.21. These results correspond to point-to-point communication in a Gaussian additive white noise channel BBAG with N0 = -111 dBm/Hz, using BPSK modulation.

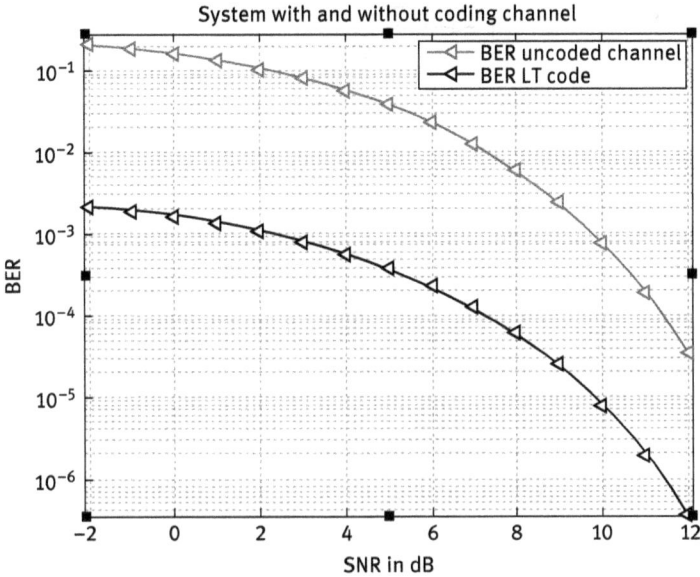

Figure 10.21: Bit Error Rate with and without LT coding.

We find that the LT coding improves the BER. In addition, it is normal to observe the degradation when the signal-to-noise ratio (SNR) increases, an interesting result for our case, concerns the optimization of energy, when applying the LT coding this is shown by the curves of Figures 10.22 and 10.23.

We have seen that wireless communication is the most energy consuming in a sensor node. This energy consumption depends on the amount of data (s) and transmission range (d). It can be modeled by the following equations:

$$E_P = E_T\,(s, d) + E_R(s) + E_{ack},$$ (10.7)

where, E_T, E_R, and E_{ack} are the energies necessary for transmission, reception, and acknowledgment, respectively. The E_T energy includes the E_{Telec} transmission consumption, and the consumption of the E_{Tamp} power amplifier.

The total energy consumed in a sensor node for an LT encoding transmitting K fragments of information is:

$$E_{LT} = (K + \varepsilon - 1) \cdot \frac{1}{\gamma dt} \cdot (E_{T_{LT}} + E_{R_{LT}}) + \frac{1}{\gamma_{ack}} \cdot (\frac{1}{\gamma_{dt}} \cdot (E_{T_{LT}} + E_{R_{LT}}) + E_{ack}\,.$$ (10.8)

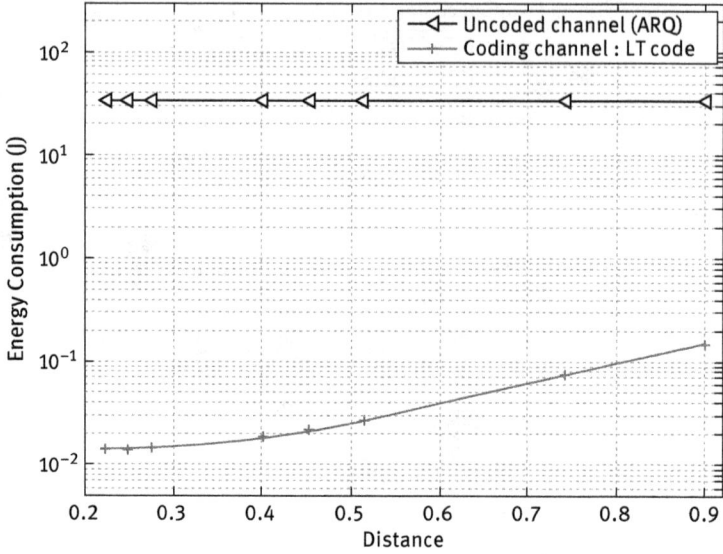

Figure 10.22: Energy optimization by LT coding as a function of the range.

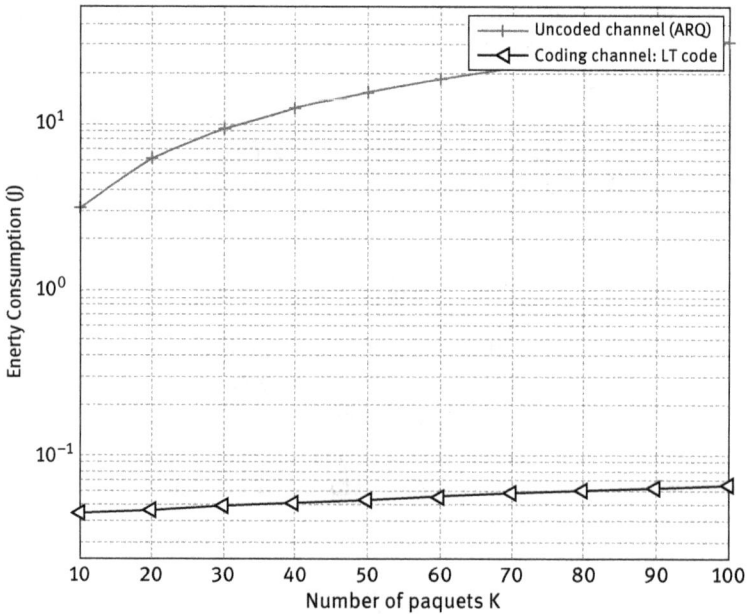

Figure 10.23: Optimization of energy by LT coding as a function of the number of packets.

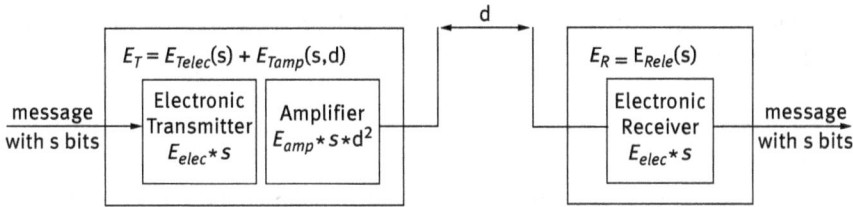

Figure 10.24: Energy block diagram.

where $E_{T_{LT}} = E_T + E_{enc}$ and $E_{R_{LT}} = E_R + E_{dec}$ are the energy consumed during transmission and reception, taking into account the consumption of the encoder (E_{enc}) and the decoder (E_{dec}).

The model was validated by deploying a seven-node BAN network on a 1.60 m person. Measurements of the consumed energies were made (Figures 10.22 and 10.23), for different distances, and for a maximum of 100 packets (Figure 10.24). We have found that the introduction of the LT encoder into a sensor node that optimizes energy consumption. In addition, this module promotes the reliability of measurements by reducing the error rate per bits.

10.5.3 Communication protocol between the nodes

10.5.3.1 Protocol strategy

To meet the different challenges of wireless sensor networks, several routing protocols have been implemented; each has its way of conveying information from the different nodes to the base station, while respecting the criterion of low consumption, which is difficult to satisfy without compromise.

Similarly, several strategies have been developed to improve routing protocols and to achieve the objective that is taken into account for reliability of transmission, and to save energy. These strategies include clustering, routing trees, aggregation, merge, and so on.

10.5.3.2 Using gateway

In our case, we propose the use of the concept of the gateway, which will minimize the energy consumption of the nodes. The gateway is a node of the network that will serve as an access point. We recall that we have 10 nodes of sensors distributed over the members of the patient. A node is initially considered normal, however, that can be selected to switch to gateway mode. The chance of a node to become a gateway node is calculated according to its proximity to the base station (BS) and its residual energy. To do this, the selection of the gateway node passes through the following algorithm (Figure 10.25):

This algorithm designates the gateway node to balance the energy consumption, to extend the life of the network. Each node tries to connect to the nearest gateway. For this purpose, the distance between the node and the gateway is

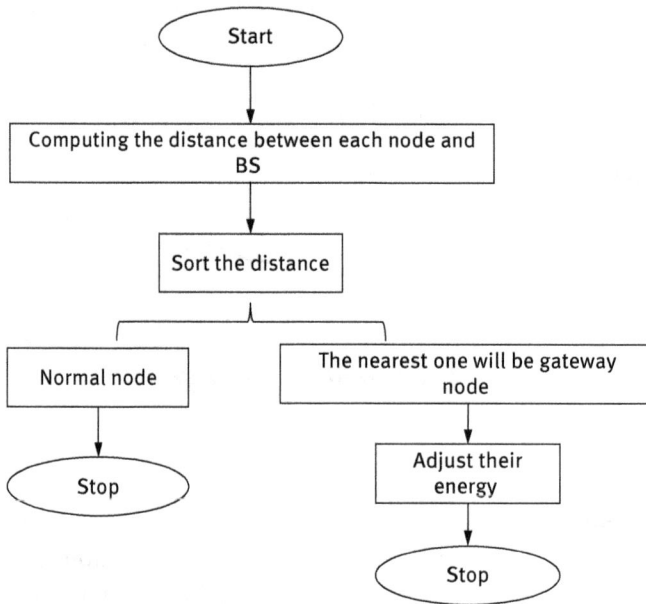

Figure 10.25: Gateway choice algorithm.

Table 10.5: Simulation settings.

Simulation Settings		
Settings	*Description*	*Value*
Eelect	Energy of the elections	50e-9
Eda	Energy for data aggregation	5e-9
Efs	Energy of the emission amplifier	10e-12
Eo	Initial energy	0.5
K	Number of transmitted bits	4000

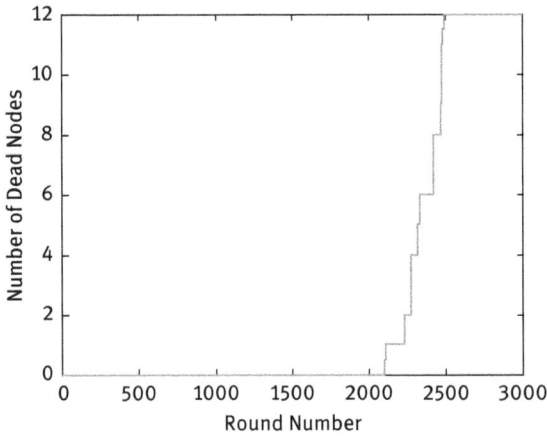

Figure 10.26: Network node lifetimes.

calculated cyclically. The gateway node merges the measurements and then sends them to the base station. The following table summarizes the character-istics taken into account for the simulation of our method (Table 10.5).

10.5.3.3 Optimization of energy

The following two curves show the evolution of the mean energy remaining in the network at each use (Figure 10.27). Using the method, we have adopted (left curve) and we can optimize the energy consumption, with respect to a traditional network (right curve).

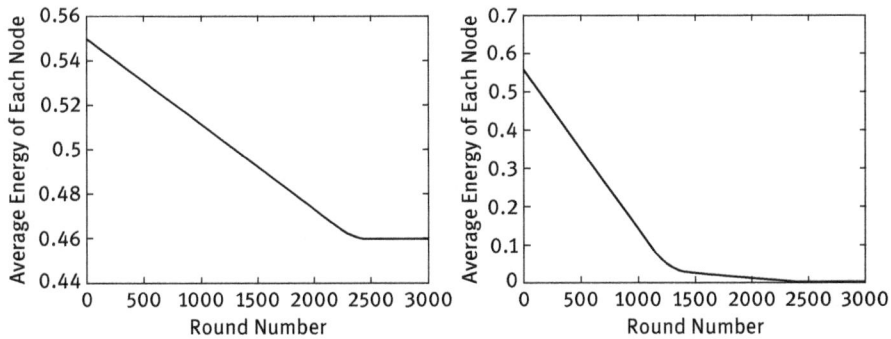

Figure 10.27: Average residual energy.

10.5.4 Data fusion

10.5.4.1 Cooperation of nodes

The use of a sensor network, in a medical context, requires particular attention to errors due to the transmission channel. The cooperative characteristics of the sensor network can be exploited to make it more robust.

Our objective, for this part, is to study the cooperation of the nodes to establish an error correction in a noisy channel. We are also looking for modeling the theoretical probabilities at the input of the main node, and the probability of frame error corresponding to a cooperative scheme.

The proposed model is subdivided into two hierarchical levels of fusion. In the first level, we applied the Central Limit Theorem (CLT) [136] and combined measurements of sensors of the same type (accelerometer, arterial pressure or electromyogram); a sequential test calculation (CUSUM) determines the patient's postural changes. The second level of the merge is based on probabilities calculated from the first level.

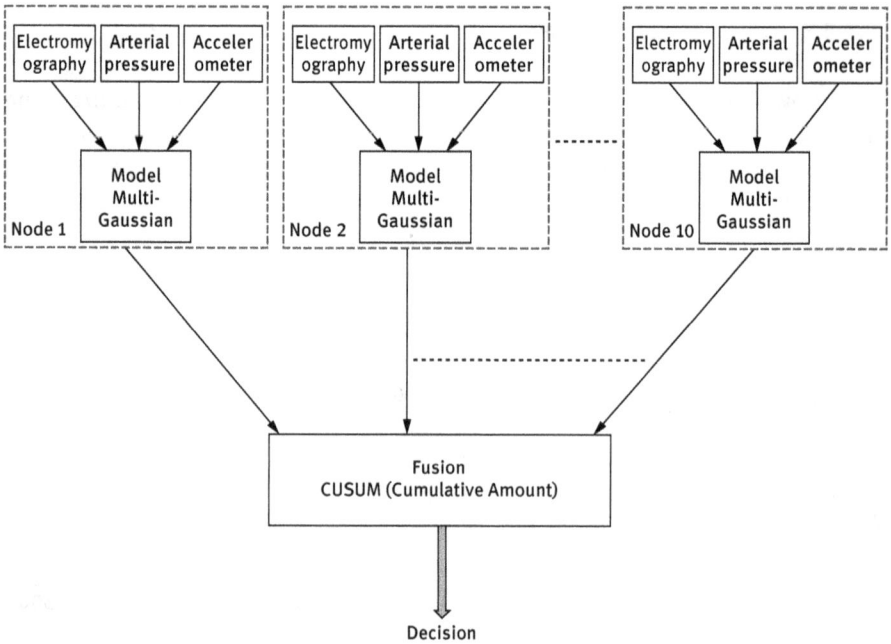

Figure 10.28: Hierarchical fusion level.

10.5.4.2 First-level of fusion

Many related works on multi-sensor fusion have been studied by several researchers [137–140]. The authors of reference [137], for example, applied the retro-propagation theorem for the classification and fusion of multi-sensor data. This algorithm is based on error correction by learning. The authors of the reference [138] quantified several local decision bits for the observations of each node. The results show that these methods can improve the capacity of the system, when the nodes are insufficient. In summary, statistical systems have improved stability, while redundancy-based systems perform better when the degree of quantification is high.

The measurements captured by the different nodes are transmitted to the Sink (Figure 10.18). It is in this node that the operations of analysis and fusion of data take place. The Sink will then pass the merged information to the embedded diagnostic system.

To detect any significant change in the state of the environment, the homogeneous observation signals are constantly combined into a single signal X_{TLC} using the following equation:

$$X_{TLC} = \sigma_{TLC}^{-2} \sum_{i=1}^{n} (\sigma_i^{-2} X_i) \tag{10.9}$$

With $\sigma_{TLC}^{2} = \sum_{i=1}^{n}(\sigma_i^{-2})$, n is the number of sensors and σ_i is the mathematical expectation of the TLC i = 1 observation X_i in the interval τ.

Then, for each homogeneous fused signal, a probability of change of state is calculated. A decision based on the likelihood ratio is affected for each category of sensors. Probabilities based on these decisions (Figure 10.28) are exploited at the second fusion level using the Chair–Varshney rule [139]. This phase increases the reliability of the network.

A quantization operation is applied to the combined observation XTLC [140]; Each local decision, denoted by "Bg," should take a binary value "0" or "1" according to the following constraints:

$$B_g = \begin{cases} 1, & si\ RG| \geq SR, \\ 0, & sinon, \end{cases} \tag{10.10}$$

Where SR is a certain threshold and RG is the likelihood ratio between the two mixing distributions H1 and H2 calculated by:

$$RG = \left| log \left[\frac{f(X_{TLC}|H_1)}{f(X_{TLC}|H_0)} \right] \right| \tag{10.11}$$

From the above results (curves of Figure 10.29: Mixing probabilities), the probability of the change of state "Pc" and that of stability "Ps" can be determined using the following equations:

$$\begin{cases} Pc = \int_S^\infty f(X|H_1) \ dX, \\ Ps = \int_S^\infty f(X|H_0) \ dX, \end{cases}$$

(10.12)

S is a fixed threshold which can be chosen appropriately from the ROC curves.

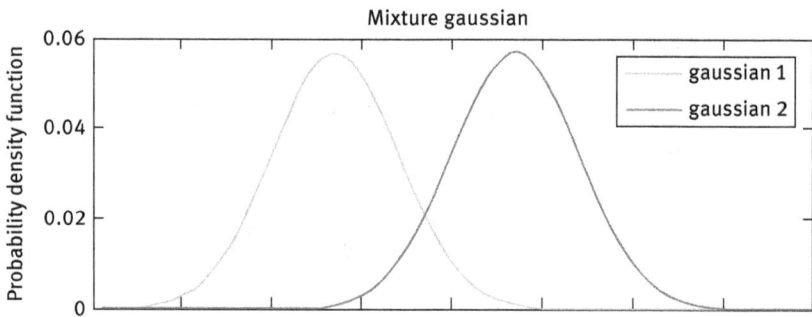

Figure 10.29: Mixing probabilities.

The calculation of the change time can be made if the decision binary value switches to "1". At this time, a cumulative sum calculation CUSUM is executed with the aim of determining the instant of the change, that is to say, the moment of passage of the distribution $f(X_{TLC}|H_0)$ to the distribution $f(X_{TLC}|H_1)$.

The CUSUM test is an algorithm for sequentially detecting state changes; it is based on the CUSUM of the instantaneous reports *RVSn* of likelihood of the two mixing distributions. The equation of this sum (CUSUM) is therefore:

$$Csum = \sum_{n=1}^k RVS_n.$$

(10.13)

The following figure shows the behavior of CUSUM when a change in *RVSn* is detected.

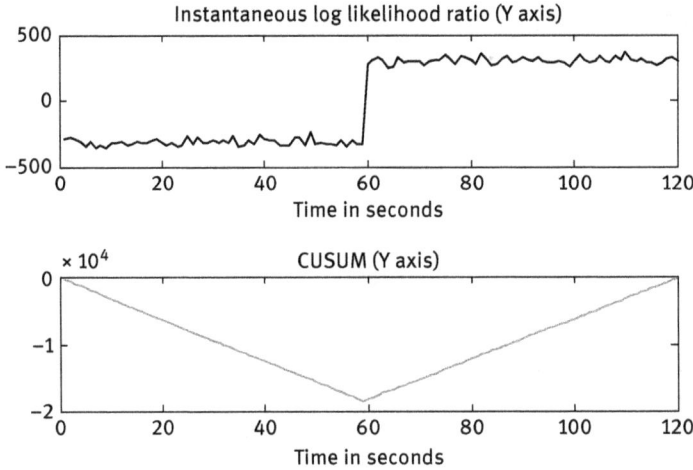

Figure 10.30: Behavior of RVS and CUSUM.

10.5.4.3 Second level of fusion

The fusion of the first level is applied to the sensors of the same type. Acceleration, arterial pressure, and electromyogram sensors are available. We will then have three different decisions: Bg_a, Bg_p, Bg_e defined by equation $Bg = \begin{cases} 1, \ si \ RG \geq SR, \\ 0, \quad sinon, \end{cases}$ in similarly the probabilities Pc_a, Ps_a; Pc_p, Ps_p; Pc_e; Ps_e are computable using equation $\begin{cases} Pc = \int_S^\infty f(X|H_1) \ dX, \\ Ps = \int_S^\infty f(X|H_0) \ dX. \end{cases}$ Then, in the second merge level, the Chair–Varshney rule [139] is applied to have a final decision DF such as:

$$D_F = \sum_{j=1}^{3} D_{Fj}, \qquad (10.14)$$

with:

$$\begin{cases} D_{F1} = \left[Bg_a ln \dfrac{Pc_a}{Ps_a} + (1 - Bg_a) ln \dfrac{1 - Pc_a}{1 - Ps_a} \right], \\[2mm] D_{F2} = \left[Bg_p \, ln \dfrac{Pc_p}{Ps_p} + (1 - Bg_p) ln \dfrac{1 - Pc_p}{1 - Ps_p} \right], \\[2mm] D_{F3} = \left[Bg_e \, ln \dfrac{Pc_e}{Ps_e} + (1 - Bg_e) ln \dfrac{1 - Pc_e}{1 - Ps_e} \right]. \end{cases} \qquad (10.15)$$

The decision D_F reflects the change in the patient's posture. This decision is based on the three types of sensors; merging this information allows for a more reliable decision.

References

[1]   Jilbab, A, Benba A, Hammouch A. Quantification system of Parkinson's disease. Int J Speech Technol 2017;20(1):143–50.
[2]   Little MA, et al. Suitability of dysphonia measurements for telemonitoring of Parkinson's disease. IEEE Trans on Biomed Eng 2009;56(4):1015–22.
[3]   Learning Repository, U.C.I.: http://archive.ics.uci.edu/ml/, June 2008
[4]   Hastie T, et al. The elements of statistical learning: data mining, inference and prediction. Math Intelligencer 2005;27(2):83–5.
[5]   Guyon I, Elisseeff A. An introduction to variable and feature selection. J Mach Learn Res 2003;3:1157–82.
[6]   Shahbaba B, Neal R. Nonlinear models using Dirichlet process mixtures. J Mach Learn Res 2009;10:1829–50.
[7]   Das R. A comparison of multiple classification methods for diagnosis of Parkinson disease. Exp Syst Appl 2010;37(2):1568–72.
[8]   Klein JP, Zhang MJ.Survival analysis, software. John Wiley & Sons, Ltd, 2005.
[9]   Singh N, Pillay V, Choonara YE. Advances in the treatment of Parkinson's disease. Prog Neurobiol 2007;81(1):29–44.
[10]   Guo P-F, Bhattacharya P, Kharma N. Advances in detecting Parkinson's disease. Med Biometrics. Springer Berlin Heidelberg, 2010;6165:306–14.
[11]   Sakar CO, Kursun O. Telediagnosis of Parkinson's disease using measurements of dysphonia. J Med Syst 2010;34(4):591–9.
[12]   Ozcift A, Gulten A. Classifier ensemble construction with rotation forest to improve medical diagnosis performance of machine learning algorithms. Comput Methods Programs Biomed 2011;104(3):443–51.
[13]   Åström F, Koker R. A parallel neural network approach to prediction of Parkinson's disease. Expert Syst Appl 2011;38(10):12470–4.
[14]   Spadoto AA, et al. Improving Parkinson's disease identification through evolutionary-based feature selection.Annual International Conference of the IEEE Engineering in Medicine and Biology Society, EMBC, 201. IEEE, 2011.
[15]   Li D-C, Liu C-W, Hu SC. A fuzzy-based data transformation for feature extraction to increase classification performance with small medical data sets. Artif Intell Med 2011;52(1):45–52.
[16]   Mandal I, Sairam N. Accurate telemonitoring of Parkinson's disease diagnosis using robust inference system. Int J Med Inf 2013;82(5):359–77.
[17]   Tenório JM, et al. Artificial intelligence techniques applied to the development of a decision–support system for diagnosing celiac disease. Int J Med Inf 2011;80(11):793–802.
[18]   Torii M, et al. An exploratory study of a text classification framework for Internet-based surveillance of emerging epidemics. Int J Med Inf 2011;80(1):56–66.

[19] Krishnapuram, B, et al. Sparse multinomial logistic regression: Fast algorithms and generalization bounds. IEEE Trans Pattern Anal Mach Intell 2005;27(6):957–68.
[20] Gutiérrez, PA, Hervás-Martínez C, Martínez-Estudillo FJ. Logistic regression by means of evolutionary radial basis function neural networks. IEEE Trans Neural Networks 2011; 22(2):246–63.
[21] Mandal I. Software reliability assessment using artificial neural network. Proceedings of the International Conference and Workshop on Emerging Trends in Technology. ACM, 2010.
[22] Rodriguez JJ, Kuncheva LI, CJ Alonso CJ. Rotation forest: A new classifier ensemble method. IEEE Trans Pattern Anal Mach Intell 2006;28(10):1619–30.
[23] Mandal I, Sairam N. Accurate prediction of coronary artery disease using reliable diagnosis system. J Med Syst 2012;36(5):3353–73.
[24] Beaudoin CE, Hong T. Health information seeking, diet and physical activity: an empirical assessment by medium and critical demographics. Int J Med Inf 2011;80(8):586–95.
[25] Sandberg K. The haar wavelet transform. Applied Math Website-Welcome to the Department of Applied Mathematics (2000) 1350001-7.
[26] Tu C-C, Juang CF. Recurrent type-2 fuzzy neural network using Haar wavelet energy and entropy features for speech detection in noisy environments. Expert Syst Appl 2012; 39(3):2479–88.
[27] Ozcift Akin. SVM feature selection based rotation forest ensemble classifiers to improve computer-aided diagnosis of Parkinson disease. J Med Syst 2012;36(4):2141–7.
[28] Zuo W-L, et al. Effective detection of Parkinson's disease using an adaptive fuzzy k-nearest neighbor approach. Biomed Signal Process Control 2013;8(4):364–73.
[29] Eberhart RC, Kennedy J. A new optimizer using particle swarm theory. Proceedings of the sixth international symposium on micro machine and human science. Vol. 1. 1995.
[30] Chen H-L, et al. An adaptive fuzzy k-nearest neighbor method based on parallel particle swarm optimization for bankruptcy prediction. Advances in Knowledge Discovery and Data Mining. Springer Berlin Heidelberg, 2011:249–64.
[31] Chen H-L, et al. A novel bankruptcy prediction model based on an adaptive fuzzy k-nearest neighbor method. Knowledge-Based Syst 2011;24(8):1348–59.
[32] Chen H-L, et al. An efficient diagnosis system for detection of Parkinson's disease using fuzzy k-nearest neighbor approach. Expert Syst Appl 2013;40(1):263–71.
[33] Keller JM, Gray MR, Givens JA. A fuzzy k-nearest neighbor algorithm. IEEE Trans Syst Man Cybern 1985;4:580–5.
[34] Hariharan M, Polat K, Sindhu R. A new hybrid intelligent system for accurate detection of Parkinson's disease. Comput Methods Programs Biomed 2014;113(3):904–13.
[35] Sakar BE, et al. Collection and analysis of a Parkinson speech dataset with multiple types of sound recordings. IEEE J Biomed Health Inf 2013;17(4):828–34.
[36] Jafari, A. Classification of Parkinson's disease patients using nonlinear phonetic features and Mel-Frequency Cepstral analysis. Biomed Eng: Appl, Basis Commun 2013;25(04): 1350001-1–1350001-10.
[37] Dongge L, et al. Classification of general audio data for content-based retrieval. Pattern Recognit Lett Elsevier Science, 2001;22:533–44.
[38] Dunn R, Reynolds D, Quatieri T. Approaches to speaker detection and tracking in conversational speech. Digital Signal Process Academic Press, 2000;10:93–112.
[39] Lamel LF, Gauvain JL. Speaker verification over the telephone, Speech Commun Elsevier, 2000;31:141–54.

[40] Gish H, Schmidt M. Text-independent speaker identification. IEEE Signal Processing Magazine, pp. 18–32, October, 1994.

[41] Campbell JP. Speaker recognition: a tutorial. Proc IEEE 1997;85(9): 1437–1462.

[42] Moore, Brian C. J. An Introduction to the Psychology of Hearing. 4th ed. San Diego (Calif.): Academic Press, 1997.

[43] Oppenheim RW. Schaffer, Digital signal processing. New Jersey: Prentice Hall, 1968.

[44] Boite R, et al. Traitement de la parole, Presses polytechniques et universitaires romandes, Lausanne, 2000.

[45] Frail R, Godino-Llorente JI, Saenz-Lechon N, Osma-Ruiz V, Fredouille C. MFCC-based remote pathology detection on speech transmitted through the telephone channel. Proc Biosignals. 2009.

[46] Fraile R, et al. MFCC-based Remote Pathology Detection on Speech Transmitted Through the Telephone Channel-Impact of Linear Distortions: Band Limitation, Frequency Response and Noise. BIOSIGNALS. 2009.

[47] Murphy PJ, Akande OO. Quantification of glottal and voiced speech harmonics-to-noise ratios using cepstral-based estimation. ISCA Tutorial and Research Workshop (ITRW) on Non-Linear Speech Processing. 2005.

[48] Hasan MdR, et al. Speaker identification using mel frequency cepstral coefficients. 3rd International Conference on Electrical & Computer Engineering ICECE.Vol. 2004. 2004.

[49] Kapoor T, Sharma RK. Parkinson's disease Diagnosis using Mel-frequency Cepstral Coefficients and Vector Quantization. Int J Comput Appl 2011;14(3):43–6.

[50] Benba A, Jilbab A, Hammouch A. Voice analysis for detecting persons with Parkinson's disease using MFCC and VQ. The 2014 International Conference on Circuits, Systems and Signal Processing. Saint Petersburg, Russia, September 23–25, 2014.

[51] Tsanas, A, et al. Objective automatic assessment of rehabilitative speech treatment in Parkinson's disease. IEEE Trans Neural Syst Rehabil Eng 2014;22(1).

[52] Teston B, Viallet F. Praticien hospitalier PhD. La dysprosodie parkinsonienne. In: Ozsancak C, Auzou P, éditors. Les troubles de la parole et de la déglutition dans la maladie de Parkinson. Marseille Solal:, 2005:161–93.

[53] Conte A, et al. Botulinum toxin A modulates afferent fibers in neurogenic detrusor over-activity. Eur J Neurol 2012;19(5):725–32.

[54] Ramig LO, et al. Intensive speech treatment for patients with Parkinson's disease Short- and long-term comparison of two techniques. Neurology 1996;47(6):1496–504.

[55] Ramig LO, et al. Changes in vocal loudness following intensive voice treatment (LSVT®) in individuals with Parkinson's disease: A comparison with untreated patients and normal age-matched controls. Mov Dis 2001;16(1):79–83.

[56] De S, Bert JM, et al. Improvement of voicing in patients with Parkinson's disease by speech therapy. Neurology 2003;60(3):498–500.

[57] Baken, RJ, Orlikoff RF. Clinical measurement of speech and voice. Cengage Learning, San Diego CA, 2000.

[58] Dejonckere PH et al. A basic protocol for functional assessment of voice pathology, especially for investigating the efficacy of (phonosurgical) treatments and evaluating new assessment techniques. Eur Arch Oto-rhino-laryngol 2001;258(2):77–82.

[59] Little MA, et al. Exploiting nonlinear recurrence and fractal scaling properties for voice disorder detection. BioMed Eng OnLine 2007;6(1):23.

[60] Alonso JB, et al. Automatic detection of pathologies in the voice by HOS based para-
      meters. EURASIP J Appl Signal Process 2001;4:275–84.
[61] Hansen JH, Gavidia-Ceballos L, Kaiser JF. A nonlinear operator-based speech feature
      analysis method with application to vocal fold pathology assessment. IEEE Trans Biomed
      Eng 1998;45(3):300–13.
[62] Cnockaert L, et al. Low-frequency vocal modulations in vowels produced by Parkinsonian
      subjects. Speech Commun 2008;50(4):288–300.
[63] Godino-Llorente, JI, Gomez-Vilda P. Automatic detection of voice impairments by means of
      short- term cepstral parameters and neural network based detectors. IEEE Trans Biomed
      Eng 2004;51(2):380–4.
[64] Boersma P. Praat, a system for doing phonetics by computer. Glot international 2002;
      5(9/10):341–5.
[65] Elemetrics K. Multi-dimensional voice program (MDVP).[Computer program.]. Pine Brook,
      NJ: Author, 1993.
[66] Tsanas, Athanasios, et al. Enhanced classical dysphonia measures and sparse regression
      for telemonitoring of Parkinson's disease progression. IEEE International Conference on
      Acoustics Speech and Signal Processing (ICASSP), 2010. IEEE, 2010.
[67] Hariharan M, Polat K, Sindhu R. A new hybrid intelligent system for accurate detection of
      Parkinson's disease. Comput Methods Programs Biomed 2014;113(3):904–13.
[68] Zwirner Petra, Murry T, Woodson GE. Phonatory function of neurologically impaired
      patients. J Commun Disord 1991;24(4):287–300.
[69] Kantz H, Schreiber T. Nonlinear time series analysis. Vol. 7. Cambridge university press,
      2004.
[70] Laver J. Principles of phonetics. Cambridge University Press, 1994.
[71] Locco Julie. La production des occlusives dans la maladie de Parkinson. Diss. Aix
      Marseille 1, 2005.
[72] Teston Bernard. L'évaluation objective des dysfonctionnements de la voix et de la parole;
      2e partie: les dysphonies. Travaux Interdisciplinaires du Laboratoire Parole et Langage
      d'Aix-en-Pro
[73] Caroline Fortin. Le visuel du corps humain: Français-anglais. Montréal, Québec Amérique,
      2009.
[74] Friedman, J, Hastie T, Tibshirani R. Additive logistic regression: a statistical view of
      boosting (with discussion and a rejoinder by the authors). Ann Stat 2000;28(2):337–407.
[75] Benba A, Jilbab A, Hammouch A. Voice analysis for detecting persons with Parkinson's
      disease using PLP and VQ. J Theor Appl Inf Technol 2014;70(3):443–450.
[76] Benba A, Jilbab A, Hammouch A. Voiceprint analysis using Perceptual Linear Prediction
      and Support Vector Machines for detecting persons with Parkinson's disease. the 3rd
      International Conference on Health Science and Biomedical Systems, Florence, Italy,
      November 22–24, 2014
[77] Benba A, Jilbab A, Hammouch A. Hybridization of best acoustic cues for detecting persons
      with Parkinson's disease, The 2nd World Conference on Complex System, Agadir,
      Morocco, 2014.
[78] Skodda S, Rinsche H, Schlegel U. Progression of dysprosody in Parkinson's disease over
      time – a longitudinal study. Mov Dis 2009;24(5):716–22.
[79] Goetz CG, et al. Testing objective measures of motor impairment in early Parkinson's
      disease: Feasibility study of an at-home testing device. Mov Disord 2009;24(4):
      551–6.

[80] Teston B. L'évaluation objective des dysfonctionnements de la voix et de la parole; 1ère partie: les dysarthries. Travaux Interdisciplinaires du Laboratoire Parole et Langage d'Aix-en-Provence (TIPA) 2000;19:115–54.

[81] Hammarberg B, et al. Perceptual and acoustic correlates of abnormal voice qualities. Acta oto- laryngologica 1980;90(1–6):441–51.

[82] Hirano M. Psycho-acoustic evaluation of voice: GRBAS scale for evaluating the hoarse voice. Clinican Examination of Voice. New York, Springer-Verlab (1981).

[83] Dejonckere PH, et al. Perceptual evaluation of dysphonia: reliability and relevance. Folia Phoniatrica et Logopaedica 1993;45(2):76–83.

[84] Fahn SE, Elton RL, Marsden CD, Calne DB, Golstein M. Recent development in Parkinson's disease. Floram Park, NJ: Macmilian Health Care Information, 1987.

[85] Weismer G. Acoustic descriptions of dysarthric speech: Perceptual correlates and physiological inferences Seminars in speech and language. Vol. 5. No. 04. © 1984 by Thieme Medical Publishers, Inc., 1984.

[86] Ramaker C, et al. Systematic evaluation of rating scales for impairment and disability in Parkinson's disease. Mov Disord 2002;17(5):867–76.

[87] Rousselot PJ. Principes de phonétique expérimentale. Vol. 1. H. Welter, Paris, 1901.

[88] Warren DW. Regulation of speech aerodynamics. Principles Exp Phonetics 1996;17:46–92.

[89] Warren DW. Aerodynamics of speech production. Contemp Issues Exp Phonetics 1976;30:105–37.

[90] Farrús M, Hernando J, Ejarque P. Jitter and shimmer measurements for speaker recognition. INTERSPEECH. 2007.

[91] Shirvan RA, Tahami E. Voice analysis for detecting Parkinson's disease using genetic algorithm and KNN classification method. 2011 18th Iranian Conference of Biomedical Engineering (ICBME). IEEE, 2011.

[92] Yumoto, E, Gould WJ, Baer T. Harmonics-to-noise ratio as an index of the degree of hoarseness. J Acoust Soc Am 1982;71(6):1544–50.

[93] Kasuya H, et al. Normalized noise energy as an acoustic measure to evaluate pathologic voice. J Acoust Soc Am 1986;80(5):1329–34.

[94] Qi Y, et al. Minimizing the effect of period determination on the computation of amplitude perturbation in voice. J Acoust Soc Am 1995;97(4):2525–32.

[95] Pouchoulin G, et al. Frequency study for the characterization of the dysphonic voices. Pro INTERSPEECH 2007, 2007:1198–201.

[96] Fraile R, et al. Use of mel-frequency cepstral coefficients for automatic pathology detection on sustained vowel phonations: mathematical and statistical justification. Proc. 4th international symposium on image/video communications over fixed and mobile networks, Bilbao, Brazil. 2008.

[97] Dibazar AA, Narayanan S, Berger TW. Feature analysis for automatic detection of pathological speech. Engineering in Medicine and Biology, 2002. 24th Annual Conference and the Annual Fall Meeting of the Biomedical Engineering Society EMBS/BMES Conference, 2002. Proceedings of the Second Joint. Vol 1. IEEE, 2002.

[98] Hermansky H. Perceptual linear predictive (PLP) analysis of speech. J Acoust Soc Am 1990;87(4):1738–52.

[99] Fletcher H, Munson WA. Loudness, its definition, measurement and calculation. Bell Labs Technical Journal. 1933 Oct 1;12(4):377–430.

[100] Robinson DW, Dadson RS. A re-determination of the equal-loudness relations for pure tones Br J Appl Phys 1956;7:166–81.

[101] ISO 226. Acoustics – Normal equal-loudness contours International Organization for Standardization, Geneva, 1987.

[102] Scheirer ED. Music Listening Systems PhD Thesis, Massachusetts Institute of Technology, June 2000.

[103] Goldstein JL. An optimum processor theory for central formation of the pitch of complex tones. J Acoust Soc Am 1973;54(6):1496–516.

[104] Licklider JC. A duplex theory of pitch perception, Experientia 7, 1951:128–34.

[105] Slaney M, Lyon RF. A perceptual pitch detector, proceedings of the IEEE International Conference on Acoustics, Speech, and Signal Processing ICASSP90, pp. 357–60, 1990.

[106] Van Den E, Stephen K, et al. Incidence of Parkinson's disease: variation by age, gender, and race/ethnicity, Am J Epidemiol 2003;157(11):1015–22.

[107] De L, Lonneke ML, Breteler M. Epidemiology of Parkinson's disease. Lancet Neurol 2006; 5(6):525–535.

[108] Huse DM, et al. Burden of illness in Parkinson's disease. Mov Disord 2005;20(11):1449–54.

[109] Lasierra N, et al. Lessons learned after a three-year store and forward teledermatology experience using internet: Strengths and limitations. Int J Med Inf 2012;81(5):332–43.

[110] Andersen T, et al. Designing for collaborative interpretation in telemonitoring: re-introducing patients as diagnostic agents. Int J Med Inf 2011;80(8):e112–e126.

[111] Bernard E, et al. Internet use for information seeking in clinical practice: a cross-sectional survey among French general practitioners. Int J Med Inf 2012;81(7):493–9.

[112] Loukas C, Brown P. A PC-based system for predicting movement from deep brain signals in Parkinson's disease. Comput Methods Programs Biomed 2012;107(1):36–44.

[113] Farnikova K, Krobot A, Kanovsky P. Musculoskeletal problems as an initial manifestation of Parkinson's disease: A retrospective study. J Neurol Sci 2012;319(1):102–4.

[114] Romenets, SR, et al. Rapid eye movement sleep behavior disorder and subtypes of Parkinson's disease. Mov Disord 2012;27(8):996–1003.

[115] Delaney M, Simpson J, Leroi I. Perceptions of cause and control of impulse control behaviours in people with Parkinson's disease. British Journal of Health Psychology 2012;17(3):522–35.

[116] Ho AK, et al. Speech impairment in a large sample of patients with Parkinson's disease. Behavioural Neurology 1999;11(3):131–7.

[117] Logemann JA, et al. Frequency and cooccurrence of vocal tract dysfunctions in the speech of a large sample of Parkinson patients. Journal of Speech and Hearing Disorders 1978; 43(1):47–57.

[118] O'Sullivan SB, Schmitz TJ. Parkinson disease. Physical Rehabilitation 2007:856–94.

[119] Sapir S, et al. Effects of intensive voice treatment (the Lee Silverman Voice Treatment [LSVT]) on vowel articulation in dysarthric individuals with idiopathic Parkinson disease: acoustic and perceptual findings. Journal of Speech, Language, and Hearing Research 2007;50(4):899–912.

[120] Rahn III DA, et al. Phonatory impairment in Parkinson's disease: evidence from nonlinear dynamic analysis and perturbation analysis. Journal of Voice 2007;21(1):64–71.

[121] Jankovic J. Parkinson's disease: clinical features and diagnosis. Journal of Neurology, Neurosurgery & Psychiatry 2008;79(4):368–76.

[122] Viallet F, Teston B. La dysarthrie dans la maladie de Parkinson. Les dysarthries 2007:169–74.

[123] Manciocco A, et al. The application of Russell and Burch 3R principle in rodent models of neurodegenerative disease: the case of Parkinson's disease. Neuroscience & Biobehavioral Reviews 2009;33(1):18–32.

[124] Wilkins EJ, et al. A DNA resequencing array for genes involved in Parkinson's disease. Parkinsonism & related disorders 2012;18(4):386–90.

[125] Niu L, et al. Effect of bilateral deep brain stimulation of the subthalamic nucleus on freezing of gait in Parkinson's disease. Journal of International Medical Research 2012; 40(3):1108–13.

[126] Lin X, et al. Conditional expression of Parkinson's disease-related mutant α-synuclein in the midbrain dopaminergic neurons causes progressive neurodegeneration and degradation of transcription factor nuclear receptor related 1. The Journal of Neuroscience 2012;32(27):9248–64.

[127] Tang L, et al. Meta-analysis of association between PITX3 gene polymorphism and Parkinson's disease. J Neurol Sci 2012;317(1):80–6.

[128] Langston JW. Parkinson's disease: current and future challenges. Neurotoxicology 2002;23(4):443–50.

[129] Saeed, A, Faezipour M, Nourani M, Banerjee S, Lee G, Gupta G, Tamil L. A scalable wireless body area network for bio-telemetry. JIPS 2009;5(2):77–86.

[130] Akyildiz IF, Su W, Sankarasubramaniam Y, Cayirci E. A survey on sensor networks, IEEE Commun Mag 2002:102–14.

[131] Chouhan S, Bose R, Balakrishnan M. A framework for energy consumption based design space exploration for wireless sensor nodes. IEEE Transaction on Computer-Aided Design Integrated Circuits System. July 2009:1017–24.

[132] Tian DF, Liang QQ. Energy efficiency analysis of error control schemes in wireless sensor networks, August 2008.

[133] Byers JW, Luby M, Mitzenmacher M, Rege A. A digital fountain approach to reliable distribution of bulk data. Conference on Applications, Technologies, Architectures, and Protocols for Computer Communication (SIG-COMM), Vancouver, BC, Canada, 1998.

[134] Samouni N, Jilbab A, Aboutajdine, D. Performance evaluation of LT codes for wireless body area network. Europe and MENA Cooperation Advances in Information and Communication Technologies. Springer International Publishing, 2017:311–20.

[135] Abidi B, Jilbab A, Haziti ME. Wireless sensor networks in biomedical: wireless body area networks. Europe and MENA Cooperation Advances in Information and Communication Technologies. Springer International Publishing, 2017:321–9.

[136] Zervas E, Mpimpoudis A, Anagnostopoulos C, Sekkas O, Hadjiefthymiades S. Multisensor data fusion for fire detection. Inf Fusion 2011;12:150–9.

[137] Sung W-T. Multi-sensors data fusion system for wireless sensors networks of factory monitoring via BPN technology, Expert Syst Appl 2010;37:2124–31.

[138] Zhou G, Zhu Z, Chen G, Zhou L. Decision fusion rules based on multi-bit knowledge of local sensors in wireless sensor networks. Inf Fusion 2011;12:187–93.

[139] Chair Z, Varshney PK. Optimal data fusion in multiple sensor detection systems, IEEE Trans Aerosp Electron Syst 1986;22:98–101.

[140] Aziz AM. A new adaptive decentralized soft decision combining rule for distributed sensor systems with data fusion. Inf Sci 2014;25:197–210.

[141] Abramson EL, et al. Physician experiences transitioning between an older versus newer electronic health record for electronic prescribing. Int J Med Inf 2012;81(8):539–48.

[142] Duffy JR. Motor speech disorders: Substrates, differential diagnosis, and management. Elsevier Health Sciences, 2012.

www.ingramcontent.com/pod-product-compliance
Lightning Source LLC
Chambersburg PA
CBHW050524190326
41458CB00005B/1649